Making Room in the Clinic

Critical Issues in Health and Medicine

Edited by Rima D. Apple, University of Wisconsin—Madison, and Janet Golden, Rutgers University, Camden

Growing criticism of the U.S. health care system is coming from consumers, politicians, the media, activists, and health care professionals. Critical Issues in Health and Medicine is a collection of books that explores these contemporary dilemmas from a variety of perspectives, among them political, legal, historical, sociological, and comparative, and with attention to crucial dimensions such as race, gender, ethnicity, sexuality, and culture.

Making Room in the Clinic

Nurse Practitioners and the Evolution of Modern Health Care

Julie Fairman

Rutgers University Press

New Brunswick, New Jersey and London

Library of Congress Cataloging-in-Publication Data

Fairman, Julie.
    Making room in the clinic : nurse practitioners and the evolution
of modern health care / Julie Fairman.
        p. ;   cm. — (Critical issues in health and medicine)
    Includes bibliographical references and index.
    ISBN-13: 978-0-8135-4319-2 (hardcover : alk. paper)
    1. Nurse practitioners—United States—History.
    [DNLM: 1. Nurse Practitioners—history—United States.
    2. History, 20th Century—United States. WY 11 AA1 F17m 2008] I. Title. II. Series.
    RT82.8.F35 2008
    610.7306'92—dc22   2007033712

A British Cataloging-in-Publication record for this book is available from the British Library.

Visit our Web site: http://rutgerspress.rutgers.edu

Manufactured in the United States of America

This book is dedicated to Barbara Bates, who left us too early, and to an old country boy who would have enjoyed my accomplishment.

Contents

Acknowledgments

I began to think about this book during my experiences teaching physical examination to undergraduate students at the School of Nursing, University of Pennsylvania, in the early 1990s. I invited physician Barbara Bates to speak to the class because we used her textbook, *Guide to Physical Examination and History Taking*. I was intrigued by her stories about the University of Rochester and her work with another colleague of mine, Joan Lynaugh, to develop one of the earliest nurse practitioner programs. I spent a great deal of time (theirs and mine) talking with them over the years and from there began to explore more fully the history of nurse practitioners.

I received valuable help from many other people as well. I am grateful to Barbara Brodie, founding director of the Center for Nursing Historical Inquiry, School of Nursing, University of Virginia, for steering me to the records of the National Association of Pediatric Nurse Associates and Practitioners and the Kathryn Jacquette Collection. Barbara is a source of great support to me and the Center provided financial support through a research fellowship. Loretta "Lee" Ford was generous with her time, personal papers, and photograph collection. She is truly an inspiration. The staff at the Howard Gotlieb Archival Research Center at Boston University, especially Diane Gallagher and Alex Rankin, helped me navigate the American Nurses' Association Collection. Richard Barry at the American Nurses' Association Library, Silver Springs, Maryland, provided access to additional documents. Nina Stoyan-Rosenzweig, archivist for the University of Florida, College of Medicine and the Health Science Center, provided generous assistance during my several visits to Florida to investigate Dorothy Smith and the College of Nursing. She steered me to the Samuel Proctor Oral History Program and its on-line collection. The digital on-line collection of the Duke University Medical Center Archives and the Society for the Preservation of Physician Assistant History special collection changed my notion of historical research, and saved me an enormous amount of time. I accessed the papers of the National Joint Practice Commission through the generosity of Dr. Shirley Smoyak of Rutgers University. She also provided her personal collection of Hildegard Peplau papers and sat for a very long and important oral history interview about her experiences with the commission. She later donated her papers to the Barbara Bates Center for the Study of the History of Nursing, School of Nursing, University of Pennsylvania.

Barbara Bates contributed her personal collection of papers, photographs, and manuscripts. Joan Lynaugh also offered her personal collection related to her work on the medical nurse practitioner program at the University of Rochester. At the Barbara Bates Center, Betsy Weiss and Gail Farr steered me to the Dorothy Smith, Doris Schwartz, and Jessie Scott Collections, and helped with reference issues. Cynthia Gurney provided access to her personal collection of papers from the Army Nurse Corp, and directed me to Karen Ballard of the New York State Nurses' Association. I also found help in the Office of the Commissioner, Bureau of Professional and Occupational Health Affairs, Commonwealth of Pennsylvania, where records (1966–1978) of the State Board of Nursing and State Board of Medicine were located.

I utilized a number of oral history interviews for the book, including those of Karen Ballard, Barbara Bates, Linda Davies, Barbara Dunn, Richard Edlick, Loretta Ford, Denise Geolot, Carol Hayes-Christiansen, Betty Hilliard, Harriet Kitzman, Joan Lynaugh, Jerome Lysaught, Carla Schissel, Jennet Wilson, and many other nurse practitioners and physicians. I conducted some of the interviews myself and others were conducted by researchers Sadie Mitchell, M. J. Murphy, Rebecca Nanansi, and Keisha Walker. I fondly remember an evening with at least thirty former faculty members from the College of Nursing, University of Florida, who offered recollections of Dorothy Smith. Barbara Resnick pointed me in the direction of a valuable collection of oral history data obtained for the Group Project, "Stories from the Early Days of Becoming a Nurse Practitioner," sponsored by the Fellowship of the American Academy of Nurse Practitioners.

This book was supported by generous grants from the National Endowment for the Humanities (FA-37223–02) and the National Library of Medicine (G13 LM007250). The University of Pennsylvania provided support through grants and fellowships from the University Research Foundation, the Trustees' Council of Penn Women Summer Fellowship, and the Class of 1940 Bicentennial Term Chair funds. I also received support from Linda Aiken, director of the Center for Health Outcomes and Policy Research, through the Claire Fagin Chair.

I am particularly fortunate to have a group of colleagues who offered advice and support. Rosemary Stevens has always guided my work and I owe her many favors. I have also been strongly influenced by Charles Rosenberg and Judith McGaw. Sarah Kagan was always willing to read. Eileen Sullivan-Marx offered expertise on nurse practitioner practice and reimbursement issues. Julie Sochalski provided advice on health policy. The seminar participants of the Barbara Bates Center Seminar Series also provided feedback on various chapters.

Cindy Connelly, Meryn Stewart, Deborah Sampson, and Joy Buck read drafts and provided comments, as did Arlene Keeling. Linda Aiken gave me access to her letters from Dorothy Smith and kept her in my sights. Michelle Han and Ira-Joel Sartorius provided research and editing assistance, along with assistants Nicole Hiti, Jennifer Hobbs, and Briana Ralston. Gina Conway masterfully assisted with manuscript preparation, and has the patience of a saint. David Proctor helped me research the incorporation documents of the National Joint Practice Commission. Sherry Morgan, research librarian at the University of Pennsylvania Biomedical Library helped me locate the Duke digital archives and other resource materials. Doreen Valentine, my editor at Rutgers University Press, helped shape the final version of this book.

My colleagues and friends in the Barbara Bates Center for the Study of the History of Nursing, Ellen Baer, Karen Buhler-Wilkerson, Patricia D'Antonio, and Jean Whelan, supported me through this long journey. Joan Lynaugh in particular has been my mentor and friend for many years. She is truly my role model and I hope I can show my students the same intellectual generosity, kindness, and compassion she shared with me.

Finally, I want to thank my husband, Ron Fairman, for his patience and support. This book could not have been written without his motivating spirit. My mother, Virginia Schauer, gave me summer space to write, and my two sons, Alex and Connor, inspired me to get this done, because, as they remind me, there is so much more in life to think about.

Portions of the following articles are used with the permission of the publishers: "The Roots of Collaborative Practice: Nurse Practitioner Pioneer Stories," *Nursing History Review* (10) (2002):159–174; Springer Publishing Company, Inc., New York, New York 10036. "Delegated by Default or Negotiated by Need: Physicians, Nurse Practitioners, and the Process of Clinical Thinking," *Medical Humanities Review* 13(1) (1999): 38–58; Medical Humanities Review, 301 University Boulevard, Galveston, Texas, 77555. "Review Essay: Not All Nurses Are Good, Not All Doctors Are Bad," *Bulletin of the History of Medicine* 78(2) (2004): 451–460; The Johns Hopkins University Press, 2715 North Charles Street, Baltimore, Maryland 21218.

List of Abbreviations

AACN	American Association of Critical Care Nurses
AAFP	American Academy of Family Physicians
AAMC	Association of American Medical Colleges
AANP	American Academy of Nurse Practitioners
AAP	American Academy of Pediatrics
ACOG	American College of Obstetricians and Gynecologists
AHA	American Heart Association
AMA	American Medical Association
ANA	American Nurses Association
AORN	Association of Operating Room Nurses
BHM	Bureau of Health Manpower
DEA	Drug Enforcement Agency
DHEW	U.S. Department of Health, Education and Welfare
DHHS	U.S. Department of Heath and Human Services
DRG	Diagnosis-related Group
IOM	Institute of Medicine
JCAH	Joint Commission on the Accreditation of Hospitals
MCHN	Maternal and Child Health Nursing Division, American Nurses Association
NAPNAP	National Association of Pediatric Nurse Associates and Practitioners
NCSNNE	National Commission for the Study of Nursing and Nursing Education
NIH	National Institutes of Health
NJPC	National Joint Practice Commission
NLN	National League for Nursing
NTA	Nurse Training Act
PHS	U.S. Public Health Service
PPS	Prospective Payment System
STTI	Sigma Theta Tau International

Making Room in the Clinic

Introduction

Let's start with a familiar story.

Mrs. Shade is a fifty-six-year-old woman with a four-year history of noninsulin-dependent diabetes mellitus. She smokes more than a pack of cigarettes per day and has done so for the last ten years. She is on a fixed income due to a past disability related to arthritis, another chronic illness. She is overweight, and she also suffers from high blood pressure. On her last visit to her health care provider, her blood glucose levels were about twenty points above normal. Her feet were warm with good pulses, and showed no signs of the typical changes accompanying uncontrolled diabetes. At this visit Mrs. Shade requested and received information about a weight-loss and exercise plan that was appropriate for someone on a fixed income. She needed a referral for county transportation resources to get to doctor appointments and to a pharmacy for medication. She also received a referral to a community-based program to quit smoking, and a demonstration on how to use a recently purchased electronic blood glucose monitor.

This story, though invented, sets up an important and realistic clinical scenario from which to consider the following questions: Which health professional or combination of professionals should provide services to meet Mrs. Shade's health care needs? How do we, as individuals and as a collective, decide who should provide particular types of care at particular times? What kind of education, knowledge, and skills should the practitioner(s) have? And, finally, how do clinicians—physicians and nurses in particular—negotiate among themselves, with patients, and with public and private interests to define the borders of responsibility and authority for clinical care? These questions all address the critical issues of both jurisdictional and cultural politics underpinning the history of health care.

The history of the nurse practitioner movement can help us think about these questions, which remain as salient today as they were for practitioners of an earlier time. The nurse practitioner movement of the 1960s and 1970s was a growing informal coalition of nurses and physicians who saw the idea of working together as a fundamental way to improve patient care. It altered professional boundaries, including both unwritten and official rules governing the use of technology and therapeutics, and perhaps most critical, access to patients.[1] During this time period, the movement helped reshape clinical practice, particularly outside of hospitals, and provided the foundation for questioning who had the authority to provide care to particular groups of patients at particular times and places. Its development from sets of isolated individual relationships to a broader national movement generously funded by federal and private initiatives illustrates how historically contingent professional prerogatives changed during a time of growing economic and political self-interest manifested by organized nursing and medicine. Local and individually determined boundaries influence health policy issues on many levels. This is where health policy strategies are put into practice, where they are molded to fit clinical practices, succeed, and fail on a minute-by-minute, patient-by-patient basis. The most effective strategies occur when local and nationally organized groups show common purpose and method. But this type of consensus is hard to achieve as heterogeneous groups and political self-interests clash with altruistic ideas. This is a major thread of the nurse practitioner story.

The nurse practitioner movement grew through the efforts of nurses and physicians as they developed a collective practice identity that challenged the traditional system of health care based on the primacy of the physician. It also confronted the professional organizations such as the American Nurses Association (ANA) and the American Medical Association (AMA). These organizations among others were indeed interested in patient care, but their focus came through a distinctly shaped lens of professional power. The nurse practitioner movement participants saw professional boundaries as more flexible and malleable than did their professional organizations. Individual nurses and physicians constantly reconstructed their practices according to patient needs and choices for the type of care they wanted. The new and entrepreneurial models of clinical practice that emerged were considered untenable by the medical organizations and initially misunderstood by the nursing organizations. Only in the early 1980s did the ANA realize how powerful nurse practitioners could be, but by that time many specialty organizations were already organized and uninterested in empowering or sharing power with the larger organization. The medical organizations from the start understood the risk these new nurse practitioners presented to the normative status of physicians, and contested them whenever they could.

The nurse practitioner movement also embraced the growing power of specialization in health care as a sort of survival strategy, although it proved to be a paradoxical one. As more physicians entered into highly complex specialties and subspecialties, nurse practitioners and their physician colleagues grasped the opportunity to develop different avenues for providing health services to address the needs of the chronically ill, elderly, and well population. But these practice areas were not centered in acute care institutions and carried less status and lower incomes than those that were. This contradictory force—greater opportunity as a trade-off for less power and smaller economic gains—somewhat tempered the movement's early impact but also kept the new models of clinical practice away from the critical eye of medical and nursing licensure boards that did not always support their innovative and boundary-crossing practice innovations.

The impact of federal funding on the nurse practitioner movement cannot be forgotten. Grounded by generous federal funding for health professional education (the Training Acts of the early 1960s), this movement gained impetus through the changes wrought by Medicare (1966) and the state-federal partnership of Medicaid (in the late 1960s). These new federal and state entitlement programs came at a time when physicians increasingly specialized and the number of those providing general medical care declined, creating shortages in poor urban and rural communities. Medicare and Medicaid created access to acute and specialty medical care, which is where the bulk of the demand for health care resided. It increased the number and type of patients receiving health care services without substantially changing the system of health delivery. Entitlement programs such as Medicare and Medicaid, among others, also had an impact on the economics and politics of health care, creating the foundation for new philanthropic ideologies and, through their failure, the later substantiation of the for-profit model of health care services. With these changes came transformations in how physicians and nurses were educated, paid, and where and how they practiced. Practically the only cost issues centered on nurse practitioners during this time stemmed from their expense to their physician colleagues and whether or not they would pay for themselves through an anticipated increase in patient flow in private offices.

Federal funding also shaped the role nurse practitioners later played in the health care system. By the late 1970s, continued and unchecked spending for health care by the states and the federal government generated various new funding solutions. A new strategy, the prospective payment system (PPS) and its payment method of diagnosis-related groups (DRGs), was eventually instigated by the federal government in 1983. It was a hospital-based solution at first, but its implementation had a large impact on outpatient services as they were extrapolated to these settings in the late 1980s and 1990s. As hospital payments were capitated (payment based on a single price for services rather than accumulated costs) and decreased, patients spent less time in hospitals and admission criteria tightened. Patients who usually received inpatient services now required care in community settings where both physician and nursing resources were in short supply. These patients needed greater amounts of focused services, including those designed to keep them away from expensive hospital care. Nurse practitioners, reconceptualized as low-cost providers, and through a growing recognition of their proficiency and efficiency, became part of the savings and health prevention measures that grew up in the 1980s. This was a new role for nurse practitioners and was paradigmatically different from that seen in the 1960s and 1970s during its developmental phase. Nurse practitioners were not originally a cost-cutting solution, and their main function had little to do with hospitals. They emerged as a way to increase access to care for underserved patients, assist busy physicians in their practices, and gain a venue and formal authority for providing nursing care to patients in the community. Shaped through the crucible of the social, political, and economic environment of the 1960s and 1970s, nurse practitioners were uniquely situated to take advantage of new opportunities for practice expansion in the aftermath of PPS and through health maintenance organizations that looked to them as inexpensive solutions for providing primary care.

In the critical period of the 1960s and 1970s, the nurse practitioner movement helped create an influential foundation for health policies that emerged in the last twenty-eight years, including health maintenance organizations, a renewed interest in health promotion and disease prevention, and consumer-based health services. There is no evidence for a direct link, but the seeds for many health policies of the last decades can be seen in this twenty-year period, from 1960 to 1980. These policies are characterized by a complex combination of public and private interests, economics, technological changes, personal relationships, and organizational politics.[2] This was also true for the nurse practitioner movement.[3]

From the beginning, I envisioned this book as a series of both parallel and interconnected historical narratives between nursing and medicine. This is not to say that other types of providers, such as social workers and physical therapists, were not important. But the territory of clinical practice that most interests me revolves around immediate and intimate patient-provider interactions. Nurses other than nurse practitioners, such as nurse midwives and nurse anesthetists, were also part of the larger movement of practice jurisdictional shift, but they have their own particular historical narratives that are at times parallel to nurse practitioners, but with longer trajectories (both types of providers existed decades before nurse practitioners). These groups of nurses are much smaller in number than nurse practitioners, and also challenged physician dominance at various times. On the other hand, physician assistants, licensed health care providers who practice medicine under physician supervision, as seen in chapter 3, are directly related to this movement.[4] Physician assistants emerged during the same time period as nurse practitioners, seemed to function identically, and were sometimes labeled the same, although both groups fought to differentiate themselves from one another.

Nurse practitioners and physician assistants formed two sides of a triangulated relationship with physicians such as pediatricians, general practice physicians, and, later, family practice physicians that flavored the debate over who had the social and cultural authority to provide health care to particular groups of patients, and how much education providers needed to adequately serve the majority of patients seeking care. This debate occurred between specialists and generalists, nurse practitioners and physicians, physician assistants and physicians, and patients and providers of all types. These groups were generally heterogeneous, and there was as much intragroup conflict over health care issues as occurred between groups. Money, status, and power issues, as well as legitimate concerns over patient care influenced how different groups and various constituents within groups tried to answer these questions.

Part of the process of addressing who should provide health care at particular times and places, and how this issue is negotiated, includes understanding how this historical nurse practitioner movement developed. This means going beyond who was first. The central issue is not *when* the first nurse practitioner program developed, but *how* these early formations and their change over time help us understand contemporary clinical practice, its authority structure, and public demands. Nurse practitioners indeed owe a great deal to early pioneer nurse Loretta Ford, who with physician colleague Henry Silver formalized the nurse practitioner role at the University of Colorado in 1965. Ford spent a great deal of her career (which is still very active) supporting and educating countless numbers of nurse practitioners. She has told her story in many important venues, including an oral history interview I was privileged to conduct in early 2006. Her recollections and thoughts are a valuable source for understanding how nurse practitioners developed. Yet hers is only one part of the history of nurse practitioners. This story is also not one of slow and steady improvement of nurses' ability to provide particular types of care. In other words, it is not a deterministic or progressive story, but one of differing cultural and temporal contexts that created the environment for providers and the public to notice the transformation going on and opportunities provided by nurses' work.

Nurse Practitioners

Nurse practitioners are nurses with graduate (master's) degrees in a nursing clinical specialty; they are licensed by each state and certified by private certification boards. They are part of a designated group of advanced-practice nurses (midwives, nurse anesthetists, and clinical specialists are also part of this group). Nurse practitioners are responsible for an enormous range of health care services, from delegated medical regimens to independent care provision in hospitals and clinics. They provide primary health care to a range of clients from the wealthy to poor, underserved, and uninsured populations, and from healthy newborns to elders and the chronically ill. They also maintain a constant presence with the acutely ill and injured in hospitals.[5] There were approximately 115,000 nurse practitioners actively practicing in the United States in 2004, and schools of nursing prepare approximately 5,000 to 6,000 new nurse practitioners each year. Sixty-six percent practiced in at least one primary care site, but 39 percent held hospital privileges. Ninety-six percent of nurse practitioners prescribed medications and wrote an average of nineteen prescriptions per day. Sixty-five percent of nurse practitioners were authorized to write prescriptions for controlled substances (such as certain types of prescription pain medications), and almost the same proportion held a Drug Enforcement Agency (DEA) number enabling them to legally prescribe certain groups of narcotics.[6]

Nurse practitioners provide a new perspective for exploring the historically contingent relationships among the social, political, and economic forces that shaped contemporary health care, which heretofore have focused primarily on diseases, physicians, and hospitals.[7] This is not a partisan or ideological approach. Nurses represent the largest health professional group in the United States today and influence all aspects of the health care system. By numbers alone, their history, including that of nurse practitioners, brings important perspectives to the surface. The profession itself is also heterogeneous and highly idiosyncratic, providing an appropriate case for reflecting upon our equally heterogeneous and idiosyncratic health care system in general. Furthermore, nurse practitioners are a recent specialization of nursing in terms of education level, practice skills, and knowledge. As such, they are emblematic of the specialization of health care in the United States.

Nurse practitioners are part of the constant change, however subtle, in who has the authority to provide health care at particular times and places. It is important to look beyond the traditional health care mainstream to understand nurse practitioners' participation and influence in patient care. Physicians traditionally were considered the normative providers of medical services, and it is their perspective that guides much of what is understood about patients, health policies, and institutions. But in fact, "alternatives"—in this case practitioners such as midwives, nurse practitioners, physician assistants, and empowered contemporary population groups—are mainstream across certain times and places. For example, independent nurses and lay providers were and are the norm in many rural clinics, but, until recently, not in urban academic institutions or in places with many physicians. Nurse practitioners might independently prescribe in one state but not another. This shifting norm is part of the historical narrative of nurse practitioners.[8]

Nurse Joan Lynaugh describes nurse practitioners as looking for an "exam room of their own"—essentially a clinical space in which to provide nursing care. This space is, indeed, a crowded one.[9] Clinical practice undeniably hinges on where and how nurses and physicians work together, but it is also structured by economics, the political circumstances, expectations, and values of the patient, other providers, and various institutions. And it encompasses much more than getting along, a concept that trivializes the most important aspect of health care—the clinical moment when provider and patient enter into a dialogue and a relationship.

Yet on the way to the clinical moment, one must unpack physicians' exclusive status as the mainstream providers of health care, and as autonomous actors. Through political rhetoric and popular ideology, physicians indeed hold cultural responsibility for those who are dependent on them—the patients. Given the enormous complexity of contemporary health care, this is a highly unrealistic expectation and an untenable position for physicians and the public. This expectation was already obsolete by the mid-twentieth century and is even more impossible to maintain in light of the contemporary knowledge explosion and changing demographic trends of aging, chronic disease, and worldwide epidemics.[10]

In general, the paradigm of health and illness has been shifting since the 1940s when lifestyle changes, new drugs, and technologies reallocated the focus from acute to chronic illness and the problems of an aging population. There is, of course, still great need for acute care resources, skills, and knowledge. Expert acute, emergency care services are critical when you or someone close to you experiences some sort of physical or mental trauma. Yet many of the instances where complex care is necessary stem from acute exacerbations of chronic illnesses, such as the heart attack experienced by the patient with coronary artery disease, or the acute pneumonia threatening the AIDS patient. There are over 100 million people in the United States suffering from chronic illness and its complications, and we might be hard-pressed to find anyone completely free of a chronic illness if persistent sinus infections, allergies, and arthritis are included.[11]

But, as the population changes, the health care system, including practitioners and educators, responds slowly. Highly scientific, reductionist, and specialized medical care remains a powerful "gold standard" or norm in our society, despite evidence indicating complex scientific knowledge will not directly meet the needs of patients similar to Mrs. Shade. Even the National Academy of Sciences recently questioned the continued need for highly scientific curricula in medical education, given our population's changing demographics.[12]

In fact, Western countries in particular are increasingly supporting behavioral strategies and individual responsibility to manage health problems such as obesity and tobacco use. These strategies do not rely on traditional sources of basic scientific evidence for treatment. Public expectations of scientific medicine as the solution for the problems of chronic illness has been shifting since the end of World War II; in many instances people can take care of themselves, undermining faith in the authority of professional medicine.[13] My patient, Mrs. Shade, could be appropriately cared for by either a physician or a nurse practitioner, but she might receive better care if a team of collaborating providers worked with her. Additionally, if her providers focused on her health needs rather than whose prerogative it is to provide care, she might avoid some of the complications associated with diabetes and arthritis.[14] In reality, it may be that clinical practice is equally effective when provided by different kinds of practitioners at different points in time, nurse practitioner and doctors becoming "one of many."[15]

Gender, Class, and Race

Nurse practitioner demographics are similar to those of nurses in general: most of them are women, white, and middle class, although a larger proportion of nurse practitioners are men compared to the general nursing population.[16] Most of the primary sources used for this book are from white, sometimes segregated schools, and organizations and leaders that were primarily white and female (class is less easy to discern).[17] All of the documents without exception use the feminine pronouns "her and she" to describe the nurse practitioner, and "he and his" to describe physicians and physician assistants.[18] The photographs

I discovered during research include white nurse practitioners with few exceptions; the Asian, Hispanic, Native American, or black subjects I found in photographs or documents were usually patients. To bring in other perspectives, my research included oral history interviews with a variety of informants, including five black nurse practitioners.[19]

This does not mean that Asian, Native American, Hispanic, or black women and men in general are not an important part of nurse practitioner history. They were and are present in nursing and have practiced as nurse practitioners. Part of the explanation for their absence in this particular time period and story centers on the choices particular schools made regarding admission strategies, as well as the types of records repositories chose to collect and preserve. Another reason may be that of politics of privilege: the characters in the stories told in this book were appointed, elected, or had the power to "sit at the table" and negotiate new types of clinical practices with others, and they were privileged to do so because they were white, middle-class women.[20]

The absence or submerged presence of a group based on race, class, and gender is a function of the highly complex power structures in health care. These structures are interrelated, making it difficult to isolate the effects of gender from those of race and class. All three are interrelated systems of historically circumscribed ideas and analytic categories. They constitute a "central piece of social imagery" around which institutions and technological systems such as health care are constructed and maintained, health policies are formulated, and crucial systems of cultural representation, such as medical authority, are or are not sustained.[21] The social status of nursing is based upon its historical perception as a woman's profession. But its social status in particular communities is also based on the intersection of its female-gendered work and its middle-class origins.

On the other hand, nurse practitioner narratives are characterized more by a complex interaction of professional interests than by male-female or race-based conflict. There are, to be sure, countless stories of conflicts between female nurses and male physicians as they tried to claim cultural authority in clinical territory (see chapter 6). But there are also stories of physicians actively courting nurses to work toward common goals. In fact, the nurse practitioner movement depended on these types of relationships. In the early 1970s, pediatricians and pediatric organizations actively courted emerging nurse practitioner organizations. And, the nurse practitioners chose to affiliate with pediatricians rather than a nursing organization, as seen in chapter 7. These relationships complicate the traditional view of medicine and nursing as a series of confrontation politics based on gender.[22]

The Hazards of Modern History

When I began to investigate the history of nurse practitioners it became clear that the project would be difficult—not because of the absence of primary sources, but because of the sheer volume of them and the number of people who were available to provide perspectives on the time period. I made choices early on about which historical episodes to include, and these choices framed the book. They make a coherent examination of the changing reinterpretations of society's health care needs and relocations of boundaries between nursing and medicine within differing contexts, ranging from individual practitioners to the larger professional organizations.

Although public interests are represented by descriptions and analysis of various federal funding programs and subjective and objective evidence of support for nurse practitioners, the individual patient voice is thinly represented. Illustrative patient letters are included, as are studies assessing public acceptance of nurse practitioners. But my aim was to use nurse practitioners as a way to understand a particular slice of the cultural institution of health care within the nexus of clinical practice at a particular time. This perspective assumes the presence of patients—it could not exist without them.

At this point it is useful to revisit Mrs. Shade. Her story, although "virtual," should not be lost on us because it is indicative of the increasing ambiguity and flexibility of roles, authority, and ownership of nursing and medical skills and of knowledge that emerged in mid-twentieth-century private practices and clinics. The ambiguity of provider roles, and in particular the onset of new types of providers, such as nurse practitioners in the 1960s, provided an opportunity for society to question more openly how and why certain professional groups, such as physicians, claimed such vast cultural authority over health care and if, indeed, these claims remained legitimate and enduring. These claims have indeed endured and are inscribed in our understanding of our health care system, but they remain contested and malleable. This book tells a small part of the story of how the negotiations over the contested terrain of clinical practice helped to shape our contemporary health care system, and continues to do so today.

Chapter 1

"Oh the Opportunities, the Possibilities . . . !"

In the 1960s, as social turmoil over women's status, equality between races, and the United States' role in Vietnam exploded into street protests, American nursing seemed superficially quite conservative. Although there were, to be sure, many nurse activists who took up various social causes, the profession itself remained rule- and tradition-bound. Nursing was a predominantly female profession, and its members came from mostly middle-class or lower-middle-class families. Almost all nurses received their training in hospital-based schools, and after graduation most worked in the institutions that provided their training or in surrounding community hospitals. During this time period, nurses were stratified more by where they took their training (e.g., the particular hospital program), their longevity in a particular job, or their race than by level of education or practice. Public health and visiting nurses or those who became teachers of nursing or administrators were the exception. These nurses entered university or college-based programs to earn degrees in areas such as education, administration, or public health. They were a small but growing handful and remained so until the end of the decade.

But nurses' seemingly conservative public image was perhaps a foil for their own assertive tendencies in clinical practice. There, they negotiated the passageways of patient care, quietly and sometimes not so quietly.[1] In these spaces, nurses grappled with physicians over competing claims of clinical authority, perhaps covertly suggesting alternative therapies, asking for permission for a particular action after the fact, or overtly refusing to follow unacceptable medical orders. Many times nurses believed they had the knowledge and expertise to make logical clinical decisions but were thwarted by institutional or tradition-based rules and roles.

Although the character of these individual interactions was shaped in part by nurses' growing empowerment as women and their commitment to patients, as a group nurses were not courted nor seen as part of this larger liberal social platform. Leaders of the women's movement showed greater interest in increasing the number of women physicians, even as they fought to combat this paternalistic medical system, than in empowering nurses.[2] Their educational level, their overtly female demographics, predominantly lower-middle and middle-class status, and lingering medical dominance historically positioned the nursing profession paradoxically in opposition to and as assistants of physicians (primarily college-educated, upper-middle to upper-class men). These qualities made most nurses invisible to leaders of the women's movement and ensured prolonged debates surrounding which practitioner—nurse or physician—should provide particular types of care at certain points in time.

The working relationships between nurses and physicians as they struggled with this question were the foundation for the shift in clinical authority in the 1960s between and within the medical and nursing profession. The contestation of practice boundaries was important because it shaped the success or failure of the larger health policy issues at the individual and local level. Legislative issues seemed static, but individual practitioners negotiated practice margins in response to fluid clinical situations. These local deliberations even determined which clinical issues came into play as policy strategies over the next two decades.

The 1960s provided the tableau for a subtle and slowly emerging reexamination of the contours of clinical practice by nurses and physicians. Changes in nursing and medical education and practice, federal entitlement policies, and economics supported more fluid movement of knowledge and skills across the practice borders through a process of negotiation rather than delegation. The word "negotiation" is chosen deliberately to characterize the newly emerging clinical practice model of the time period. The term implies agency, volition, and participation of all parties involved in the process of constructing practice boundaries. Agency is a requirement for negotiation even when one party holds greater power, and it assumes each party has the authority and the ability to make choices of some kind.[3] The everyday agency evoked by nurses and physicians in practice settings in turn contributes to the tension between the realities of clinical practice and larger societal structures of power.

At the local level, at the point of care, rules and policies are not definitive; they can be flexible, and some degree of uncertainty exists.[4] It is here that both nurses and physicians practicing in the 1960s and 1970s made choices to relinquish traditional tasks and the knowledge embedded in them or to take on new ones that redefined their immediate practice boundaries. It was a two-way process involving several ingredients, as physician Barbara Bates suggested: "First, a nurse with competence and with courage. Second, a doctor with the willingness to experiment and to learn from a nurse. Third, continuity of these two people over a sufficient time so that they can learn to know and trust each other, to give and take. And, fourth, a specific goal in patient care."[5] Bringing these components together, in turn, supported experimentation with practice boundaries.

But these choices also led to competing claims of knowledge and power surrounding the patient encounter. It was here, in a particular and peculiar political space of the clinical moment, that nurses reimagined their clinical practice. This process, as both a political and practice movement, represented the accumulated weight of individual actions, and these actions were, at times, at odds with the positions taken by national and state organizations and, in many instances, their individual colleagues.[6] As one physician noted, "Now that we are entering the pressure cooker of inflation and government regulation, it is time to serve notice that the 'health care team' consists only of the physician and his patient."[7] Perspectives of this kind, which were and remain conspicuous, flavored the negotiations surrounding clinical practice, making necessary the individualistic and personal nature of the merging models of patient care.

Dialogue over professional borders was not singular in tone and ranged from respectful to hostile. But, in order for patient care to move smoothly along, common ground needed to be found between the work nurses thought they could do, physicians' perceptions, and patients' needs. This triangular formation was not easily maneuvered. Sometimes the negotiations were polarized to the point that the two professions talked about themselves and one another using the language of exclusion and victimization. The medical profession was (and somewhat remains) normative and exclusive, prioritizing the skills of medical diagnosis and prescription of treatment (rather than the combined efforts of several professions) as the most essential and rigorous components of health care. In turn, many nurses publicly proclaimed their victimization by physicians, suggesting that nursing's claims for autonomy and authority required toppling medicine from its lofty pedestal of cultural authority.[8]

There were components of truth in each of these perspectives. During acute illness crises, patients indeed required exquisite medical attention and knowledge, such as those cases requiring surgery. And nurses were often treated unfairly—or frankly abused—in clinical practice, especially when working among the chronically ill and older populations.[9] Yet, as most nurses and physicians recognized, relationships at the clinical moment in the patient's space were much more complicated than simple exclusionist and victimization narratives suggested. Many clinical associations were saturated with close, respectful, and collaborative experiences.[10] Studies of critical care nurses, nurses in battle, and dialysis nurses, for example, suggest the mutuality nurses and physicians shared as they struggled to comprehend the meaning of new clinical data and technologies to shape patient care.[11]

In other contexts, nurses used active resistance as well as other strategies of implicit noncooperation with both physicians and patients to control their behavior. "The doctor-nurse game" came to mean the subtle (and not so subtle) ways nurses controlled the behaviors of the physicians with whom they disagreed or found inexperienced.[12] In settings such as obstetric wards, nurses and their patients struggled between two gendered systems—the domestic world of the home and women's values, and the exceedingly structured, scientific, and highly masculine world of hospital and medical authority, which included nurses' own strict behavioral codes. Nurses straddled these worlds, vulnerable to gender expectations, age, and class differences, oftentimes behaving boorishly toward their women patients who might have been natural allies.[13]

Part of the complexity of the questions surrounding clinical authority stemmed from the shifting meaning of medicine's normative status. Since the mid-nineteenth century, medicine assumed this position and described all other providers in language that established hierarchical relationships.[14] The media, medicine, and sometimes nurses themselves used terms such as "secondary provider," "nonphysician," "paramedical," or "midlevel provider" to describe practitioners who were not physicians. This language devalued the services provided by others and supported systems of payment tied to medical control. From this position, physicians claimed not only economic power but also the power to control the knowledge and skills associated with medicine.

Yet on closer examination, physicians' claims were not naturally constructed—they were socially constructed by contextual forces—by physicians themselves and by nurses' complicity. Because of physicians' cultural authority, class, race, and gender, they held the power to create and re-create the boundaries of medical knowledge and skills. The nursing profession may have indirectly perpetuated this. By standing in opposition to the medical ideal, nurses came to require it for their identity.[15] Medicine conceptualized as an oppressive force could just as well serve as a powerful unifying factor, as a "rhetorical force-multiplier" for nursing during times of conflict within the nursing profession itself.[16] And, nurses' disinclination to confront physician authority structures may have also indicated their sense of the reflected authority and power they gained from physicians. In many instances—nurse practitioners constituting just one example—physicians smoothed the way and supported nursing practice.

Even so, skills and knowledge informally passed back and forth between nursing and medicine. Most of these skills, such as the use of the thermometer or stethoscope, transferred quietly from doctors to nurses when they were no longer considered of high status or when they became a nuisance.[17] On the other hand, sharing of knowledge became a common occurrence in the practice of public health nurses in the early twentieth century, in the first critical care units of the 1950s, and during wars, as nurses and physicians in close quarters taught each other how to care for acutely and chronically ill patients.[18]

During the 1960s and into the 1970s, informal negotiations were structured by "nurse and physician identity crises."[19] Physicians struggled with ballooning patient loads, dwindling physician interest in primary care (physicians who are the first point of contact for patients, such as family practice and general practice physicians and pediatricians), information overload provided by new technology, and desperately needed educated allies.[20] Nurses, meanwhile, looked for ways to use the skills and knowledge they already had and to take on those they believed they could handle. Unable to find this opportunity, some were so discouraged with their practice limitations that they considered leaving the profession. One nurse described her journey to nurse practitioner training. "I was looking for a way out of the nursing profession after less than ten years as a registered nurse," she remarked. "A colleague in the family planning clinic where I worked heard about a one-year training program for women's health care nurse practitioners in California and urged me to apply. I didn't even know any nurse practitioners at that time; however, before I gave up on nursing and became a clinical psychologist, I thought I should give nursing one more chance."[21]

Perhaps nurses also sensed opportunity in medicine's unfulfilled promises to a growing public demand for general (rather than specialized) health services, and they boldly expanded their practices in new and exciting dimensions. Physicians themselves were open to the possibilities of educated allies. "If he [the physician] is to have an associate capable of thinking and making judgments," pioneer physician-nurse practitioner team Barbara Bates and Joan Lynaugh wrote, "he must allow it to happen, even encourage it."[22] In this environment, the clinical practice boundaries were opening to cultural and political negotiation.

During this period, nursing and medicine, although separate in their professional philosophies, moved in both parallel and intersecting paths to restructure patient care. Indeed, the changes both professions experienced were pivotal to the shape of later practices, as was the mutual dependency of medicine and nursing in the provision of patient care.[23] The 1960s were a time of crucial change for American health care. The ramifications of the strategies national leaders and local practitioners devised during this time to cope with change continue to influence health care provision, contemporary practice, and relationships between nurses and physicians to this day.

Reports and Opportunities

Preserving physicians' normative status was predicated on an adequate supply of physicians in clinical settings. This was not the case in smaller communities or for general practitioners. As primary care physicians at the local level complained about their overwhelming workload, national commissions perpetuated the perceptions of a generalized physician manpower shortage and suggested solutions that focused primarily on methods to support physician practice rather than any restructuring of medical care provision. Physicians continued to move primarily into highly specialized areas of medical practice. In 1952, the President's Commission on the Health Needs of the Nation documented a severe technician shortage (the technician category included nurses, as the largest group, along with health aides and practical nurses) and suggested the development of schools of auxiliary medical services under medical control.[24] In 1956, the report on paramedical personnel of the surgeon general's consultant group on medical education also noted a shortage of paramedical personnel (nurses, health aides, technicians, and practical nurses) to meet the needs of chronically ill patients.[25]

In 1959, the Bane committee (part of the surgeon general's consultant group on medical education) moved closer to acknowledging the interrelationship of medicine and other health professions. The committee conceded that physicians could not carry out their increasingly complex responsibilities without the collaboration of other health professionals.[26] These findings were echoed in the 1965 report of the president's commission on heart disease, cancer, and stroke, and in the 1965 Coggeshall report of the executive committee of the Association of American Medical Colleges, which also recommended that medical schools assume responsibility for evaluating and training allied health professionals.[27]

For more than ten years, these reports shared common themes: essentially, the health of American citizens was threatened by a physician shortage. And, the threat was even more serious because there was also a shortage and underutilization of other types of health personnel who supported physicians' practices. All of these reports, although innovative in recognizing the interrelationships of the health professions, were quite traditional because they failed to propose new strategies for providing more accessible services and perpetuated the primacy of physicians in health care. Considering the continuity of common themes, it is not surprising that few innovative strategies emerged from these reports. Most of them recommended increased funding for physician education in general and strengthening medicine's control over the training of auxiliary personnel, including nurses. Yet in one sense, the reports provided an unintended opening and an avenue for other health professionals to broaden their roles by taking on functions traditionally considered within the realm of medicine. Physicians, as the reports reminded policy makers and other professional groups, needed relief from the more mundane and less complex portions of practice (such as duties ranging from filling out forms to well-child care and employment physicals), and clearly affirmed that physicians should allocate these tasks to other professionals.

More importantly, many of these reports were after-the-fact and merely documented the stresses and complexities physicians such as general practitioners and pediatricians had been facing for several years. In fact, in many cases they had been devising their own sometimes less-than-effective, private strategies for relief. By the early 1960s, most of these strategies involved delegation of responsibilities to nurses and allied health professionals for primarily administrative and clerical tasks such as completion of insurance forms, stocking of clinics, inventory of supplies, and answering phones.[28] Yet giving these responsibilities to nurses barely scratched the surface of their capabilities, and was a fairly poor use of their time.

Using nurses in expanded clinical roles was already the norm in many private practices, but, for the most part, their work was shaped by sexism and paternalism. "If you have a secretary or nurse who is too old, too fat, too sour, domineering, possessive, dictatorial," one physician wrote, "who pushes patients around and generally behaves as if it is her practice, fire her tomorrow."[29] In general, physicians were reluctant to see their office employees as more than "their girls," similar to a housewife or a domestic worker.[30] Many physicians refused to delegate services such as patient education, counseling, and advising to nurses. They were more comfortable assigning these things to the ladies auxiliary, composed mostly of physicians' wives and daughters. AMA president Wesley Hall in his 1970 inaugural address proposed a greater role for this group. He suggested the auxiliary might be utilized to help busy physicians in their practices by helping to educate poor women about prenatal care and teens about drug abuse and addiction.[31]

But in some areas grassroots physicians, perhaps taking to heart the openings provided by the reports, sought relief in other ways and recognized the

importance of nurses' clinical skills. These physicians, perhaps more liberal
minded or innovative than some of their colleagues, began to negotiate and
offered to train nurses to perform certain skills that were key parts of clinical
practice.[32] In return, some nurses agreed and welcomed the opportunity to
incorporate new knowledge into their practice and to perform new skills, with
the proviso that physicians were available for support when needed. As one
nurse practitioner noted, "He [the physician] taught us to do things that needed
to be done when he couldn't get there, like suture lacerations. . . . He wanted us
to do everything we could to help him, but he was always there to make the
decision. . . . It was a teaching/learning situation you [had] to go through with
each physician, . . . we probably taught them a lot about how to get along with
people that they didn't get in their training."[33]

The most formative discussions concerning knowledge claims and skills
were played out at the parochial level in informal conversations between nurses,
physicians, and patients. At the grassroots level, in clinics and private practices, nurses and physicians negotiated responsibility and authority according
to the needs of the community, the practice, and their own personal prerogatives. In rural areas, for example, a physician may have had responsibility for
several clinics in different counties but was unable to hire or afford a partner;
both the practice area and salary may have been uncompetitive with urban or
suburban practices. A nurse practitioner described a similar practice relationship: "He [the physician] was in the one clinic one day and another clinic
another day. He had a private practice too. But he was always available by
phone and always responded immediately. . . . I was with him two and a half
days [per week] and really learned an awful lot from him. . . . He didn't have a
problem with nurses learning to do this [contraceptive care] and he really
taught me to take care of a lot of abnormal patients."[34] The nurse practitioner
provided coverage for patients when the physician could not physically be at
the clinic—and, significantly, at a cheaper rate. Practice economics were critical issues for many physicians and a major reason they chose to enlarge their
work with nurses.

The specific location of the patients was also pivotal in the development of
the nurse practitioner role. Public health nurses providing services in the community typically practiced beyond the traditional boundaries of practice in
hospitals or private practices. They were quite independent and less bound by
institutional rules. In 1965 nurse and educator Loretta "Lee" Ford developed
the nurse practitioner certificate program at the University of Colorado with her
colleague Henry Silver, a pediatrician at the university. Ford explained how the
nurse practitioner role segued from her previous work. "I had at least twelve

years of visiting nurse service and public health nursing services," she noted, "and in Colorado particularly in [rural] public health, we would have the whole county to cover in terms of schools, maternal and child health follow up. We would have classes that we taught for the Red Cross. We would have crippled children's clinics, tuberculosis clinics, school clinics, immunization clinics, the child health nursing conferences, and child health conferences. So we were doing generalized services and lots of it."[35]

Ford was interested in expanding the nurse's role "not because there was a shortage of physicians . . . maybe it provided the opportunity, but to tell you the truth, I wasn't even aware of it. It wasn't in my frame to help medicine out."[36] She saw the nurse practitioner role as a way to legitimize what she and her public health colleagues were already doing. "When it came right down to it," she noted, "we were making decisions. And the more I worked with people like the orthopedist in the crippled children's clinics or the physicians in the child health conference, it was very obvious that the things that we were identifying were also what the physician was identifying, in terms of growth and development. And indeed, we knew more about the generalized care, and mothering and parenting. Or were more concerned about it than the physicians were, because they were looking for defects, and we were looking for strengths, and for prevention and promotion of health in families."[37] The setting and the particular individual participants determined the flavor of the negotiations, as did the economic status of the patients. Ford noted, "You practiced clandestinely so nobody knew what you were doing, I mean, you had to do it. . . . There was nobody else, and, the poor families . . . frankly expected you to make those kinds of decisions anyway."[38]

Ford described the nurse practitioner movement as an outgrowth of her work on community health practice and curriculum development, and Silver's somewhat serendipitous attendance at the same state conference. Ford remembered, "We couldn't get enough of them [general practitioners and pediatricians] to man our nursing child health conferences [clinics]. So the state health department called this conference of both practitioners and educators together . . . , and Henry Silver went to that conference. I did not know him."[39]

Silver was not initially enthusiastic about the ideas generated at the conference, such as independent nursing practice and nurse-physician partnerships, but he became intrigued after talking to his department chair, C. Henry Kemp. He then tried to draw support from pediatric nurses, but he received little interest. "He couldn't get anyone to follow up," Ford remembered. "He was very cordial, he said, and all that, but he couldn't get anybody to work with him."[40] In fact, Silver was looking in the wrong direction. He went to a familiar group, to hospital

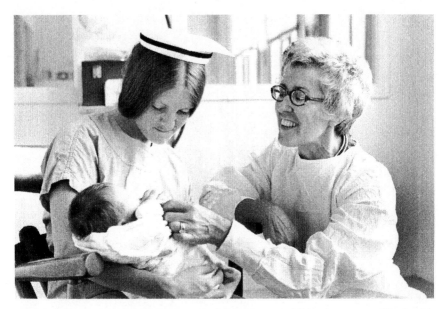

Photo 1 Nurse Practitioner Loretta Ford examines a child, circa 1975. (Used with permission from Loretta Ford, personal collection.) Ford developed the first nurse practitioner program in 1965 at the University of Colorado with physician Henry Silver. She was the first dean at the University of Rochester School of Nursing in 1972, and served until 1985.

nurses, who had little experience with primary care or with collaborative practice. After several discussions, Ford reported, Kemp said to Silver, "Henry, you look up Lee Ford. Now she's in community health, and the things that you're talking about are community health."[41] Kemp knew of Ford's work and understood what she and other nurses were doing and how they could work with Silver.

As Ford and Silver developed their program, others across the country were also doing the same. At first, no consultation occurred as each group worked according to its own motives and experience. The diversity of the practice context precluded consistently shaped negotiations that could be packaged and replicated across the country. And even when the numbers of nurse practitioner training programs exploded in the early 1970s, physicians and nurses found common ground on an ad hoc basis, one by one by one.

Re-creating Clinical Practice and Fragmentation of Clinical Thinking

Within this contested territory of the clinical space, individual nurses and physicians reconstructed their practice realities. This process was both entrepreneurial and highly ambiguous. Some nurses had to consider their role of primary health care provider in the context of previous positions as office assistants or staff nurses—and many were still responsible for those duties after their nurse practitioner training. They also struggled to integrate a medical role into a nursing role, at first operating in two separate spheres. One nurse complained during the early stages of her nurse practitioner training, "I didn't know if I should examine the patient or clean him up."[42] This nurse keenly understood but had no solution yet for the unresolved dichotomy many nurse practitioners experienced as they stood in both the nursing and medical realm.

Eventually, nurses and physicians settled into an integrated and more balanced professional approach. Physicians themselves, although understanding the need to learn to work collaboratively, constructed elaborate systems to verify the competence of their new nurse colleagues that went beyond those established for physicians themselves. One nurse practitioner noted, "In the beginning he was real gentle in letting me do things. Don't even make a referral without him, don't do this. Don't do that. But soon he [knew] you well enough."[43] Physicians, in turn, also struggled as they relinquished a portion of the "emotional heart of medicine," realizing they had to share their relationships with patients.[44]

As practitioners reconfigured the boundaries of practice and learning, they indirectly segmented and fragmented clinical thinking skills, which were physicians' traditional source of authority. The process of clinical thinking is a dynamic entity of patient data collection and generation of treatment in the social, political, and experiential construction of the individual physician and the profession itself. Clinical thinking consists of the skills and knowledge that physicians traditionally used to organize and collect data. It includes eliciting a patient history, performing a physical examination, ordering diagnostic tests, creating a diagnosis, formulating treatment options, prescribing treatments, and making decisions about prognoses.[45] It is a dynamic process that incorporates technology and the intellectual and experiential part of medicine. Physicians used clinical thinking to define themselves and give coherence and validity to the medical role. Their position—their authority and power—was traditionally predicated on these skills. And, in fact, contemporary health services, including diagnostic tests and procedures, admitting privileges, and collection of patient services, are organized around the clinical thinking process of physicians.[46]

Clinical thinking is, then, more than a functional process: it is the foundation upon which physicians legitimize and define their social and professional status and authority and through which they claim ownership of the patient. Through its strategic data organizing function and its ability to harness linguistic forces inherent in labeling and naming patient problems, it is an incredibly powerful process as a seamless whole.[47] In general, physicians' sense of ownership is infused with an overwhelming sense of personal and professional responsibility for each step of clinical thinking. Relinquishing part of the process—even to colleagues—would have broken its integrity and required physicians to disregard powerful medical school socialization. Even into the 1970s, medical school teachers specifically warned against sharing any portion of the physician's traditional role, and most physicians heard their professors preach that all good consultants do the history and physical exam themselves no matter how many times it was previously performed.[48] This sense of individual responsibility (e.g., in order to be responsible for patient care I have to verify the data collected by another physician) extended to a culturally derived suspicion of others' judgment—including other physicians—especially those not trained at the same institution or profession.

Until the mid-twentieth century, physicians claimed the formal process of and secured responsibility for clinical thinking, but many instances can be cited of nurses, in particular, informally and temporarily participating in parts of the process. Nurses, for example, performed various technical skills for data collection, informally engaged in circumspect diagnosing of patients, prescribed, made treatment decisions during emergencies, and even coached interns and residents through routine procedures and treatment decisions.[49] Turn-of-the-century visiting nurses at Henry Street Settlement House in New York City staffed the first aid room.[50] Farm Security Administration nurses working with the rural poor during the Depression prescribed medications, referred sick migrant workers to hospitals, and developed childhood immunization programs.[51] In black communities in the South, "back porch nursing" provided maternal and child health care and basic health services in churches, back rooms of stores, and homes. This type of health care proved enduring even when local hospitals opened because many new institutions did not support outpatient medical services.[52]

Even so, physicians legally and situationally controlled the process of clinical thinking. Despite unacknowledged and informal participation from nurses and other professionals over the decades, physicians remained responsible for and made the final decisions about interpretation of data and medical treatment of patients until the health care environment of the 1960s supported loosening of their control. As other practitioners expertly used these skills to care for appreciative patients, they exposed the political character and permeability of legally and socially constructed practice barriers.[53] Nurse practitioners personified this situation.

Shifts and Breaks

In the last half of the twentieth century, an ideological, linguistic, and epidemiologic shift occurred that opened the process of clinical thinking to inspection and negotiation. Chronic illnesses and the problems of both a baby boom and an aging population transformed the patient profile in exam rooms, clinics, and in hospitals in general, which saw their acuity steadily increase. The prevailing diseases of the time—heart disease, cancer, arthritis, and stroke—were not, as New York physician Walsh McDermott noted, "susceptible to treatment, because substantial changes would be required in an individual's lifestyle."[54] And, as many clinicians realized, lifestyle changes and their immediate effects were difficult to quantify, and even more difficult to persuade patients to execute. It was becoming impossible to measure the impact of medicine "because the traditional indicators of mortality and disease rate no longer captured the real picture of population health."[55] Influenced by changing demographics and epidemiological trends, the whole paradigm of health and illness was changing, and traditional ways of defining clinical success, such as morbidity and mortality rates, were losing their relevance.[56]

Not only were the skills and knowledge in medical curricula increasing in complexity and mismatched to the needs of most patients, but clinical advances and sheer numbers of patients in both hospitals and clinics supported a shift in the importance and symbolic meaning of traditional key data collection methods embedded in clinical thinking, such as the physical exam and patient history. These components, through the meaning bestowed upon them by the patient and public in general, were traditionally therapeutic in themselves as their performance provided a sense of well-being to patients. One writer noted of these personal interactions, "Patients once experienced a catharsis in being able to tell their stories at their own pace, and felt a thorough physical examination to be an expression of the doctor's concern for them."[57]

But this process was time consuming, and physicians spent many tedious hours performing periodic physical examinations. The medical history, too, became downplayed, and physicians grew less tolerant of long, detailed patient reflections especially when a reception room full of patients was waiting for them. By the mid-1960s, many physicians devised strategies to economize their time by using self-administered history forms and referring patients to the newly emerging multiphasic screening centers.[58] And, more sophisticated understandings of the relationship of X-ray images and laboratory results to patient signs and symptoms sometimes made percussion, palpation, and auscultation seem redundant and even old-fashioned. Although physicians continued to use these tools, they increasingly relied more heavily on scientific findings, especially in the larger urban academic settings. It was, as one physician aptly noted of the 1960s, the "measurable driving out the significant."[59]

A crack in the wall appeared, so to speak, in the cultural myth of the therapeutic power of physicians' authority. Perhaps physicians, nurses, and consumers all sensed the subtle shift in meaning of these traditional personal interactions. Growing alienation of patients from their physician providers created an opportunity for educated allies such as nurses to gain knowledge and the public's permission to apply it. Also to be considered here was an empowered, increasingly educated public that now had the foundation to question an authority—the physician—who was once considered unquestionable. A pre–World War II middle-class family might have used the same general practitioner for years. But a growing sense of dissatisfaction, stemming perhaps from less attentive and busy family physicians, along with a more knowledgeable public provided a shaky foundation for loyalty. By the 1970s, patient surveys captured the public's sentiments, indicating that two-thirds of patients polled would be willing to change their provider if they found one that listened better and showed more interest in their complaints.[60]

From a slightly different perspective, physicians probably sensed the economic and professional promise of educated allies during a time of both increased demand and declining patient loyalty and trust. If they could find a competent and economic collaborator who listened to patients and answered their questions, and who could provide some of the personal, hands-on care that required so much time, they might be able, by proxy, to gain back some of the public's trust. Nurses, some of them working in physicians' own offices, provided the possibility and prophecy for reorganizing and renegotiating medical borderlands. As one physician told me, "I have not looked historically at nurse practitioners and the people who chanced it, but I think that we had a crisis and I've always looked for allies. One of my mentors always said, 'When your head is in the guillotine for extended periods of time, ask for help.'"[61] It was, it seemed for some, time to ask for help.

Negotiating Clinical Thinking

Clinical practice negotiations centered on clinical thinking because they occurred at the bedside or in the exam room between individual nurses, physicians, and patients. This is where clinical thinking was used most intensely and the opportunity for dialogue was most likely. At this point, the negotiations were continuous and involved informal and sometimes tacit social interactions framed by the personalities of the doctors and nurses and the local community's needs. They were supported and nourished by the mutual dependency of medical and nursing professionals as they struggled together to provide health care for their patients and create meaningful practices for themselves.

In fact, and perhaps most germane, negotiations were not mandated from above by the edicts of national organizations, such as the American Medical Association (AMA) or the American Nurses' Association (ANA), or by educational institutions. They happened in a seemingly disconnected way in many different places, and only later came together as a fortified movement. A nurse practitioner astutely noted, "This all [nurse practitioners working with physicians] occurred because [the] physicians knew us and felt that we had good judgment—we had worked with them before."[62] The process was personal—individualistic rather than institutional—and served the needs of doctors, nurses, and patients.

Although imbalances in power existed between the nurse and physician negotiators—and each party may have held different perspectives of how the negotiations proceeded—this imbalance did not stymie the process because both physicians and nurses obtained something they needed or wanted.[63] Among other things, physicians received less-costly help in their busy practices and the freedom to pursue more interesting cases by teaching nurses to perform various parts (such as physical examination, history taking, decision making based on the data collected) of the clinical thinking process. "Our insurance carrier came out and said 'Don't do that,'" one nurse reported, "but he [the physician] wanted us to do everything we could to help him."[64]

For doctors, working with nurses in new types of practices was not always without risk because many of their physician colleagues could only see challenges to their traditional authority and not the potential benefits. Physicians who taught in the early nurse practitioner programs were chastised by their less enlightened colleagues and labeled as collaborators in a very negative sense. A nurse practitioner from Texas noted, "These physicians, since these were our first preceptors (clinical teachers), had to go against the mind-set of the medical community and risk being professionally shunned."[65] The same nurse practitioner recalled a panel presentation at a state conference that included both nurse practitioners and their physician colleagues, although the physician members were difficult to recruit because they were fearful of their colleagues' reaction. "On the surface," she noted, "the program was received in an amicable demeanor and questions about the practices followed the presentation. However, on the following day, conversations among physicians were overheard with statements of 'getting these doctors' through the medical board to get them out of practice."[66]

The early nurse practitioners were highly dependent upon like-minded, liberal-thinking physicians who—though unsure of the breadth of nurses' contributions and wary of their less liberal colleagues—nevertheless were willing to experiment. A nurse practitioner noted, "I was lucky back then to have a very supportive MD collaborator. He never worked with a nurse practitioner before—I was the first in a three-county rural area. However, he was impressed with what I had learned. I can still hear him say, 'You really do know what you are doing.' He stood side by side with me for awhile, but soon gave me the independence I had always wanted as a professional. And he always backed me up. . . . Not all the physicians in these three counties were thrilled to have a nurse doing what I was doing—prescribing pills, putting in IUDs, and diagnosing problems. That is where my supportive physician collaborator came in. He told those skeptical physicians that I did know what I was doing."[67] Another nurse reported, "I almost never saw [another] physician. It [contact with physicians] was almost always on the phone. There was more antagonism. 'A nurse practitioner? What is that, what did you do? Who did the exam? You did the exam? Well, was there a doctor there?' "[68]

Nurses were not always willing collaborators. Physicians sometimes had to convince nurses to seize the new opportunities the nurse practitioner role offered. But taking on new skills and responsibilities and forging more independent roles was daunting to nurses who were already experts in a particular clinical field. Nurse Denise Geolot remembered how physician Richard Edlick approached her with the idea of entering the emergency nurse practitioner program at the University of Virginia. "He came to me and he said, 'I want you to work with me on this opportunity,' and I said to him, 'I'm very happy doing what I'm doing.' I was working in critical care and teaching it. . . . And, I absolutely loved what I was doing. And I said, 'I really have no interest in changing.' And he said, 'Oh the opportunities, the possibilities, and what you could do if you did this—the challenge!' "[69]

Participating nurses, both cautious and eager, chose to enter into new practice arrangements that moved them to borderlands of both medical and nursing worlds. As they reshaped their practice, nurse practitioners reaped the benefits of status linked to their new skills and the ability to work in new and more meaningful ways that corresponded with their experience and education. The sense of rediscovery and relocation comes through in one nurse's recollection: "I didn't have to rely on what the physicians said. I had my parameters and I could treat a patient within them. I had my own decision-making. I was a lot more independent, autonomous, and it did a lot to help me realize that hey, I can do this, I'm not dumb. I can do this, and then as I learned more and more, I really was able to do the things for patients that I had always wanted to do for years and had to wait for a physician to agree. I could take care of the problems I saw. It relieved frustration."[70]

But with authority came responsibility and the loss of a safe space provided by the more encapsulated, circumscribed nursing position. Even though physicians provided much-needed support, nurse practitioners still had broader areas of responsibility and expectations that required emotional adjustment—both self-imposed and external. "After twenty years as a pediatric nurse in a tertiary pediatric hospital setting, I returned to the University for my MSN [master's degree in nursing] and jumped into the role of a pediatric nurse practitioner in primary care that seemed like a whole new world to me," one nurse practitioner noted. "Gone was the security of always knowing what to do, enter the new world of discovery."[71] Denise Geolot, who became a nurse practitioner in the early 1970s, noted, "It was very exciting and unsettling at the same time. . . . Now I was dealing with the whole person as opposed to just the cardiac system. You're responsible for managing a much broader base of care. In the CCU [Coronary Care Unit] you're working under protocols, but again, you're an expert so that you know exactly what to do. And all of a sudden, you're a learner and a novice."[72]

As nurse practitioners took on new roles, so did their physician partners. One nurse astutely described this joint learning process:

> Any of my independent jobs, I went in with a physician who had never worked with a nurse practitioner before and so I always started out very, very slowly, very cautiously. [I] would start out with, "These are the things I can do, but you tell me what you want me to do." And I generally started out pretty restrictive. Self-restrictive because I wanted them to feel comfortable with my decision-making and I wanted them to feel comfortable with how I did things, and then slowly show them that I knew how to do some other things and that I would be glad to do it. You know, tell them that "this woman has a big mass on the right side, it's pretty tender, I think we need to get an ultrasound. Is that what you want me to do?" And then, pretty soon, it was just—"Oh, you didn't need to call, just go ahead and do that."[73]

Negotiation was a time-intensive and sometimes painful process. As this same nurse noted, "There were times when I would come home and say to my husband, 'Do I have holes in my head? Why am I doing this [educating a new physician about her role] again?' "[74] But the process repeatedly led to mutually beneficial practice and patient care, as this nurse practitioner noted: "Although I was in the community, I was not working with any physicians from the community because the physician that worked in the clinic was from another town. So recognizing that we had patients that lived in this town, we felt the need to refer them, if they needed additional help, to a physician in the vicinity. So it was kind of hard getting those physicians to not grumble and growl, and to take you serious, recognize that you were doing something worthwhile and that you were not stupid." She went on, "But then as we were there longer and longer, when we sent a patient to them, that patient did in fact have an accurate diagnosis, had been treated well, things sort of settled down."[75]

In turn, nurse practitioners also had to trust their physician colleagues not to expect or force them to go beyond mutually established boundaries. "I just trusted the physician I was working with that what he told me to do was ethical, proper, and legal," another nurse practitioner described.[76] Relying upon state practice acts to help define practice boundaries was difficult in the 1960s and even into the 1970s as most were unchanged from earlier decades.[77] Until the states revised the acts in the mid- to late 1970s to keep up with practice (see chapter 6), there was room for contingency and flexibility within the framework of individual negotiations between nurse practitioners and physicians. Even so, physicians were cautious because their medical colleagues sometimes reported their more collaborative activities to the state licensure boards. In Pennsylvania, for example, the medical board investigated complaints lodged by physicians that certain nurse practitioners were diagnosing patients and practicing medicine. These complaints ranged from the general (e.g., that nurses were practicing medicine) to the specific (e.g., they were performing physical assessment and collecting health history data).[78]

Although the lack of defined roles could have been quite liberating in a sense, many nurse practitioners entering their first posttraining roles—especially when the practice focus differed from earlier positions—wanted and needed physician colleagues to understand their ability to contribute to the practice and to support them during their initial work experience. In one example, a group of physicians hired a newly graduated nurse practitioner in the late 1960s to work in a north Philadelphia pediatric clinic that had received funding from the Model Cities Program (a part of President Lyndon Johnson's war on poverty that began in 1964). This nurse practitioner described the difficulty: "They [the physicians] weren't familiar with it [the nurse practitioner role]. They had gotten health education and welfare [department] funding to hire such a person. They had no clue, and I had almost no clue myself. I had a little more information than they did, but I was kind of looking for somebody to help me implement the thing, and they were like kinda filling a position because the government said 'hire such a person and pay them x salary.' So it wasn't really clear what I was to do."[79]

The fledgling nurse practitioners were in general uncertain and untrusting of their own abilities and needed support from their physician colleagues, which was not always available. If the nurse practitioners could not trust their physician colleagues to back them up when problems arose, collaborative practice was insupportable. "I let them know in the beginning that this was my first job and what I would need is a lot of checking things out with them, them becoming familiar with what I knew, learning from them because this was my first job. [But that] fell on deaf ears. They didn't seem to quite understand that it wasn't OK just to go to lunch if I had a patient with a 104 temp who possibly had meningitis. I would have to go find them in the lunchroom. They'd forget to turn their pagers on. . . . I didn't know whether they thought I could do it or if they just weren't on top of things."[80] In the absence of useful and adequate support, nurse practitioners felt isolated and their contributions to the care of patients in the clinic or practice was unacknowledged or diminished. Patient care was not compromised at its most basic level as access continued, but the potential for expanded availability and more in-depth services nurse practitioners might have offered was limited.

Part of the discrepancy between what nurse practitioners wanted from their physician colleagues and the kind of support they received stemmed from a paradox confronting nurse practitioners. During their educational programs, nurse practitioners learned a great deal about particular skills and clinical facts, but they also gained knowledge not shared by their nursing and physician colleagues. This was hybrid disciplinary information achieved by integrating medicine with nursing, and it produced a subtle but acknowledged practice paradigm shift. As practice roles changed, physicians and nurses alike questioned which practitioner—general nurse (non-nurse practitioner) or physician—was the appropriate supervisor to most effectively train and mentor new nurse practitioners.[81] The answer, more and more frequently, particularly from nursing, was an experienced nurse practitioner. In the decades of the 1960s and 1970s and even later, there were not enough of them qualified to oversee the education of or provide basic mentorship and socialization for those new to the role. In the breach, many groups claimed authority for nurse practitioner supervision. Too many supervisors created problems of scale and detail for developing practices, as nursing and medicine, state and federal governments all attempted to control nurse practitioner education and practice.

As these complications arose, nurse practitioners began seeking sources of support beyond their physician colleagues. One nurse explained: "I don't have any good memory of them [the physicians] being very informative. I don't know if it just wasn't a great fit, but they sort of left me on my own. They didn't want to seem to make it fit. To find more of a support group, I used to go up to St. Christopher's [a children's hospital in Philadelphia, Pennsylvania]. There were nurse practitioners up there I could hang with. . . . I could work with those nurses and . . . discuss common concerns that we had in clinical practice, what we were doing, how we were sorting things out. It was useful."[82]

Other sources of validation and support helped nurse practitioners during their negotiations with physician colleagues. These ranged from peer-to-peer relationships with other nurse practitioners to satisfied groups of patients receiving care. A pediatric nurse practitioner working in the same practice over several years noted a familiar duality early on in her practice. "I was not the first nurse practitioner in the [clinic] practice . . . so it was already geared for them. It was harder in the hospital. We used to go on nursery rounds to convince them [nurses, hospital residents and other physicians] of our expertise."[83] The nurse continued, "Now . . . , the nurses are so happy we're there. They think kids get better care on weekends and every baby gets examined. Every mother can see we are doing this. They always feel issues get dealt with more comprehensively when we are there. So it's a full 180 from not having any backup to completely having a fan club."[84]

In short, for early nurse practitioners and physicians, collaborative clinical practice was a complex and individually negotiated process. It involved exquisite timing, making adventuresome choices, recognizing opportunities for dialogue, however limited, and generally applying artful and creative strategies to carve out significant and satisfying clinical practices.[85] In this ambiguous environment, all practitioners could claim something.

Many astute physicians understood and anticipated opportunities and challenges. George Ferrar Jr., president of the Pennsylvania Medical Society in 1969, keenly realized the importance these kinds of practice relationships held for all kinds of providers. "Right now," he questioned his constituents, "how many of you are willing to supervise—from, say ten miles away—a satellite office staffed by a medical corpsman or a registered nurse with several months of additional training . . . who will be a screening practitioner and at the same time treat the emergency and less complicated conditions with nothing more than the availability of telephone advice from you? You say it will never happen?"

He went on to assure the membership, "Such a person *will* come into being with or without your cooperation and guidance, and if such an assistant comes into being without our [physicians] active direction, this health professional someday could become *the single greatest opposing force* that medical doctors have ever faced."[86] His warning, although clearly directed toward maintaining medicine's control over practice, articulated the rapidly changing clinical milieu. Nurse practitioners and their physician colleagues took advantage of this fluidity as they reimagined and reconstructed new kinds of clinical practices, or legitimized already established relationship to meet their own and their patients' needs. They, like Richard Edlich could declare, "Oh the possibilities, the opportunities . . . !"[87]

Chapter 2

Following the Money

While individual nurses and physicians together reconfigured local clinical practices, larger collectives such as professional organizations and academic institutions responded to their own sorts of challenges. As early as the 1950s, vociferous policy and ideological debates raged through medical and nursing schools. The discussions occurring both between and within professional groups focused on three important issues: how many and what type of practitioners were needed to adequately provide patient care in the contemporary health care environment; how educational institutions, not known for their flexibility, might produce the faculty leadership and appropriately trained clinicians to take on this challenge; and finally, how strong linkages could be created between disciplinary knowledge and socially relevant health care.

Medicine and nursing in the 1960s and 1970s responded to these challenges in ways that had profound consequences for both professions. For nursing in particular, a major paradigmatic shift in education was needed, moving from one that defined excellence as skillful manipulation of equipment and patients to another that required a more humanities- and science-based curriculum. This approach provided nurses with the tools to think about patients in a radically different way in a rapidly changing system of medical care. Nursing was not the only group facing issues of this kind as the engineering, accounting, and library science occupations experienced similar internal struggles.[1] And similar to these groups, nursing was neither prepared for the shift nor at times willing to make the change. The profession slowly experimented with new curricula and practice models as it tried to make sense of "what it actually meant to take care of patients."[2]

Medical education experienced these stresses in tandem with nursing, although the flavor and direction were slightly different. General practice physicians' satisfaction with the relationships they built with patients and their traditionally broad preparation could not compete with the cultural and economic opportunities offered by training in the increasingly popular medical specialties (e.g., surgery and its subspecialties, cardiology and dermatology), thus contributing to the shrinking numbers of physicians in community-based primary care practices. Medical school curricula, postgraduate training (e.g., clinical training after medical school), and the interests of powerful academic hospitals focused on research and highly complex patients also directed physicians into specialty practices. But although physicians were trained in the increasingly acute academic hospital environment where they took care of patients after heart valve surgery or giving them toxic chemotherapies, they were less likely to be employed there after their training. This education/practice incongruence required newly minted physicians to meet head-on the culture clash between academic medicine and community practice. These coalescing factors obligated physicians to reexamine clinical practice models and think, albeit reluctantly at times, about including different kinds of practitioners.

Spurred by streams of federal money, nursing and medical professional organizations reacted to the changes already occurring in clinical practice. If the government or the organizations had established some sort of broad strategic planning process backed by their financial resources and social power to respond to the nation's health care needs, a more balanced and organized foundation of education and training might have emerged. Instead, most of the federal largesse supported (and still does) basic science research, academic-based hospitals, and medical specialty training, as efforts to equilibrate the acute care focus with that for the "the well and the well but worried" met with much resistance.[3] Academic medicine and nursing magnificently prepared clinicians to care for hospital patients who were receiving new, complicated surgical procedures or medical treatments, as this is where the funding and the political and social power of health care intersected. But most physician and nurse educators found that creating new practice models and educational programs to care for patients outside hospitals and in clinics was only marginally interesting, until an influx of federal money and a growing cadre of nurses and physicians in collaborative primary care practices created momentum in the 1960s and 1970s.

Medical Education and Practice

Medical practice and education were also going through tremendous changes that accelerated after World War II. These changes were more market driven (the market being the institutions, government agencies, and third-party insurers who compensated and employed physicians), rather than an "intellectual movement concerned with bodies of knowledge."[4] The changes reflected choices about the focus of education and practice that were driven in part by a great deal of federal and private investment that prioritized basic research over clinical education.

Generous federal investment post–World War II supported enormous scientific research efforts at university medical schools. These programs contributed a great deal of new knowledge and techniques, reciprocally fueling already present and newly emerging specialties, high-tech hospitals, and empowered specialty certifying boards. Lured by the excitement of the research endeavor and socialized by professors to seek out intriguing, groundbreaking cases, physicians were trained, for the most part, to practice in a severely limited setting—the acute care hospital.

Although steered by a highly specialized and bureaucratic marketplace, medicine was an essential part of the social fabric of American identity and status. Medicine's powerful social authority was embedded not only in the way individual citizens and their physicians created a personal social contract, but in how medicine itself, as part of a broader social phenomenon, became part of the "public interest." As such, a forceful combination of private and public institutions for research and education, professional organization oversight, and medical school missions funded, encouraged, and cajoled medicine to respond to public needs while addressing the interests of the marketplace.[5]

By the end of the 1950s, most middle-class Americans considered health care a basic right earned through employer-financed or privately purchased insurance supported by middle-class prosperity. Increased popularity and affordability of hospital insurance supported greater utilization of hospitals and the medical and surgical specialists who practiced there.[6] In contrast, there was also a growing population of citizens who were unemployed or working in low-paying nonunion jobs, especially in rural and poor urban areas, who were ineligible for federal assistance and could not afford physician fees. To meet their health needs, this group of patients began to seek care in overburdened and underserviced city and county health clinics, hospital walk-in clinics, and emergency rooms.

These urban and rural centers were places where medical practice was at its thinnest and perhaps farthest removed from the research and practice agenda of the urban academic centers. Urban hospitals and rural providers alike felt the crunch, as federal support for medical training focused more on specialty practice rather than general medical practice and yielded fewer professionals staffing emergency rooms and outpatient clinics.[7] One physician noted, "The emergency room was a very important part of educating residents, but they did not have adequate faculty supervision and [we] had no trained emergency physicians, and basically the quality of care being given to the patients was not acceptable. . . . There was no trained rescue squad and no consistent operation of a poison control center."[8] Inevitably, the clinics were a hard sell for medical students and residents compared to the excitement of the operating theater or general units. Their experiences helped shape the growing specialization trend.

At the same time, many authorities predicted a physician shortage. Depending upon the source, the number of physicians between 1950 and 1960 seemed to decrease, from 141 to 140 per 100,000 population.[9] The mobilization and health manpower report of 1955, the Bayne-Jones Report in 1958, and the Bane Report in 1959 all forecasted a dire shortage of physicians in the ensuing ten to twelve years.[10] Similar to the effect of the later 1963 surgeon general's consultant group report on nursing, the reports mobilized both medical schools and Congress to work toward increasing the supply of physicians. Other compelling arguments to grow the physician supply came from public hearings, such as the Senate Subcommittee on Aging in 1958 that exposed the lack of access to care for older adults, the inability of community hospitals to fill their labor needs with interns and residents, and a growing perception by the American public that they were losing their community practitioners.[11] But unlike the ANA, which strongly supported federal funding across the board for nursing education, the AMA responded with a "preconditioned set of attitudinal responses" against government influence and control over practice, and was unenthusiastic, to say the least, about federal support for medical education, including money for student scholarships.[12]

Despite the AMA's tepid support, Congress enacted the Health Professions Education Assistance Act (P.L. 88–129) in 1963 to expand teaching facilities and increase enrollments in schools of medicine via loan guarantees.[13] The influx of large amounts of federal dollars supported growth in the numbers of schools and students. Between 1964 and 1970 alone, thirteen new medical schools opened, and the number of graduates increased at a faster pace than in the previous decade.[14] The number of physicians per 100,000 population grew from 140 in 1960 to 151 in 1971.[15]

But rather than increasing the number of physicians across the board, the funding supported a shift from one area to another that was part of a growing decades-old trend. Manpower drained away from lower-paying and less-prestigious areas, such as general practice and primary care, and rapidly flooded the more glamorous medical and surgical subspecialties.[16] The number of sub-specialists grew as the number of general practitioners dropped from 120,000 in 1931 to 56,000 in 1971.[17] In 1955, 44 percent of active practicing physicians reported themselves to be full-time specialists. This proportion increased to 55 percent in 1960, and to 70 percent in 1965.[18] The number of specialty boards also grew. By 1940 there were sixteen specialty boards, nineteen by 1949, and twenty-three by 1984.[19]

As the number of physicians increased with the infusion of federal monies, general practitioners faced enormous demands for their services, especially from growing families with children, and from older adults. Even the combined force of general practitioners and pediatricians (whose number was growing in tandem with other medical specialists) could not keep up with the demand for children's services in particular. As the ratio of pediatricians per thousand children under the age of fifteen rose from 7 to 16 per thousand over a period of twenty-one years from 1940 to 1960, the ratio of the combination of pediatricians and general practitioners decreased from 352 to 151 per thousand children.[20] Additionally, most of the newly trained physicians practiced in urban academic or suburban area hospitals, contributing to a growing shortage of physicians providing primary care in rural and inner-city areas.[21]

Advertisements for physicians in rural Pennsylvania in the late 1960s captured the dilemma, but they could easily have been drawn from any other areas in the country. Between 1965 and 1970 at least 50 percent of practice opportunities noted in *Pennsylvania Medicine* (the journal of the Pennsylvania Medical Society) were for general practitioners. For example, three communities in northeastern Pennsylvania with a combined population of seven thousand and a trade-area population of thirty thousand (surrounding industry and worker population) had only one practicing physician in the area, and were advertising for another. Another town searching for a physician had a population of two thousand and a trade-area of six thousand. The town had two physicians, but one was in "advanced age." The nearest hospital was twenty-eight miles from the town.[22]

These shortages were troubling to the medical societies in particular, who decried them not only from the standpoint of service to patients, but understood the opportunities physician shortages in these areas gave newly emerging health providers. Pennsylvania Medical Society president George Ferrar Jr. addressed these issues as he noted in 1969:

Even now such groups are functioning in our city health departments, in the infirmaries of large industries, in the neighborhood health centers under Office of Economic Opportunity supervision. Which do you want? And if you think the problem is not with us now and growing you are

mistaken. . . . The State society's Physician Placement Service has registered with it more than seventy communities with varying degrees of need
for additional medical coverage, and it is growing month by month.[23]

The situation worsened by the 1970s. In 1971, the number of physicians
per 100,000 population varied from 195 physicians in the largest metropolitan
areas to 42 in some rural areas. In 1963, 98 counties in the United States were
without active physicians, and by 1971 this number had reached 133 counties.
The result was a net loss of care providers during a critical period of increasing
demand for primary care services. A larger number of older adults and poorer
families won access to health services through President Lyndon Johnson's Great
Society programs, the social initiative that produced Medicare and Medicaid.
An expanding population of children produced by the baby boom and a period
of relative prosperity that allowed a larger population to afford private physician
services contributed to the demand.

Piecemeal initiatives defined much of the public policy decisions in
primary health care during this time. The initiatives were typically crisis and
demonstration-oriented, highly fragmented approaches, the "try it and see"
approach, and lacked a steady unifying sense of strategic planning to address
primary care demands.[24] Congress increased access to health care through a series
of initiatives aimed at delivering services to targeted constituent groups and
areas. The Economic Opportunity Act of 1964 (P.L. 88–452) increased access
to neighborhood health centers. The number of health stations and community
clinics in low-income urban or special designation areas increased with the
Housing and Development Act of 1962 (P.L. 89–117) and the Appalachian
Regional Development Act of 1965 (P.L. 89–4). Access to clinics for migrant
workers and Cuban refugees increased with the Migration and Refugee Assistance
Act of 1962 (P.L. 87–510). These initiatives provided some relief for particular
groups but were not an overall solution to the primary care needs of the nation.
Additionally, these centers, at times, lacked qualified physicians and were some
of the first to experiment with providers such as nurse practitioners.

Until the mid- to late 1960s, medical educators responded slowly and somewhat ineffectually to the demographic and political changes taking place in the
United States. This was in part because patients in hospitals—where most learning and training took place, and where most federal funds for medical education
were directed—were acutely ill, unlike the majority of patients in the community,
where chronic problems associated with aging and childhood development
reigned. Following the large infusion of money post–World War II to medical
schools to ramp up the research endeavor, curriculums focused primarily on the

natural sciences, a base of which was obviously needed to care for complex, hospitalized acutely ill patients. Many medical experts rationalized the focus on the natural sciences because they believed this type of knowledge was key to prescribing and understanding the new pharmacotherapeutics. But one practitioner noted the difference between rhetoric and reality when he reasoned, "This sensible rationale ignored the realities that, first, it is not at all necessary to understand basic metabolic pathways in order to prescribe successfully; and second, most doctors forget this information anyway after they leave medical school."[25]

There were, however, pockets of reform despite prioritization of funding to basic science research and education. New types of academic health centers— the University of Florida and the University of Kentucky in the late 1950s, the University of Rochester, Case Western, and Rush in the late 1960s—redesigned themselves during an incredibly active period of social, medical, and nursing education reforms.[26] These academic health centers reflected the times, developing as they did amid the mounting belief in the right to health care, the civil and women's rights movements, community activism, and a growing realization by states that a primary-care physician shortage limited access to care for the citizens.

Not to be forgotten was a growing movement to "regionalize," as actualized through the regional medical programs of the mid-1960s. Policy makers assumed that regional academic health centers would provide guidance for fulfilling the health needs of rural, suburban, or small city populations, as well as becoming regional service commodities.[27] These centers emphasized the availability of better-quality care and a more efficient response to the increased access to care created by the passage of Medicare and Medicaid legislation in 1965. Their philosophy and approach of integrated medical and nursing education within the university, and their interest in restructuring patient care through the collaborative nexus of medicine and nursing, produced more activist, community-centered institutions.

Unlike most other academic health centers at elite institutions where medicine and nursing operated as separate and disparate pursuits, these centers, true to their reform character, were experiments in collaborative practice. They generated new models of clinical thinking and for cross-disciplinary care, such as the nurse practitioner–primary care physician team, and a renewed emphasis on primary, comprehensive care.[28] They redefined the traditional hierarchy in academic health centers by models of shared governance and encouraging a "best mix" of disciplinary and professional talents to increase productivity and access to health services. Private entities such as the Robert Wood Johnson Foundation and Kellogg Foundation provided support for these centers.

Other types of reform programs emerged during this time. Albert Einstein Medical Center in Philadelphia, offered a doctor of comprehensive medicine program in the late 1960s. This curriculum produced physicians who began their preparation in high school by taking all of their premedical science courses there, and afterwards were admitted to a special medical school for education in general practice. These physicians were ready to begin their practice at twenty-two years of age and practiced for at least one year under a general practitioner before becoming certified. They could, as one writer noted, "take a good history and make a thorough exam."[29]

The community-based medical center was another exception and emerged in part through the largesse of federal and state funding initiatives in the mid-1960s. Similar to shared-governance academic centers emerging on the scene in the late 1950s, the community-based medical schools also built upon earlier ideals of activism and advocacy. Created as independent entities both with and without formal linkages to major academic medical centers, these schools were less expensive to build and run. They used local colleges and universities for basic science courses and included heavy doses of social science and humanities courses. They also focused on secondary and primary care rather than tertiary care, and used community hospitals and their medical staffs for clinical education. The community-based schools did not eschew research; they focused their attention on clinical rather than basic science research. Schools such as the College of Human Medicine of Michigan State University, the University of North Dakota, and the Rockford School of Medicine of the University of Illinois experimented with new curricula developed to be blatantly untraditional. A broad clinical experience for students, a team approach to health care, and the provision of regional service were just a few of several common goals.[30]

Most of these innovative schools and programs struggled to survive. With their untraditional approach to the curriculum, the use of community clinicians for supervision, and the dismal results their students sometimes earned on the national board exams, these schools failed to impress accrediting bodies. Additionally, professional organizations gave little support for these nontraditional approaches to medical education. Nevertheless, their existence illustrated the problematic piecemeal attempts by both medical-education leaders and smaller nonelite schools to develop strategies to address clinical practice issues. Despite the presence of a handful of innovative schools and programs, much of professional medicine remained tied to traditional models of education and practice that were decidedly hierarchical in their scientific focus and their relative parochial approach to patient care. These philosophical standpoints created the foundation for a powerful socialization of those who entered medical school, and indirectly contributed to the growing space between patient needs and physician practice.

These approaches helped maintain medicine's powerful hold on health services, but they created enormous difficulties for new physicians when they entered into actual practice outside of the academic cocoon. For example, most medical students in academic centers had little opportunity to consider other health professionals outside the traditional, captain-of-the-ship model that underpinned medical care during the last century. "The student physician has relatively little formal contact with members of other health professions," physician Barbara Bates noted, "and thus has little opportunity to widen his perceptions of what others may contribute to patient care. He sees few practitioners skilled in the team approach whom he can emulate. The medical resident . . . has become a teller, not a listener; an authority in his own field, not a questioner in others. When frustrated by failure in a team enterprise, he retreats to his own territory: medical knowledge and authoritarianism. There he feels safe."[31] When physicians practiced from this framework, they struggled to envision new models of care and the potential other providers held, such as nurses, to complement their practices. Of course, not all physicians were so highly self-conscious, as demonstrated by the significant numbers of those who began to experiment with new practice models, but many were.

Adding to the dilemma was incongruence between hospital experiences during training and the type of patients newly minted physicians encountered in their practices. Most students' clinical experiences took place in acute-care settings where patients were complex and unique, but that was not the case in practice. As such, recently graduated pediatricians experienced a culture shock in their new practices. Comments such as "I had anticipated practicing pediatrics, not placating parents," and "I trained long and well. . . . Yet, the knowledge gained in medical school and residency is very seldom used," were indicative of the challenges new physicians faced, and for which they were unprepared.[32] The unchallenged assumption that physicians knew what was best for their patients ran through much of medical education, but was unjustified because very few students and clinical teachers had experience with the problems of health and disease in the community. Most medical education did not match the skills and knowledge of the students with the needs of the communities they were to eventually enter because the physicians and teachers in the medical centers did not actually see most of the community.

Nor, it seems, were students necessarily becoming facile with the skills they would need in practice after medical school and residency. A highly critical 1984 report by the Association of American Medical Colleges, which cited studies as early as the 1960s, pointed out deficiencies in physical examination, history taking, and critical thinking skills of medical students, interns, and residents.[33] These skills were in theory highly prized, and their use by others, such as nurse practitioners, contested by physicians. Reasons for this deficiency included specialization and loss of generalized skills, the failure to reinforce or supervise skill acquisition, and the probable downgrading by both students and faculty of the value of basic skills. On the contrary, many faculties were simply unskilled in these areas.

For the most part, much of the community did not require the sophisticated diagnostic and therapeutic techniques taught in most academic center medical schools or practiced by academically trained physicians in their offices. A 1961 study captured the dilemma of conflicting educational priorities and patient needs. Within an average month in Great Britain or the United States, for every 1,000 adults sixteen years of age or older, about 750 experienced what they recognized or recalled as an episode of illness or injury. Some 250 of the 750 consulted a physician at least once within the month. Only 9 of these patients were hospitalized.[34] Most care, it seemed, took place outside of the hospital, in the clinics and offices of individual practitioners, where they saw primarily uncomplicated cases. Of every 10 patients under the continuing care of New York State internists in the early 1960s, one patient came to the office for a physical examination, 7 for continuing management of a known clinical condition (an existing problem), and only 2 came to present new complaints.[35] Whatever the case, the disparity between what physicians were taught and how and where they practiced, and their maldistribution, opened a gap large enough for other practitioners, such as nurse practitioners, to step in and reshape patient care and their own practices in many different ways.

Nursing Education and Practice

Physicians' normative position in clinical practice was reasonable before midcentury. Until then, most nurses lacked education in the basic or applied sciences and the support of the profession itself to systematically broaden nursing roles by taking on new responsibilities such as clinical thinking. Most nurses were trained under a task-based paradigm of care and later worked in hospitals and their associated training schools where physicians held jurisdictional dominance.[36] The combination of advanced, academic-based clinical education that supported expanded nursing practice was a difficult proposition for professional nursing to undertake on a large scale as its clinical roots were more pragmatically planted and process based.

The regimentation of nursing care was an early phenomenon of nurse training perhaps most closely associated with elite nurse educators such as Isabel
Stewart at Teachers College, Columbia University, in New York. In the late
1920s, Stewart developed a popular efficiency method of nursing based on scientific management principles derived from time and motion studies of industrial workers. Most hospital training schools (also called diploma programs)
used this model as a basis for their curricula from the 1930s until the late 1960s.[37]
Nurses who were trained in this method certainly gained scientifically based
technical competence (procedural information on how to bandage wounds,
insert different types of catheters) but lacked an intellectual understanding of
the knowledge needed for larger patient-focused principles or goals. As a result,
much of nursing training and practice was rule based, activity oriented, and relied
heavily on the repetition of procedures rather than scientific or social theory-
based decision making. To be sure, nurses continued to attend to the basic comfort needs of patients, providing back rubs and soothing therapeutic baths. But
nurse educators increasingly believed these female-gendered skills could be made
more scientific and regimented to increase efficiency.

By the 1950s, many schools included courses in basic and behavioral sciences, but they did not always follow through to teach students how to apply this
information in clinical practice.[38] As a result, nursing competence continued to
be judged by technical expertise rather than the intellectual component of patient
care. "The emphasis, in my nursing education," nurse M. Lucille Kinlein noted,
"was on the set of activities, the procedures or techniques, to be carried out for
the patient in accordance with a medical regimen. The criterion of what was to
be learned was the sufficiency of the knowledge to prevent a mistake or to
avoid injury and trauma—but not sufficiency of the knowledge to bring about a
desirable health state."[39]

During this time, sociologist Esther Lucille Brown and nurse educators
Hildegard Peplau and Virginia Henderson also developed their critiques of nursing education and reformulated their ideologies of nursing care.[40] After she left
Columbia University's Teachers College in the early 1950s, Virginia Henderson
refined her scientifically based, patient-oriented philosophy of clinical nursing
that continues to influence modern nursing care. She believed that knowing
how to do a procedure was only a small part of nursing practice. The nurse then
had the responsibility to pass this information on to patients so they could be as
self-reliant and participate in their care as much as possible.[41] This philosophy
was the underpinning for a very different approach to nursing care, incorporating what the care meant to patients and how they partnered with nurses.

In the 1950s and 1960s, nurse educators and scholars more vocally acknowledged the discrepancy between the needs of patients and nurse training and practice. Peplau, Henderson, and Brown all wrote about the connection between patients' emotions, their physical conditions, and the importance of patients as active agents in nursing care. [42] Their writings contained other common threads. First, nursing education and practice should be based on the individual needs and problems of patients. Second, nurse education and patient care should be framed by theories and ideas from the basic and social sciences. And third, nurses best received this foundation in academic institutions rather than hospital-based training schools.

Nursing education had, indeed, been moving into colleges by the early 1950s. At Teachers College, Columbia University, nurse educator Mildred Montag was concerned about registered nurses' delegation of basic nursing tasks (like bathing and toileting) to less-educated aides, practical nurses, and students. She believed that the skills patients required ranged from the professional skills of registered nurses (monitoring and evaluating patients) to assistive skills (such as personal care). In between was a range of hands-on technical skills that a worker with more education than an aide but less than a registered nurse could safely perform. Her perceptions grounded her 1952 model of nurse education that took place outside of hospital training schools without the service requirement (e.g., the use of students to staff hospital wards). She reasoned that the program, based in community colleges over two years (instead of the traditional three years in diploma programs), more appropriately prepared a new type of nurse, the associate degree nurse, to perform technical tasks. Three-year diploma graduates who increasingly specialized by clinical focus and role (e.g., education and administration), were in short supply and were hard pressed to perform these duties.[43]

Montag's research showed that these programs were reasonably successful and resonated with students and educators alike, as they easily gained in popularity throughout the 1950s and 1960s (and are still somewhat popular today) as a solution to the loss of registered nurses at the bedside. Over one hundred associate degree programs existed in 1960 only eight years after the first associate degree program opened in 1952, and by 1970 there were more associate graduates than those from baccalaureate and diploma programs.[44] The community college programs contributed to an increasingly class-conscious nurse workforce. Nurse training was an economically priced path to upward mobility for lower-middle and middle-class women during this time, as the training schools charged tuition rates affordable for middle-class families.[45] Community college education required a financial commitment similar to, and in some places, less than training schools, over a shorter time period, and was much cheaper but not as in-depth as the higher-level baccalaureate programs.[46] Although class is a term with many connotations, the development of a new level of worker, although college educated, compounded an already hierarchical workforce stratified by education level, place of training (e.g., elite versus nonelite training schools), family income, and class. But layering was difficult for the public to differentiate and appreciate. The associate, baccalaureate, and diploma graduates were (and are) all labeled nurses, and all looked the same with the same type of uniforms. Status was implicitly made clear, however, to nurses working in hospitals and clinics through the nursing pin, name tag, and cap (each school had a trademark style). The registered nurse was at the top of the nursing pyramid, and one who specialized pushed workforce boundaries toward even more hierarchical differentiations.

Montag's technical nurse could, indeed, be considered a specialty worker. The type of specialization Henderson, Brown, and Peplau had in mind was based on clinical rather than technical expertise or experience, and could only occur in graduate level programs. Peplau developed her ideas about psychiatric clinical nurse specialists earning graduate degrees as early as 1956 (this was an extraordinary proposal as most nurses did not hold baccalaureate degrees at this point), and envisioned them providing a therapeutic one-on-one relationship with the patient.[47] Nurses should develop this kind of relationship, she believed, as long they received the educational foundation to apply the appropriate theories and interpret patient data. When clinical experience and knowledge were coupled with a strong theoretical foundation, nurses had the tacit authority to interpret data rather than merely report it for the use of other professional workers (e.g., physicians). In fact, nurses had the obligation to do this. Her theory went on to suggest that the process of interpretation, not dissimilar to clinical thinking, required analytical reasoning and data organization to move to the next logical stage to prescribe interventions. Peplau summed up her beliefs in a speech before the Nebraska Psychiatric Institute, College of Medicine, in 1958. She noted, "In my opinion, a work situation which forbids the nurse to make interpretations is one which places obstacles in the way of the development of nursing as a profession. . . . Such a situation also restricts the growth of nurses as persons of the use of their capacities for reason[ing]."[48]

Individualized and patient-empowered care concepts might have been idealized, but they were undeniably more germane to the care of patients both in and out of hospitals than the procedure-based, functional method. In hospitals, patients had more complicated medical problems, typically life-threatening acute episodes of chronic illnesses rather than the infectious diseases seen in earlier decades. The nursing care required by patients undergoing new procedures, such as mitral valve surgery and large-scale operations for cancer, and taking new, more potent medications had to be based upon their physiological and psychosocial needs rather than traditional routines or procedures. Patient conditions changed rapidly and required nurses who could make detailed and knowledgeable assessments and decisions.

By the early 1960s, nurse educators who were aware of the clinical realities in hospitals and the lack of care in rural and urban clinics began to pay greater attention to the writings of Brown, Henderson, and Peplau. These nurses began to conceptualize new clinical practice models and innovative academic clinical education programs. Their goal was to provide nurses with an intellectual foundation based on a liberal arts education in universities and colleges that supported broader clinical practice roles for nurses.[49] For example, nurse educator Francis Reiter devised the nurse clinician graduate curriculum at New York Medical College in the early 1960s. This program taught nurse clinicians to examine patients' responses to their illnesses rather than categorize patients by the number and type of procedures needed. It also trained nurses to provide care based on a rational, analytical decision-making process similar to clinical thinking, but without using the language of diagnosis and treatment.[50]

While Reiter developed her program in New York, Dorothy Smith, previously of New York University and the first nursing dean at the University of Florida in 1957, also experimented with the idea of a nurse clinician—a nurse with responsibility for a particular patient area—who was on call twenty-four hours a day for consultation with nurses and physicians (see chapter 3).[51] University of Colorado public health nurse Loretta Ford designed a postbaccalaureate curriculum for pediatric nurses providing preventive ambulatory health services to children in poor, rural areas of Colorado. This program included courses rarely found in nurse training schools at the time—pathophysiology, child development, and health promotion—and taught students to understand the underlying principles of healthy child care and patient education. The program also prepared students to provide preventive nursing services outside of the hospital in collaborative practices with physicians.[52] And at Cornell University–New York Hospital School of Nursing, Laura Simms developed the clinical nurse specialist role to utilize expert clinicians as consultants to generalist nurses. The concept of an expert clinician (rather than an expert of procedures) spread across nursing specialties and emerged in oncology, mental health, nephrology, and the intensive care unit.[53]

These experiments were not attempts to make nursing more like medicine, but were intended to paradigmatically shift and expand nursing practice to its fullest capabilities. Although in many hospitals less educated nurses' aides increasingly took on the more mundane and lower-status skills such as bathing patients and emptying bedpans, nurses were still responsible. The difference for nurses was that their thinking about these skills enlarged and was better integrated into practice. As they bathed patients, nurses assessed skin condition and emotional status, or evaluated the patient's response to medications as they measured urine production. In the clinics, nurses collected more detailed information from patients and developed treatment and referral plans. Nurses had a better sense of what the data meant; they could relate their findings to the patient condition, formulate clinical judgments, and adjust treatment plans. Patients and their responses to their illnesses, families, and lifestyles, rather than the task at hand, were the focus of care. This change in clinical thinking was both the foundation and the justification for the expanded practice experiments that culminated in the nurse practitioner role.

The expert clinical practice movement provided nurses with a bigger window of possibility through which they could formulate patient care questions, make decisions about treatment, and take action. But this was not the dominant educational paradigm for nurses in the 1960s and 1970s. Most still received training in traditional, hospital-based schools, and the proportion of nurses with college degrees during this time period ranged from 12 to 20 percent. The degrees were not typically clinically focused and were granted primarily from schools of education and administration after nurses completed training school.[54] Although the shift toward patient-focused education and practice began to accelerate in the early 1960s (as seen in the growth in popularity of innovative clinical decision-making texts such as Bertha Harmer and Virginia Henderson's *The Principles and Practices of Nursing*), institutional resistance and reluctance from the nursing profession in general counterbalanced and slowed these new practice and education ideas from taking root.[55] Many nursing educators were not yet convinced of nurses' ability to think. They loudly debated the safety of teaching nurses these skills. Nurses themselves were self-conscious about "thinking," as can be seen in the numerous nursing theories that emerged during this time period, many of which were formulaic and provided highly structured formats for approaching patient care.[56]

Convention was one of the strongest reasons for resistance from nurse educators. Most nurses were socialized in training schools to believe their practice was dependent on the orders of physicians and that there was little they should do independently. Traditional patterns of authority and discipline discouraged many nurses from challenging the status quo and kept most nurses from moving beyond conformist practice patterns.[57] A more broad-based academic preparation and expanded practice also presented a risk to many nurses who were unprepared to take on new challenges. Fear and misunderstanding by nurses themselves presented a formidable obstacle to shifting education and practice paradigms. Many influential nursing education leaders, including Dorothy Mereness, Peplau's colleague in psychiatric nursing, and Martha Rogers, head of the Department of Nursing at New York University, even though based in academic institutions, resisted forays into broadened clinical practice because they believed such nurses were practicing medicine.[58] Mereness, unlike Rogers, eventually realized the need for nurses in expanded and advanced practice, writing in 1970 that organized nursing moved too slowly to embrace these ideas.[59]

Other professional groups felt threatened by the implications of broader clinical education and practice roles. Jerome Lysaught, director of the national commission for the study of nursing and nursing education, recalled a conversation he had with a National League for Nursing (NLN) executive in the late 1960s. While the commission recommended closing diploma schools in favor of baccalaureate programs (this action was the usual subtext surrounding discussions of advanced education), the league, which accredited nursing schools of all types (most of which were diploma schools), felt extremely threatened by this proposal. The NLN executive noted, "Do you realize the income that we make from diploma schools of nursing [from accreditation fees]?"[60] Many constituencies on both medical and nursing sides could not understand the value of more educated nurses nor wanted to pay for them. The loss of income and of a source of workers anticipated from the possible closure of diploma schools was a powerful incentive for many different groups to challenge the new paradigms of education and practice.[61]

Nursing's position within higher education also slowed the acceptance of the new education and practice approaches. Although nursing education began to move into colleges and universities in the early twentieth century, only a handful of clinically based baccalaureate and graduate programs existed in the early 1960s. Most collegiate programs taught nurses to be educators and supervisors rather than clinical experts, and offered courses that focused on educational theories and management styles rather than human development and pathophysiology.[62] Part of the problem was the lack of nurses with advanced degrees who could teach in clinically focused baccalaureate programs. "We found," one educator noted, "that most nursing faculty . . . were clinically inept. I know that sounds harsh. That's what the truth was."[63] In many places, the baccalaureate and diploma programs existed side-by-side, sharing clinical placements and teaching staff, but maintaining separate humanities and science faculties and teaching space. Many of these arrangements were steeped in conflict as each program infused different values into their students and institutions.[64]

At the same time, the federal government and private foundations began investing in nursing education, and the number of clinically based academic programs grew. The stimulus for federal funding was threefold: numerous reports predicted a nursing shortage (such as the surgeon general's report by the consultant group on nursing in 1963); analysts outside of nursing began to understand that many nurses trained in hospital schools were unprepared to care for complex patients; and the population of chronically ill patients who needed care outside of the hospitals continued to expand.[65] Federal funds through the Nurse Training Act (NTA) in 1964 supported the construction of teaching facilities, student loans and traineeships, and faculty training at elite academic institutions such as Yale, University of Rochester, University of Pennsylvania, and Case Western. The greatest impact, however, came through federal support of de novo free-standing baccalaureate programs associated with smaller colleges and universities.[66] These schools, rather than the elite, were responsible for the increased numbers of nurses with a baccalaureate education.

In addition to the funding, professional nursing needed a combined, concerted effort to enlarge nursing roles and to begin moving nursing education into baccalaureate programs. This was one of the recommendations of the 1963 surgeon general's report. It also proposed a national investigation on nursing education to study how this might most efficaciously happen. The NLN and the ANA took the lead to establish a joint commission to study, among other things, how to finance and conduct such an encompassing national investigation. These organizations, and a mix of private and public interests groups such as the American Nurses' Foundation, the Avalon and Kellogg Foundations, and an anonymous donor funded the commission, which was then mandated to conduct a study akin to the early twentieth century Flexner Report that helped reshape medical education.[67]

The commission for the study of nursing and nursing education (or the Lysaught Commission, named after the director Jerome Lysaught), commenced in October 1967 and was only one of many groups examining nursing at the time. During its preliminary work, the Lysaught Commission found more than forty reports completed between 1960 and 1969 that addressed nursing supply, practice, and education. These studies came from twenty-nine states and twelve national and regional conferences or research groups. Nine of them were published in 1967 and 1968 alone.[68] The multiple interest groups addressing the problems of nursing education illuminated the growing dissatisfaction of legislators, academics, professional organizations, practicing nurses, and physicians with the direction of national health care, of which nursing was a critical part.

This renewed attention was important because it illustrated the vital place nursing held in both public and private health care agendas. The hard part was capitalizing on the power of this strategic position without alienating groups such as nonelite nursing educators, physicians, hospitals, and practicing nurses themselves, whose approval, both tacit and formal, was necessary for any type of change. The commission members acknowledged that a shift in the basic philosophic approach to the education of nurses was needed, but they also realized this perspective would be politically sensitive, difficult to articulate, and to implement without alienating the aforementioned groups whose support was critical for later execution.

In 1970, the Lysaught Commission report, *Abstract for Action*, offered more than fifteen innovative recommendations addressing nursing roles, education, and careers. It initially invoked a flurry of controversy and excitement.[69] The more controversial recommendations received the most attention from critics and supporters alike. They included a major shift in the language of practice (e.g., into "episodic" or "distributive" care), a rapid change in the philosophy of nursing practice, and relocation of the place of nursing education, from hospitals to academic institutions. The concepts of episodic and distributive care, which categorized work by setting and skill level (thus negating a traditional ideology that a diploma nurse was appropriately trained to function in any setting), never gained support.[70] The recommendations that focused directly on practice, including strategies to improve the relationships between nurses and physicians, found greater acceptance. The national joint practice commission, a ten-year experiment that brought nurses and physicians together to work out collaborative strategies for better patient care (see chapter 6), was one recommendation that was quickly implemented and endured longer than most.

Based on Esther Lucille Brown's classic descriptive and sociologic methods, and reinforced by the expertise of another prominent sociologist, Robert Merton, the report was comparable in method and recommendations for change to the 1965 study of medical education, *Planning for Medical Progress through Education*, by Lowell Coggeshall, a University of Chicago physician and former special assistant to the secretary of the Department of Health, Education and Welfare in 1956, and also a member of the commission. Coggeshall's study, however, served as a blueprint for change in the medical profession because it had the strong support of the Association of American Medical Colleges, and multiple medical specialty organizations moved its proposals forward.[71] But conditions surrounding the Lysaught Commission were more complex. Physicians and hospitals still held a strong grip on nursing education. The AMA in particular continued to support diploma schools until the mid-1970s and actively lobbied against the recommendations from the commission report. It also received a tepid hearing by the ANA and NLN, two organizations that helped fund the study and could have added their constituency weight to proposals.[72]

Another problem may have been the organizational politics of the Lysaught Commission itself. Although it produced an innovative report, it did little to ensure the wholesale buy-in by major professional and hospital organizations. Nine of the twelve commission members, including the director and commission president, were educators, sociologists, physicians, or hospital administrators, not nurses. Eleanor Lambertson, who held the position of secretary of the com-mission, was joined by only two other nurses, and all three came from major academic or administrative positions. Margaret Dolan and Lambertson were heads of nursing departments in elite universities, and Mary Jane McCarthy was the director of nursing service at the Veterans Administration in Washington, D.C.

Although small in numbers, the nurses on the main commission were pow-erful leaders and accustomed to working and negotiating with male colleagues. The meager representation of nurses was somewhat equalized by higher repre-sentation on the various advisory and regional boards (e.g., the nursing advi-sory board) that generated the actual data and responses upon which the report, and later the appendices, were based.[73] Of the other members, Merton and Lysaught had different political agendas than the physicians and nurses, and were interested in reshaping clinical practice from a broader, sociological per-spective. The absence of high-level representatives from powerful professional organizations such as the AMA, the ANA, and the American Hospital Association (AHA) was significant (although the medical and nursing members all belonged to and were quite active in their respective organizations). Given the member-ship and composition of the main board, the report was extremely innovative and forward thinking and probably a function of members highly skilled in political negotiations.

The report recommendations, although receiving wide distribution in jour-nals, books, and in a series of pamphlets, hardly filtered down to midlevel leaders, educators, and the rank-and-file practitioners (many of whom were conservative and loyal to traditional nursing practice and education). In contrast, the typi-cally training-school-friendly board of the AHA actually passed a resolution in support of the recommendations, much to the horror of a particular class A con-stituent, the membership group for the hospital schools of nursing. The hospi-tal schools were not, however, a homogeneous collection. As Lysaught noted, "Many of them were very supportive. . . . I met with people from the Catholic Hospitals Associations group of hospital schools of nursing. And essentially they were saying they had no problems with the recommendations to close the [training] schools [and move to baccalaureate programs]."[74] The association just wanted time for a reasonable process to phase out the schools, as they realized the occupational view of nursing was no longer relevant.

The report was indeed controversial and, as nursing journal editor Edith Lewis noted, "paved the way for a sort of displacement phenomenon. Whether we hail [it] as gleefully as a taxi in the rain or see it as a tumbrel coming along to take the nursing profession to the guillotine, it becomes easy to react [to the report]."[75] She cautioned her readers, and indirectly the professional nursing organizations, to remember the considerable amount of time and effort put into the report by nurses and many others, and that nurses asked for this appraisal. She called for critical attention and, simultaneously, for patience and reflection until some time could be given to the implementation phase. Lewis seemed fairly optimistic about the report, but many years later admitted to the transient excitement the report generated. "Only those in my generation and a few students of nursing history," she noted, ". . . will remember the Lysaught report."[76]

In the end, the commission reiterated messages that had been in play since the controversial report of the committee for the study of nursing education (the Goldmark report) of 1923 recommended collegiate education for nurses and broadened clinical expertise.[77] Other studies of nursing education and practice, such as the Brown report of 1948, the Ginzberg report of the same year, the Bridgman report of 1953, the report on nursing education and Catholic institutions in 1963, and finally the 1963 surgeon general's report, all reiterated the same themes: nurses needed professional, university-based generalist education and clinically focused graduate education to meet the challenges of patient care. In 1971 these recommendations still elicited enormous controversy, but rang true. Until nursing fixed basic nursing education by creating a unified standard for entry into the profession (rather then the three levels of diploma, associate, and baccalaureate degree), graduate education for clinical nursing specialization could not advance.[78]

As the Lysaught report stirred up debate about the amount and type of education nurses needed in particular settings, many failed to acknowledge nursing already had a fairly successful track record of obtaining federal support for the growth of college-based training programs, specifically through the 1964 NTA and through the military.[79] Additionally, the nurse workforce was already stratified by clinical specialization and level of education, although not quite as standardized as the committee recommended through closure of diploma programs and manufactured hierarchies of episodic and distributive care. In other words, some of the major recommendations of the Lysaught report were already in place during the commission's lifespan. The difference between what was already occurring in education and practice and the principles put forward by the report was that it formalized these issues in a very broad national public forum.

As it was, more and more nurses were receiving more and more education. By the late 1960s a growing number of nurses were educated in collegiate programs or went back to school for a baccalaureate degree, creating a viable pool of nurses who could advance to clinical practice-focused graduate education and who were then competent to teach advanced clinical skills in baccalaureate programs.[80] Even before the 1964 NTA, the division of nursing began to fund advanced clinical education in master's programs beyond public health and psychiatric nursing through the Health Professions Education Assistance Act (P.L. 88–129) in 1963. This program was one of many forces that spurred the growth of graduates focusing on advanced clinical practice from 14 percent in 1964 to 57 percent in 1974.[81]

At the same time, the division of nursing of the Public Health Service funded university-based pre- and postdoctoral fellowships for graduate study, offering traineeships for professional nurses to prepare for "specialized clinical practice," language reflected in the 1964 NTA.[82] Among others, the children's bureau of the U.S. Department of Health, Education and Welfare in 1964 funded short programs in the care of premature infants via state public health services and supported programs at the Institute for Premature Care at New York Hospital, New York City, and a similar program at the University of Colorado's School of Nursing.[83]

These somewhat vague and flexible federal programs provided some of the first funding streams for advanced clinical practice education. Both the certificate program to train nurse practitioners at the University of Colorado and the physician assistant program at Duke University in 1965 were supported by a combination of federal and private funding. Moreover, many of these federal programs, such as Title X, eventually paid for the training and practice of nurse practitioners in rural and urban health clinics.[84] At the same time, the regional medical programs funded continuing-education programs for nurses and doctors focusing primarily on heart disease, cancer, and strokes. The Great Society programs of the Johnson administration provided support for postgraduate clinical training for both physicians and nurses committed to work with disadvantaged patients in urban and rural health clinics.[85]

Until these nationally funded programs came about, few other avenues existed for nurses who wanted to increase their clinical expertise after their general training. Later legislation such as the NTA and Comprehensive Manpower Act of 1971 (P.L. 92–158), and the amendment of the Public Health Service Act in 1971 (P.L. 92–52) included more specific language for special projects, typically the code word for nurse practitioner training programs. For example, the 1971 PRIMEX program was funded by the National Center for Health Services Research and Development through the manpower program. The term "PRIMEX" was coined by University of Washington School of Nursing dean Madeline Leininger in 1969 and was promoted by nurse faculty at the school to reflect nurse practitioners' emphasis on primary care and preventive services.[86] Designated and specific authority for funding for advanced clinical practice via nurse practitioner programs came later with passage of the 1975 NTA.[87] But until then, an entrepreneurial approach to gaining advanced clinical education was necessary, as innovative schools of nursing and medicine, along with community and public health organizations, took advantage of funding flexibility to create new models of education and practice.

In the meantime, practicing nurses were developing parallel clinical philosophies similar to those generated by a handful of nursing leaders in colleges and universities. Nurses specializing in critical care, public health, midwifery, urban and rural clinics, and other emerging areas (oncology and nephrology, to name two) responded to daily clinical realities. These nurses, in the absence of formal-education opportunities, relied on experience, self-education, entrepreneurial spirit, and physician teachers. These settings in particular may have more easily supported broader nursing roles because physicians' jurisdictional boundaries were more porous, and institutional control was weaker or absent. Physicians may have felt less restricted to try new practice arrangements themselves.[88] Architecturally discrete areas, such as intensive care, cardiac care, and dialysis units, limited institutional interference. And in urban and rural health clinics and hospital emergency rooms, an increasing patient load and shortage of physicians provided the opportunity for both nurses and physicians to lay aside traditional relationships and ways of communicating and forge ahead into new ways of relating to each other and to their patients. In these areas, at the bedside or in the examination room, nurses and physicians negotiated practice boundaries and traded knowledge.

In both public clinics and intensive care units, nurses spent a great deal of time with their patients and were able to more broadly inform and teach physicians about the patients' emotional and clinical conditions. This process represented a cross-pollination of medical and nursing knowledge and technical science. One nurse explained, "Once I learned, I taught a million of them [physicians] how to do dialysis . . . and I learned about renal disease from them . . . there was never anything written down [about learning], just an unspoken agreement."[89] One Arkansas intensive care nurse glibly noted, "Doctors and nurses trained each other, and after a year or so, nurses were smarter than the doctors."[90] Nurses also learned to use the language of clinical thinking, for example, how to describe particular skin lesions, frame the patient's complaints in an organized manner, or talk about changes in laboratory studies. Nurses received implicit permission to engage higher-status physicians in the politically important process of communicating more effectively about patients using a common language.

The trajectory of changes in education and practice occurred in such a way that it is difficult and even unnecessary to discern which came first—better education for nurses or changes in practice. Perhaps it isn't useful to think about this, but rather the influence these changes together had on patient care. Practice changes required adventuresome nurses and physicians who could learn together and communicate. This was a singularly local phenomenon, difficult to replicate. On the other hand, key nursing leaders' perceptions that expert clinical practice was the key to better patient care, and their willingness to experiment in academic centers as well as push the federal government for funding, jostled the education system for nursing. The combination of these multidirectional forces was a powerful impetus and medium for the nurse practitioner movement.

The incongruence between the health care needs of the American public and the traditional focus on science and highly complex patient care in medical schools and residency programs created an opportunity for different kinds of practitioners. Nursing was poised to take advantage of tensions in the traditional relationships of physicians and patients. A growing number of nurses were eager to do and know more, stepping into the breach with their experience as a talisman for success. Education slowly followed, although it is unclear at times who was leading whom. But it was clear that a growing cadre of nurses, physicians, and patients were looking for something different as a solution to their patient care problems.

Chapter 3

Psychology Girls and Clandestine Groups

Rethinking Specialization in Nursing

Academic health centers in the 1960s and 1970s were located at the nexus of socially relevant medical care and scientifically advanced treatments and procedures. These institutions were ground zero for the proliferation of specialist nurses and physicians. They were also both politically and socially charged with producing the practitioners who served the larger community. Two academic health centers, the University of Florida in Gainesville and the University of Rochester in New York, serve as exemplars to illustrate the difficulties and opportunities that arose when practice and education merged, influencing each other within the context of specialization at the institutional level. These cases also demonstrate the importance of individual relationships and local organizational politics, as well as the need to meld larger health policy strategies with them. In fact, the success of the programs at Florida and Rochester was predicated not only by institutional policies but by the presence of compatible people and ideas.

Academic Health Centers

The academic health center is a contemporary concept with important distinctions. The more traditional label, "academic medical center," typically described the alliance between a medical school, teaching hospital, and its medical staff. Academic health centers encompassed the particular university, the teaching hospital, various professional schools, health care providers, administrators, insurers, suppliers, and patients. This model is analogous to large technological systems.[1] These centers were and are more than hospitals associated with university medical schools that happen to train residents. They function as large-scale organizations with interdependent parts, and are of decisive importance in American health care. They show the potential value of concerted participation—shared governance—of medicine and nursing in the mission of the university and the provision of services. The University of Florida in the late 1950s, Case Western Reserve University in Cleveland, Ohio, in the late 1960s, and Rush University Medical Center in Chicago, Illinois, and the University of Rochester in the early 1970s all redesigned themselves as academic health centers during an incredibly active period of social, medical, and nursing education reforms.[2] They were particularly good at both self-examining their larger mission and harnessing federal funding. These characteristics ensured change in both system and function across large groups of people and services encompassed by the centers. Of course, the larger-scale changes needed to start somewhere, and these opportunities usually occurred between individuals who shared visions of better health care and who managed to get along in highly structured environments not always amenable to change.

Nursing Education in the Academic Health Centers

The hospitals and clinics of the academic health centers, similar to community practices, provided the room for adventuresome nurses and physician colleagues to experiment with collaborative clinical practice and education models that crossed health care systems and professional schools. Some nurses in academic institutions took their enlarged roles a step farther and began to try out new ways of teaching other nurses to do the same. This new material was truly exciting, and gave entrepreneurial nurses the opportunity to teach something interesting instead of the traditional education and administration courses. Many partnered with equally enlightened nursing and medical educators, taking what they learned from their practice experiments and developing clinically focused graduate programs or even new baccalaureate program models. In a sense, they brought nursing education structurally closer to a medical model by emulating its tradition of teacher-practitioners.[3]

Few nurses were prepared to teach students the new skills and knowledge they needed, such as physical examination, pathophysiology, and clinical decision making, to function in expanded roles. The shortage of faculty and researchers to take on this work was troublesome, and it took some time before supply caught up with the need. One report noted 1,657 nursing faculty vacancies in the United States in 1968.[4] Universities in general and academic health centers in particular were the institutions best positioned to help solve the faculty shortage because of the unique relationships between the professional schools and the rest of the campus. But few financial incentives existed for them to expand expensive graduate programs, nor to develop clinically focused ones to produce the needed faculty until the passage of the Nurse Training Act (NTA) in 1964, followed by a second act in 1971.

The pace of graduate education entrepreneurship quickened after the landmark report of the secretary's committee to study extended roles for nurses in November 1971, *Extending the Scope of Nursing Practice*. The report recommended moving nursing education to academic institutions, developing curriculum innovations to encourage collaborative and comprehensive care, and establishing education and legislative environments to support the expanded role for nurses.[5] It provided the impetus for the 1971 NTA that directed millions of dollars to support certificate and graduate programs that would teach nurses to fill nurse practitioner educator and practice roles.

But problems at the baccalaureate level set an unsteady foundation for graduate programs. Federal funding, although welcomed by universities and contributing to the production of needed clinically expert faculty, was somewhat off target. The 1964 NTA also pumped substantial funding into hospital training schools, thus helping to sustain at least for another decade an educational model slowly losing its clinical and educational relevance. The funding policy did not solve the historic larger problem of finding the best place to educate nurses in general, or provide incentives for a single point of entry into practice (e.g., diploma program, baccalaureate, or associate degree program graduates could all be registered nurses). These issues had to be resolved before clinically based graduate programs could be assured of the high quality of the students they admitted. In effect, the funding policies ensured the confusion surrounding nursing education in the 1960s and 1970s.

Supported by such diverse organizations as the armed forces, the federal government, and private foundations, nurse educators in academic health centers shifted the paradigm to focus on patient care and, in the process, developed a new type of unification based on clinical practice.[6] It brought together academic and institutional leadership within the clinical field to create innovative education models that included clinical research and faculty-based practice without the labor requirements for students. The success of these endeavors varied, with entrepreneurial zeal sometimes outstripping organized planning and strategies, and conceptualization advancing beyond accomplishment.[7] And although they lacked uniform structure and purpose and were undermined by personality clashes, professional suspicion, and administrative resistance, in general, efforts to redefine the practice and education field were fairly successful.

The University of Florida

In 1956, the leadership of the health center at the University of Florida, Gainesville, was a deliberately organized group of like-minded individuals who believed in the promise of shared governance and the integrated education model proposed for the new institution. This group consisted of nurse Dorothy Smith, along with colleagues George Harrell, dean of medicine; J. Wayne Reitz, president of the university; and Russell Poor, provost of the health center (followed later by Sam Martin). They comprised the core of one of the earliest academic health centers.[8] Together, they created something akin to a corporate notion of skunk works, pockets of highly innovative people involved in slightly eccentric activity, having fun, enthusiastically experimenting.[9]

Named after the late university president J. Hillis Miller, the health center was a novel idea for the time. Although other university hospitals and medical and nursing schools experimented with different facets of education and practice, this health center was not designed to deal "solely with the abnormalities of man—his illnesses . . . but on consideration of the total man, his environment, his emotions, and his daily life as a citizen of Florida."[10] The health center mandate also included the education of leaders in all of the professional fields, including medicine, nursing, pharmacy, allied health, and dentistry.

Smith and her colleagues thrived in this environment, and they genuinely seemed to get along quite well. Reitz accompanied her to the Florida state board of nursing to get her program approved—no small task given its innovative nature. Poor insisted that all health center deans and the hospital administrator have equal votes on the health center council, and Harrell believed strongly in the idea of "human biology," which called for integrating nursing and the biomedical and pharmaceutical sciences into professional education programs and clinical practice. His support and attitude influenced medical students and medical faculty.[11] As the only woman in the group, she more than held her own in the discussion and planning sessions—Smith was tall, perhaps over six feet, thin, and exceedingly charming. Her presence and intellect helped her hold her place. "Everyone here has been very nice," she noted in a letter to her friends left behind in Hartford, Connecticut, "and I'm enjoying *all* my men but it will be nice to get some faculty here to talk about nursing."[12]

With the support of her fellow deans and the university president, Smith implemented exciting new plans that reflected values the rest of the nursing profession was only beginning to discuss. At Gainesville, the nursing college was integrated into the mainstream of university life at all levels. The nursing students took the same courses as other university students; there was no special "chemistry for nurses."[13] Smith also believed the courses in the arts and sciences provided the foundation for training nurses to think in creative ways. She incorporated a broad humanities-based curriculum, similar to George Harrell's ideas for the medical school.[14] Nursing students took classes with Sidney Jourard, a University of Florida psychologist, to help them learn and adjust to their role as student nurses and cope with outside resistance; Carol Taylor, an anthropologist who helped the nurses understand health systems; and Howard Wooden, an art historian, who helped the students understand the value of merging creative thinking and social issues.[15]

These ideas were phenomenal for American health care at midcentury. "I'm reminded of something one of our psychiatrists told me," Smith later wrote, " He said we were turning out students who would be frustrated professionally because they would not see what we had—or what we were trying to do outside of the University of Florida. I told him that rightly or wrongly I would rather have our graduates know what is possible or what could be possible, even if they did get frustrated."[16] Smith, along with Hildegard Peplau at Rutgers University and Francis Reiter and Marguerite E. Kakosh at New York Medical College, perhaps more than any other nurse leaders during this period, steered nursing education toward producing intellectually capable and expert clinical practitioners.[17]

The cornerstone of Smith's program was shared responsibility for patient care in the health center between nursing service in the teaching hospital and nursing education in the College of Nursing, including mutually developed quality measures, staffing, student education experiences, faculty practice, and patient care philosophy. The unification program also assumed shared control for patient care between nursing and medicine, with each recognizing the strengths they brought to support patient recovery. Smith's model influenced the thinking of many important nursing leaders and laid the foundation for numerous clinical advances in nursing over the next fifty years, including evidence-based care and advanced practice nursing.[18]

But there was also a substantial group of physicians and staff nurses that was unconverted and unconvinced. Hilliard noted, "I think they [Martin and Harrell] had to run interference, too. There were a lot of doctors, a lot of people, but particularly, the doctors, were vocal."[19] Even the local press weighed in. *The Florida Times-Union* labeled the students, "psychology girls," reporting they used "brains rather than bedpans."[20] Some medical specialties, especially those based in part in primary care, more easily bought into Smith's ideas. Physicians in obstetrics and gynecology, pediatrics, and psychiatry were more open to innovation and collaboration, while surgeons and general medicine physicians (after Martin became provost) were sometimes reluctant participants who saw Smith's ideas for clinical integration, with its underlying principle of independent thinking, as challenges to their authority and control.

Smith insisted on and was awarded the positions of dean of the college as well as chief of nursing practice in the hospital, and her broad influence also contributed to the insecurity of those who did not share her vision for integration.[21] She had at least three main reasons for taking on this large responsibility. First, she wanted to secure practice privileges for her faculty so they could cooperatively and collaboratively engage with staff nurses and physicians. The faculty would then be able to "model" the expert clinical care she wanted the staff nurses and her students to emulate.[22] She recognized the pervasive friction between practicing nurses and educators, and believed faculty practice was one way to overcome this obstacle to improve patient care. She noted, "While our faculty controls nursing education at the university, we nevertheless believe that our control is effective only insofar as we ourselves become more proficient in the practice of that which we are trying to teach, namely nursing."[23] Second, she wanted to be able to speak for all of nursing at health center council meetings, the governing body composed of the deans, provost, and the hospital administrator.[24] "If I couldn't do this," she believed, "I would be speaking only for nursing education while the hospital administrators or physicians would be speaking for nursing service."[25]

A third reason surfaced in her writings. She believed the organization of medical education in academic centers was a useful framework for integrating nursing education and practice. To reproduce this structure, her faculty needed admitting privileges so they could serve as practitioner-teacher role models. One of her faculty noted, "What she wanted to do was set up nursing [education] more like medicine. . . . Where you have your faculty and you have your residents and interns and the medical students, and they both practice [and learn]."[26] This model included specialization of practice in areas such as pediatrics and medical and surgical nursing, with decentralized administrative functions. To make this work, nursing faculty section chiefs had to have authority equivalent to these positions in the school of medicine. This was an important model, Smith wrote, because it was the "only way to get department status (university) within the college. . . . This was the way doctors and patients were placed, and the university understood this model and accepted it."[27]

When Smith arrived at Florida, difficulties quickly surfaced. Hiring nurses to work in the health center was a challenge. She tried to employ an all-baccalaureate staff, but because of scarcity of nurses with degrees and the salary restraints imposed by the state system (the health center pay rate was almost the lowest in the state), this was a tremendous, and in the end, a futile task.

Smith believed the staff nurses she could engage, in general, were unprepared to assume the clinical professor roles she envisioned as part of the unification strategy. Instead, she placed faculty, most of whom had masters or doctoral degrees, in the roles.[28] She described the transition: "On the 4th floor, each of us took a service. . . . At first we were attending and residents and everything—all for 24 hours. Then we began to get a few of our graduates to help."[29]

Smith herself followed the model in her own practice and eventually established a medical psychiatric nurse consultation service. "Today, me, a nurse, received a consultation sheet requesting me to see a patient for Dr. M.," Smith wrote. "It seems the entire medical staff met last night and discussed me and my philosophy. Some said that up to last night, most of them had been quite suspicious—wondering what my 'gimmick' was. Several gave examples of what I had done for patients and [how I had] contributed to patient care. So they decided to use me formally on a problem patient."[30]

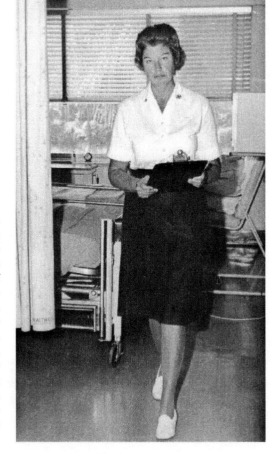

Photo 2. Dean Dorothy Smith at work in the hospital, circa 1965. (Personal collection of the author.) Smith was dean of the College of Nursing, University of Florida, Gainesville, from 1956 to 1971. This print is a reproduction of an image in the Harrell History Archives, Health Science Center, University of Florida, Gainesville, and was presented to the author in honor of her participation in the University of Florida College of Nursing Dorothy M. Smith Nursing Leadership Conference in 2004.

The model seemed a curiosity to many in the health center, but proved quite enticing to others outside the state, in particular. Smith and her colleagues wrote extensively and traveled around the country describing the work in Florida. Other health centers followed her lead and "were experimenting with the same model—Yale, Western Reserve, Pittsburgh, Rochester, and others wish to do so if they can find willing nurse leaders."[31] In fact, people came from around the world, from as far as Australia, to see this system at work.

Smith's success as a dean and in her practice was partly due to the compatibility of her ideas with those of George Harrell, and her ability to convey to like-minded faculty and students her beliefs about care organized around the primacy of patient needs rather than medical diagnosis or particular tasks. Although this model may seem unremarkable now, for the 1950s, 1960s, and 1970s it was innovative and novel and tied to her beliefs about research and clinical evidence. As one of her instructors explained, Smith believed "nurses should be more autonomous and have a basis for their practice rather than the old book we used to run by, the procedure book, that we had a brain and we should use it. The problem was finding a place where they would let you use it."[32]

Above all, with the support of her health system colleagues, Smith constantly fought for the idea and the reality of nursing as a practice profession and an academic discipline. "The academic nature of clinical nursing practice was intellectually challenging," Smith said, "perhaps even more challenging than administration and teaching, an almost heretical thought (in the 1950s)."[33] In other words, she strongly believed critical thought should be the basis for practice. She spoke to this philosophy in lectures and papers from the 1950s on. "To me, the distinguishing characteristic of professional nursing is clinical thinking," she noted in a later speech. "Every patient, whether well, getting sick, being sick, or being well has the right to a nurse who, by virtue of this clinical nursing thinking, manages the nursing care and is accountable for that care."[34]

None of this made a difference if nurses failed to record or analyze the information they derived from it. Smith noted the importance of nursing data in a speech to the Florida State Nurses' Association in 1957. Nursing, she wrote, "must be constantly seeking to improve its own practice . . . but we are not yet disciplined ourselves to the necessity for constant study and research. . . . We cannot say with any certainty which way is the most effective until we try many ways, tabulate our results and get some data."[35] This part of the process was critical because it provided the foundation to measure the effectiveness of nursing practice. "Nurses must be able to . . . discuss and to act, and think about why it [a particular practice] worked," she wrote to a colleague. Otherwise, "this kind of nursing cannot be taught, replicated or improved. And, all of this is hard thinking and takes lots of basic science, both social and biological and not many nurses are used to applying this, able to show it, to write it."[36]

Smith's appreciation for not only the process of clinical practice but the collection of evidence developed very early in her career. She completed her first study of clinical practice as an affiliating student at Bellevue Hospital in New York City in the early 1940s. She wrote, "I figured how long it would take to take and record temperatures on 75+ patients with only 3 rectal thermometers, using prescribed safe technique. This had to be done between 5 and 7 am. I sent the results to the mayor of New York City, with a request for more thermometers and more help. I had previously sent the results to both nursing and hospital administration with no effect. I never heard from the mayor either."[37] She kept asking questions. How could educators and practicing nurses improve their ability to think intellectually about their patients? How could the nursing paradigm shift from training to education so nurses could provide patients with the kind of care they needed? Where could nurses find or use the evidence to support the changes she believed had to be made?

Smith also thought a great deal about these questions as she drove through the South as a consultant for the National League for Nursing (NLN) from 1952 to 1956. She was quite disturbed by the conditions she found in many of the schools, which were largely hospital dependent and emblematic of the state of nursing education as a whole. In a 1956 letter to a close friend she noted, "This has been a very bad week for me as the schools have been quite poor—perfectly ghastly exploitation of students. . . . And actually, I know that it isn't entirely their fault—at least some of them—for they just don't know any better. But it is frustrating for they are just turning out nurses who will carry on the vicious practice of taking out their hostility on patients and students."[38] Reflecting on another school, she wrote, "I was very disturbed today . . . [they] have 37 graduate nurses and 4 psychiatrists for 7,000 patients so you can imagine the kind of care the students see given. The students do all the 3–11, 11–7 [shifts]. . . . According to the records most of the students had an IQ of 85–95. A real mess."[39]

At the university, Smith provided students with the permission and support to think intellectually about nursing practice and to take the time to document the findings in the chart, activities that students in schools she visited for the NLN could not imagine. In addition to its importance to nursing practice, this process made visible the work of nurses and helped other professions understand that nurses had something important to say and could contribute to patient care decisions. One of the early innovations Smith initiated for capturing clinical practice information was the nursing history. This simple technology—a patient data form—documented information derived from a nursing assessment and created a record for all providers to access. The basic underlying principle was the assumption of significance—first, that nurses had the intelligence to collect appropriate data; and second, that the nursing data were important enough in the larger care scheme of the patient to be integrated into the patient record, where all caregivers could consult.

But to Smith, the data were most important to the nurses themselves and their development as expert practitioners. The evidence nurses collected not only helped organize patient care but also served as a vehicle for other nurses to see illustrations of expertise. Some of the recordings by nurses "were not particularly helpful," nurse Lucille Mercadante explained. A typical nursing entry—"sleeping, no problems"—was a frequently encountered example.[40] Most nurses were untrained in the clinical thinking skills Smith considered key to data collection and collaborative care, and the nursing history and care plan served as a teaching tool for nurses who were just beginning to understand their ability to contribute to the larger patient care vision.

Although simple, the nursing history proved somewhat controversial and probably mirrored the larger problems that plagued the concept of practice and education unification and integration. A small but acutely symbolic issue—nurses writing in the patient chart—actually stirred great debate. Mercadante noted some of the difficulties. "The care plan in many, many ways really told the story about the patient and the patient care program. We struggled. We struggled to keep the medical records [department] from removing nursing care plans."[41] This idea of charting data, especially on the newly created history and Cardex forms Smith, her colleagues, and students developed, was quite unique for the time period. In many places, nurses had no authority to write notes on patient charts, and most hospitals discarded nurses' notes (usually collected on a clipboard or separate notebook) when doctors discharged patients.[42] Sometimes physicians destroyed the nursing history form themselves because they saw the patient chart as medicine's domain, as a way of controlling patient access and information. Many believed the nursing data were superfluous and cluttered the chart. At the bedside, where power and authority over patient care was most local and critical, the paradigm of patient care on many units had not yet shifted from "my patient" to "our patient."

Nurses themselves were not always convinced. Smith often spoke of the diploma mentality, meaning a nurse who focused primarily on the procedures and medications a patient needed rather than the patient's psychological and emotional needs. Despite her best efforts, an unofficial hierarchy developed in the hospital that prioritized the faculty with the degrees. Mercadante explained, "You would get graduates from the diploma schools who would have had ten, twelve, fifteen years' experience, practicing, taking care of patients. And along comes a faculty person with a master's degree, maybe one year of experience. There was this feeling of, you are going to tell me what to do? This is my patient; I have the experience."[43]

Smith's belief in the need for expert practitioners necessitated new, clinically focused graduate-level programs. She realized that although generalist nurses at the baccalaureate level could think critically about patients, they required higher and more complex skills to become more effective clinicians, collaborators, and role models. And frankly, she believed, "The staff nurse could not do it alone; she needed help from someone who understood nursing and its potential."[44] Building on the strengths of the baccalaureate program, Smith envisioned nurses who developed advanced critical-thinking skills, who could diagnose, prescribe, and treat complex nursing problems. These nurses combined the essential elements of experience and advanced thinking about clinical phenomena to develop, collect, and analyze data to establish the evidence base for practice. She began to think about expert, expanded practice and operationalize it in the programs at the college much earlier than many other recognized programs.

Smith's model of practice was based on collaboration and planning rather than skill transfer from physician to nurse. The difference can be seen in her later ambivalent stance about nurse practitioners, but not about nursing. "I don't object to doctors giving over some of their tasks—but I suspect that nurse technicians could be taught to do most of them. When I take a history on a patient I'm looking for things I can do—or need to attend to—and when I observe the patient it is for the same reason."[45] If the expert nurse clinician integrated traditional medical skills into practice, Smith believed they should only be used to support nursing care.

Innovative ideas required, at the least, the space and time to be discussed and tested. But, like most skunk works, Smith and her colleagues and their ideas survived and prospered only as long as the leadership circle stayed intact or other like-minded individuals joined them. As members left Florida for other places, new colleagues were not always receptive to the ground breaking models found there. There were organizational and economic changes that couldn't support the original philosophy. Additionally, her thinking and that of her other colleagues was perhaps so pathbreaking that their goals weren't realistically achievable together, let alone individually without the support of a broad array of people and professions. In fact, George Harrell never had the full support of his medical school faculty or the larger university to truly implement his original proposals for an integrated medical curriculum.[46]

By 1968, Sam Martin, George Harrell, and Russell Poor moved on to other challenges while Smith tried to maintain the model of shared governance and unification the founding group created.[47] She tried to remain optimistic, but there were problems at many levels. As in other parts of the country in the late 1960s, south Florida experienced a severe nursing shortage and the health center faced growing financial problems. The hospital struggled with the state to get paid for the care of indigent patients, and there were high-level discussions about the ethics of transferring poor maternity patients to surrounding community institutions such as Alachua General Hospital to reduce costs.[48]

Money was tight in the health system, but like many other hospitals it spent a great deal on new technologies and complex services rather than basic care. "It will be a catastrophe in my mind," Smith wrote to Provost Edmund Ackell, "if this Health Center does not try to demonstrate both aspects of healing (care and cure) through some kind of equitable funding. More and more machines, more acute beds, more and more emergency admissions—without the care aspect—make this place a poor environment for students to learn the fundamentals of a supposedly service profession."[49] The public was beginning to notice some of the conditions as well, and the provost received letters describing patient care problems. One family wrote to Ackell after their child's hospitalization that "the nursing care was non-existent. Had one or the other of us not [have been] able to be with the child at all times, we wonder who would have performed such tasks as refilling the croupette water dispenser, administering fluids, obtaining blankets and sheets for a bed that was continually saturated."[50]

In early 1970, Smith laid out her frustrations to the provost. "This memorandum is a protest," she wrote, "against the steady decline in support services for nursing. It is not a strike, a sit-in, a placard-carrying demonstration. Neither does it present unconditional demands. I submit, however, that the situation is serious."[51] By this time, Smith no longer enjoyed the same level of support from her colleagues across the university, and she was unprotected from both administrators and physicians who did not believe in shared governance or collaborative practice, nor nurses who did not support unification principles. These forces were free to disrupt and to sabotage, and develop their own alliances more in tune to the administration change. And although her faculty remained fairly loyal, she gradually lost many of the original group who moved on to other challenges, taking her ideas with them. Another factor was the developmental phase of the health center. A ten-year entrepreneurial period laced with optimism and enthusiasm gave way to a season of routine business and continuity. Although Smith and her colleagues gave a mighty effort and extensively published and promoted their ideas, the original creativity could not be sustained.

Perhaps the reality of overseeing both the school and the hospital nursing service finally took its toll on Smith. It seemed she had to fight for everything she needed as well as for maintaining the systems already in place. She voiced her frustration in a 1970 memo to health system provost Ackell. She needed "additional faculty lines (as requested in the last two budgets) and competitive salaries for three. . . . If we could just *once* get the number of new lines requested we might find enough hope and courage to continue our 60 hour work weeks."[52] Many of these systems were expensive—the unit manager system, the nurse consultants, and a decentralized organization in general. While they freed nurses to provide patient care, additional employees were needed to perform duties hospitals typically got for free from the nursing staff, such as preparing time cards, payroll, equipment maintenance, and surveillance. As the health system moved toward a more corporate model, the paradigm of care shifted to that of large health systems facing economic realities in the struggle to survive.

Ironically, as the health center reconsidered its commitment to its original governance and unification structure, the national commission for the study of nursing and nursing education (the Lysaught report) recommended some of the same strategies Smith and her colleagues implemented several years earlier. Many other health centers, such as Yale, Western Reserve, and Pittsburgh, were experimenting with the same ideas. In contrast, the University of Florida health center was moving away from the structure many other places were finding interesting and innovative.[53] As other institutions embraced her ideas, Smith fought for their survival at the health center.

Smith felt increasingly frustrated and devalued as she became more and more isolated from the main decision-making structures of the health system. In a December 1969 memo to the faculty, she noted, "We have made much progress this year and this is evident even to some of those in the Health Center who would divide us or prefer that we be organized differently . . . [including] the collection of data to answer threatening or blaming memos, the use of rational behavior in contrast to defensive or uninformed behavior."[54] She was having particular difficulty with the director of patient services at the health center who believed he, rather than the College of Nursing, had responsibility for nursing services.

Smith clashed with him over many things, including a 1969 grant proposal Smith's faculty submitted for the development of a graduate nurse specialist program at the health center. In a detailed letter he asked to be read at a public meeting, the director wrote that he found the proposal totally unacceptable, noting that although he supported the idea of nursing specialists, he "did not consider that we have excellent specialized patient care in this hospital."[55] Shortly after the meeting, Smith wrote to Provost Ackell to protest the tone and content of the letter. Although she agreed with some of the criticism, she wrote, "I do not expect you to do anything about this, but I do think you ought to know that this is the kind of behavior to which nursing is subjected day in and day out."[56] This episode, one of many, kept Smith and her faculty preoccupied with the politics rather than the practice of patient care.

Smith increasingly found her situation at the health center untenable, as the power struggle between the hospital administration and the College of Nursing was emotionally draining. In early July 1970, she lost her battle to keep the college and hospital nursing services unified. Instead, the provost offered her a "six-month trial period" for the college to be involved in (rather than control) administration of nursing services. She declined the offer, noting, "We do not wish to take advantage of this trial period . . . it has been made very clear that the hospital director and the chief of staff are opposed to the College of Nursing involvement [in the health center], and we no longer wish to be engaged in this kind of power struggle."[57]

On July 13, 1970, Smith received a vote of approval for a memo she wrote to Provost Ackell, which "essentially turned the hospital over to 'whom it may concern.'"[58] It was, as Smith noted, "a pretty good letter," laying out her frustrations with the lack of funds to accomplish her goals of unification and to keep the nursing service functioning. Ackell, although not always supportive, realized the damage possible in an abrupt change in the hospital nursing structure and leadership, and the difficulty he might have finding a new director of nursing service in a short period of time given the hostile conditions in the health center. He convinced Smith to reconsider, and the nursing faculty rescinded the memo on August 3, 1970, believing the negotiations went on in good faith.

By February 1971, however, Smith again believed she could make no further progress with the provost and the hospital administration and shortly thereafter, she resigned as dean, believing she rather than the College of Nursing or its ideas had become the issue. Smith could not successfully negotiate her vision for nursing within the health system with the replacements for "her men" and her "women," and her position became untenable. Consensus was impossible, and there remained little room for experimentation and discussion. With her departure from the position (she remained on the faculty for several years), the health system continued to grow and prosper, but in ways and directions different from what Smith envisioned or approved. The context had changed, and in the realities and challenges of place and time the university moved in a different direction. Meanwhile, others elsewhere across the country continued to experiment with the concepts and practice of unification, shared governance, and clinical-practice models with greater or lesser success.

The University of Rochester

The University of Rochester, similar to the University of Florida at its founding, had a unique blend of nurse and physician leaders and practitioners who, because of personality, vision, and leadership skills, established a fine sense of mutual responsibility for patient care. Eleanor Hall, chair of the Department of Nursing from 1957 to 1971; J. Lowell Orbison, dean of the School of Medicine and Dentistry; internist Barbara Bates, pediatricians Evan Charney and Robert Hoekelman, psychiatrist George Engel, and chair of medicine Lawrence Young, to name a few, were all fairly liberal-minded and energetic faculty members who supported inventive practice and education models. Since 1961, some of these leaders were part of an effort to develop an autonomous School of Nursing, and in 1968, with the promise of W. K. Kellogg Foundation support if a substantial plan developed, university president William A. Wallis appointed an ad hoc committee to explore the possibility.[59] The interdisciplinary committee released a report almost a year later, in January 1969.[60]

Innovative in both its scope and its intellectual approach, the report acknowledged the interrelated nature of patient care and the disorder within nursing at the university. "No profession can care for patients itself," the committee noted, "Each is dependent upon the others, and the patient upon them all."[61] But before nursing could think of its interrelated role with medicine, it first had to get its own house in order and identify leaders who shared philosophy and vision. As the committee noted, "They [nursing] must heal the wounds within their own profession."[62] The closure of the diploma school in the early 1960s still incited strong feelings from alumni, and the turf battles between nursing education and service channeled a great deal of creative energy away from patient care issues.

Most important, the committee recommended a School of Nursing on par with the School of Medicine and Dentistry, and a single position of both dean and director of nursing. The dean of nursing, in turn, appointed chairs of practice, research, and education, again paralleling the organization of the School of Medicine and Dentistry; these chairs also needed secondary appointments in the appropriate School of Medicine departments. This arrangement provided the foundation and the opportunity for interdisciplinary research collaboration, education, and development of new practice models.

To support nursing's place alongside the dental and medical school, the members of the committee also recommended stronger integration of nursing education into the academy. Nursing, the committee noted, must "recognize and encourage academic study," essentially realizing, more than ten years after the advocacy of Dorothy Smith and her colleagues at the University of Florida, that nursing indeed was an intellectual discipline. The major implication of this ideological stance was that nursing education programs across all levels, especially at the graduate level, needed to reflect and sustain their legitimate place in the university.[63]

The committee's support for nursing's integration into the academy was subtly informed by the sometimes covert clinical practice experimentation already going on in hospital clinics where some committee members worked, and by experiences of committee members for whom interdisciplinary practice was the norm. Barbara Bates, chair of the committee, came from the University of Kentucky, which during the 1960s developed a medical center model based on systemwide interdisciplinary practice and a focus on primary care and public health.[64] She understood the importance of working with other health professionals as well as the need for generalist and specialist collaboration to improve access and the quality of patient care. Perhaps equally as important, informal changes were already under way in hospital clinics, and the opportune hiring of several young energetic nursing faculty at the school only fueled these changes.

"These are some patients I would like to follow,"[65] wrote nursing faculty member Joan Lynaugh to physician Nate Lassman in late 1968. Lassman was a medical resident in U-wing medical clinic and Lynaugh knew him previously from her own practice in critical care. So began a seemingly simple arrangement

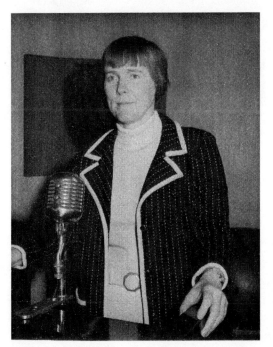

Photo 3. Physician Barbara Bates, circa 1970. (Joan Lynaugh personal collection, Bryn Mawr, Pennsylvania.) Bates and colleague Joan Lynaugh developed the medical nurse practitioner program at the University of Rochester in the early 1970s.

around the time of the school of nursing committee. Lynaugh recalled, "I had
been working with Nate Lassman for several months. . . . We agreed that I—he
had already started work with some of the clinic nurses to see chronically ill
patients—would join that group. There were two, the head nurse and one of the
staff nurses in the clinic, developing a small practice. . . . And I said I'd like to
start seeing some patients with him and just see what I could do with them."[66]

Lynaugh saw this opportunity not as a way to learn medical skills, but "primarily [as] a modification and reorganization of nursing practice, to improve
[my] capacity to evaluate patients' response to illness/therapy and/or to evaluate their level of health."[67] These skills were value-added for her nursing practice. Over the next year, Lynaugh worked with Lassman in the clinic evaluating
patients and adding to her array of clinical skills as part of an informal experiment involving three nurse-physician teams. This was a highly entrepreneurial
endeavor, with each group developing its roles within its frame of professional
competence and personal comfort.

Every six months the teams met to discuss their experiences, and a common pattern emerged surrounding the nursing role. At first, the nurse joined
the doctor in his interview and examination of patients to get acquainted with
the style of practice. Gradually a sense of trust and security developed, and the
nurse took on increasing responsibilities for interviewing, focusing especially
on areas of personal and family problems, medication review, health teaching,
and guidance.[68] Lynaugh's clinical notes illustrate her efforts:[69]

> Patient R.G., "Lives with unmarried daughter, RX for VPC's with
> digoxin—<VPCs, c/o palpitations, EKG, urine, mini chest, return
> for visit, controlled cardiac with fleeting arthritis, not working.
> Patient R.H., "Valve repair, blood spec. inadequate, repeat ordered,
> OK, making little progress in work rehab, Nate says ok.
> protime <10%
> hct decreased, pro 10%, hospitalize.

Her notes document the chronicity of the patients she saw, and her progres-
sively increasing comfort in her evaluation skills, including her ability to incorporate patient-centered information into patient care, decide when to perform
particular examinations, make referrals, and interpret laboratory values.

Physician team members were very positive. They reported increased
knowledge about their patients and a greater sense of continuity as nurses
cemented links to the community by referring patients to public health and visiting nurse agencies. Some physicians reported the ability to see more patients,
while others reported qualitative, rather than quantitative, changes. Both

nurses and physicians reported easier detection of medication errors when they worked together.[70] Patients also seemed to recognize that the nurse and the physician were working together. "My dear Nurse Lynaugh and Dr. Lassman," began a letter in 1970 to the team. "I thank you both very much for all you have done and all you have ahead of you with mother!"[71] This type of practice was happening in other parts of the medical center, as nurse and physician leaders (in internal medicine and pediatrics, at least) supported a generous amount of clinical practice innovation and collaboration. It was a matter of the right people being in the right place at the right time rather than any type of strategic policy planning.

New types of programs began in other parts of New York State. In 1971, Cornell–New York Hospital and Medical Center (CUNY) began its PRIMEX program.[72] This curriculum was designed to focus specifically on educating nurses to provide primary care and preventive services in the community. The PRIMEX program was the culmination of a ten-year-long experiment that began in 1962 under the direction of internist George Reader. This earlier program used an extended nursing role particularly for the care of poor, elderly clinic patients.[73] The PRIMEX program was designed to extend the reach of this program by teaching more nurses the advanced skills they needed to provide care to this particular population.

In the children's clinics at Rochester in 1968, pediatrician Evan Charney and pediatric nurse Harriet Kitzman developed a collaborative practice model, incorporating skills that nurses already had but were underutilized. Kitzman remembered: "We were all in situations where the expectation of clinical decision-making, and taking leadership in clinical decisions, was present. . . . There already was a tremendous amount of responsibility being assumed, although it was not recognized as such."[74] Kitzman began to work with Charney almost accidentally. "I had the fortuitous opportunity," she noted, "[to] be contacted by someone about the kinds of exciting things that were going on in the department of pediatrics, particularly the new way of training residents, pediatric residents, in continuity of care."[75] Nurses were key to the community pediatrics model developed by chair of pediatrics Robert Haggerty as part of a new model medical curriculum focusing on comprehensive patient-centered and primary care.

Haggerty also supported a climate of collaborative care that strongly influenced the socialization and acculturation of medical students and residents. Although nurses unofficially participated in medical education, the formalization of nurses' role and the two-way learning aspect was a key piece that the pediatric leadership supported and deemed crucial to quality patient care. Kitzman described the nurses' contribution: "It became easy to see how a team of a nurse and a physician together, at that point in time, could really provide both exceptional care for the families, but also that the nurse could learn more about the ongoing clinical dimensions of care, and that the residents could learn much more about how to help families live with developing children."[76]

The medical center focused on providing comprehensive and primary care while regionalizing itself, and therefore looked outward to the health needs of the community. This strategy, while improving access to care for people in both urban and rural areas, also created a foundation for new practice models. Charney and Kitzman began to think about the type of practitioners needed to support this type of primary care outreach, and with funding from the Public Health Service and the Children's Health Bureau, they began a child health nurse pilot program in 1968. The program tapped an underdeveloped resource and helped inactive nurses return to the workforce in a broadened primary care role. It included a four-month training program of advanced clinical education, clinical experience, and eventually practice in a nurse-physician team to provide well-child care.[77] Kitzman and Charney planned the program and selected the pediatricians and nurses to participate in the project, choosing the most influential and largest pediatric practices known to be friendly to the ideas of collaboration. As Kitzman remembered, "They [community pediatricians] had a number of patients that we knew, and could accommodate additional partners in terms of the nurses. Rochester pediatrics always had a very close relationship to pediatricians in the community. And so they were [already] doing clinical teaching, et cetera, within the medical center. So these were people who had a very positive standing within the medical center, in collaborative relationships to start with."[78]

Kitzman and Charney met with the physicians over several months in a sort of acculturation and socialization process. Some of the physicians had concerns about changing relationships with patients, and needed support to develop communication strategies to assure patients that the quality of care they received from the nurse-physician team would not be less than they expected from the physician alone. Kitzman recalled, "What was resolved during that time were all the worries of what if something is missed, what would happen. . . . And what happens to relationships with patients, and [they] would work with someone with different kinds of skills. And it was very important to do it at that point in time because we were also developing these same kinds of roles in the health department, in new neighborhood health centers. And it was important to be clear that the kind of care that can be provided in teams, with nurses and pediatricians, is all the care that anyone needs. . . . And this is not as though it's care for the poor when pediatricians are not available."[79]

Meanwhile, in the medical clinics, Lynaugh found similar collaborative opportunities, but she realized that although she was learning new types of skills to supplement her own nursing knowledge, she still needed greater expertise in clinical judgment and more practice responsibilities beyond the traditional nursing practice boundaries. Working in an interdisciplinary team gave her a clearer sense of the care she had the potential to provide as a nurse, along with the skills and knowledge she knew she could master but did not yet have. "Barbara [Bates] and I kept talking about what else I needed to know in order to make decisions about [patients]," she remembered. "What I needed to know, basically, was how to evaluate their congestive failure, how to evaluate their peripheral edema, how to decide about their acute and subacute complaints, how to examine their eyes because they all had hypertension. . . . After lots of discussion, we came to the conclusion, it was probably just the two of us, mostly, although other people must have been involved, that we would teach a course in physical assessment and ultimately in history taking. What we decided to start with was physical assessment."[80]

Out of these and other discussions came the idea of the "clandestine group" in March 1971. This was a clinic in the traditional sense—a physician expert and a student learning how to take care of particular patients. Except, of course, the students were fully trained nurses rather than medical students or residents, which was why the planners kept the group under the radar. There was a handful of physicians who disapproved of nurses learning how to take histories, perform physical examinations, and essentially develop a certain level of clinical judgment. Thorough exploration of the patient history, communication skills practice, as well as supervision of students performing clinical examinations by expert senior practitioners also formed the foundation of a new third-year clerkship developed for medical students during this same time period. Some of the physicians who diligently developed and sustained the program were somewhat reluctant to share the implicit authority of these skills with practitioners other than physicians.[81]

Some physicians eventually changed their perspective. George Engel, for example, later came to appreciate the integration of the nursing and medical perspective in these skills. He wrote to Barbara Bates and Joan Lynaugh:

The language of nursing is in my judgment the proper language of medicine and indeed a major part of our efforts with the medical students is to inculcate the attitudes implicit in that language. We do reasonably well through the second year but thereafter students to varying degrees succumb to the powerful impact of the physician's cultural milieu in

which they find themselves. For some it becomes the ticket of entry to
the magic circle to be able to refer to a patient as 'this 33 year-old white
female.' 'Female what' is my usual rejoinder if any student is forgetful
enough to present a patient to me in that fashion.[82]

The clandestine group was, as a January 1971 memo noted, to be "confined
to a selected group of nurses on an experimental basis."[83] The organizers
wanted to keep the group small, as a pilot project, and minimize the publicity
that might emerge from those unable or unwilling to participate. The nurses
were also practicing on each other, another similarity to the unique third-year
medical clerkship. But for those who agreed to join the group, this was an
adventure, with an underlying tension of expectations. It was fun and exciting to
learn in this way, and as Lynaugh noted, "We were somewhat amused by it all."[84]

The ten nurses and five physicians who took part in the Wednesday evening
group were a diverse collection of practitioners. Several came from intensive care
units, others came from the emergency room or general medical floors. All of the
nurses were looking for something new to regenerate their practices. Lynaugh
noted: "I really wanted to get back in [practice] in a way to what I had done before,
when I was a medical nurse. Where you really got to know your patients . . .
people stayed in the hospital for a couple weeks. And you sort of saw them either
not get better or get better. But in ICU it wasn't like that. So I thought it would be
much more interesting to work with people with congestive failure and hypertension and diabetes and general failure to thrive as adults and see them over a
long period of time. And so the medical clinic was perfect for that."[85]

The physicians had to be equally comfortable providing the teaching.
"Nate was like that," Lynaugh noted. "He was in his skin, he didn't have any
trouble with that. And of course Barbara [Bates] had no trouble with it. The
other thing about it is you had to have a physician who could give up his
patients."[86] Lynaugh remembered one superb physician who invested heavily
in the relationships he had with his patients. "He [took] his own blood pres-
sures. . . . He always did. I could support him in that because he didn't want to
make his patients think that he didn't care about them any more. For [him] it
was the real thing. . . . He loved teaching the house staff. You really had to have
somebody, especially then, who was able to be comfortable with himself and
also put up with a certain level of suspicion from his colleagues."[87]

All of the physicians involved were familiar with the role of professor or
teacher, as they were all academic physicians involved in resident education.
This type of teaching, however, was somewhat different. Medical students and
residents were supposed to learn these skills, and there was an assumption that

they had the appropriate foundational knowledge to integrate them into their practice. In contrast, the physicians had to believe that teaching nurses physical examination skills was an appropriate thing to do, and they had to be sure enough of their own status in the medical center to downplay dissent from their colleagues. Because physicians traditionally were involved in nursing education as well, this kind of teaching has occurred constantly throughout nursing and medicine's history. The difference was that nurses were learning in a more formalized way the heretofore professionally guarded skills of clinical judgment and physical assessment.

The whole endeavor raised enormous questions: Were clinical thinking and physical assessment inseparable from their basic science background, or were they part of a routine that was more experience based? Could nurses be taught and learn clinical judgment? And could they safely take care of patients when applying these skills? Although physicians made mistakes, how many mistakes by nurses would people tolerate? And was it legal? These were unresolved questions for all involved. Physicians needed answers to these questions before they could comfortably participate, and some seemed to come to this point earlier and easier than others.

Bates understood the history and the challenge from the beginning and was probably one of the few physicians who actually thoroughly thought through the process. She knew there were uneasy tensions involved in teaching complex diagnostic reasoning and physical examination based on anatomy and physiology to nurses who lacked a basic science background. For physicians, "diagnostic reasoning led to possibilities." For nurses, it became out of necessity a "matching process, albeit an exquisitely complex one, where clinical findings were matched with those within the range of normal" or recognized as deviations.[88] Lynaugh agreed, noting some physicians involved in the clinic believed "this [physical examination and clinical thinking] was something, not that anyone could do, but could be taught and learned and that it was safe and that there was a certain familiarity and routine about this whole business of data collection and clinical thinking."[89]

Ten nurses and five physicians met in the Wednesday night group. Some volunteered and some were deliberately chosen by Joan Lynaugh and Dorothy Taylor, assistant director of nursing services for ambulatory care, who also had a hand in the formation of the nursing clinic. Lynaugh and Bates developed a curriculum, schedule of classes, and generally set the overall tone of the group, which ran for twelve weeks in early 1971. "We had to do it all," Bates remembered.[90] They weren't thinking of "clerkship lite" but of a different paradigm for learning a complex set of skills. Despite this, the whole course was planned in a fairly casual way. "And so what we did basically," Lynaugh noted, "was Barbara and I sat on the porch in the fall and we drew up a curriculum. It was all about physical diagnosis. Trying to decide what to teach."[91]

Almost immediately, Lynaugh and Bates encountered problems finding quality physical examination texts. Most of them at the time were in narrative form without photographs, or included drawings that were unclear, confusing, or too small. There were no texts for the beginning practitioner, and none combined all elements into the step-by-step guide Lynaugh and Bates wanted for nurses. Most were missing content on patient relations, recording data, and presenting clinical findings. Barbara Bates was quite fond of using pencil illustrations of her points, both on her manuscript drafts and while teaching residents. She was also an avid birdwatcher. She began to illustrate the system modules she and Lynaugh developed, based on the series of drawings she was keenly familiar with from *Peterson's Field Guide* for birds.[92]

Lynaugh and Bates gave portions of the modules to students each week. Their popularity grew exponentially, and by late 1971 even medical students in the general clerkship at the university were using them to supplement, and at one point replace the text developed by physicians Engel and Morgan for the

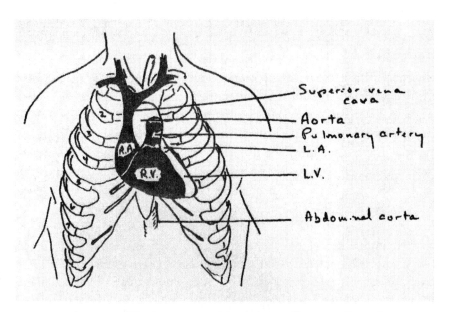

Photo 4. Diagram of the heart, original hand-drawn illustration by Barbara Bates. These illustrations were used by Bates and Lynaugh in their nurse practitioner program, and they were later incorporated into the textbook *Guide to Physical Examination and History-Taking* published in 1974. (Joan Lynaugh personal collection, Bryn Mawr, Pennsylvania.)

same purposes. Pediatrician Robert Hoekelman worked with Bates to develop a pediatric assessment section that was integrated into the module collection and eventually used by pediatric residents. The Rochester regional medical program funded publication of the modules, and eventually, in 1974, the Lippincott publishing company took over.[93] This physical-examination booklet, developed for nurses and marketed for both nurses and physicians, eventually became one of the best-selling texts on Lippincott's publication list.

As the group continued, Congress debated, and, in November, President Nixon signed the 1971 NTA. Although nurse practitioners were not mentioned specifically ("expanded roles" is one example of the terminology used in the legislation), at least some of the $83 million proposed for special projects ended up supporting nurse practitioner programs.[94] But even before the 1971 NTA, funding was available. Jesse Scott, director of the division of nursing of the Public Health Service and her division colleague Margaret Sheehan (who was also an acquaintance of school head Eleanor Hall), encouraged Bates and Lynaugh, and Kitzman and Hoekelman, to apply for funding to formalize their programs. On-the-job-training was important for beginning practitioners, but there was a serious need for more structured ways to provide the essential skills and knowledge nurses needed to continue to expand their role.

To help actualize their ideas, both groups developed proposals for the division. Kitzman and Hoekelman's pediatric nurse practitioner project was funded in 1970.[95] In early 1971, Bates and Lynaugh received their own funding to plan more formalized behavior objectives for the program, as well as to train nurses who could then teach these skills to other nurses. They had in fact been developing their teaching skills not only with the physical examination course in the Wednesday night group, but they also consulted and shared teaching materials with Rochester neighborhood health centers and the medical department at Kodak. Their experiences helped them move beyond the singular focus on physical examination and onto the broader areas of physical diagnosis, clinical thinking, and nurse-physician collaboration.[96] These linguistic changes may, indeed, be subtle, but they are symbolic of the progressive changes taking place in nursing and medical practice, of the efforts of collaborative pairs of practitioners, exemplified by Bates and Lynaugh, and of their efforts to situate the dialogue and intellectual process surrounding practice in the clinics where it occurred.

One of the key concepts of this project was the nurse-physician team. This idea, honed and polished in the hospital clinics, was extended into the community and included physician preceptors and nurses who agreed not only to work together as participants in the planning process and development of teaching modules (the nurse would also complete the training program), but also later as a unit to support more students when the program ended. Underlying this concept of the team were the assumptions that, first, changes in nursing and physician practice function and philosophy were needed to make the nurse practitioner role successful, and second, that nurses had a substantial role in ambulatory care. This group of thirteen nurses and twelve physicians, the participant planning group, was established to develop the curriculum, begin to define the role of the nurse practitioner, identify models to facilitate practice and teaching through clinical preceptorships, work through the realignment of the nurse-physician team, and identify means of evaluating practitioner performance.[97]

To identify and select the collaborative teams, Lynaugh and Bates developed background materials and took to the road to identify compatible nurse-physician pairs that would have the important job of both creating and trying out the curriculum. Essentially they needed groups that could eventually function similarly to those in the medical clinic. They learned early in their search that their practice relationships were unique and not easily replicated. In one of their meetings with a potential nurse-physician team in mid-1971, Lynaugh noted, "The initial phase of the meeting began with an exchange between Dr. K and Barbara [Bates], and after a few minutes, myself. . . . With no questions from the nurse . . . it seemed evident and worries were expressed around the lack of knowledge about one another that existed between the physician, the nurse, and the administrator . . . not enough basic trust or understanding in the group to come to some conclusion about participating."[98] At another local community hospital, the physician initially met with Lynaugh and Bates, and then invited the nurse into the meeting—she apparently had not been previously notified. A medical resident next joined the meeting, "launching into a brief dissertation on the value of allied health personnel in primary care, and what he construed as the appropriate relationship between the nurse and the physician."[99]

After Lynaugh and Bates chose the groups in the fall of 1971, the nurses of the planning teams participated in a five-week curriculum pilot and continued a half-day weekly training session until May 1972. This program included interviewing and history taking, physical examination of the adult, medical nursing content emphasizing common problems in ambulatory care, issues in role change, collaborative professional development, as well as a clinical experience portion.[100] The medical nursing portion of the curriculum was important, as from the beginning this was a nursing program with a nursing identity. It was not meant to provide nurses with knowledge that set up competition with physicians—this was a frequently discussed and dismissed idea. All the participants were firmly of one mind in this, as they were chosen because of their understanding of the potential for nurses to have greater participation in primary care.

The program did not mimic physician extender programs also proliferating during this time (e.g., physician assistant programs), but built on and enlarged the strategies already implemented in places such as Denver and Kansas City, Kansas. Bates and Lynaugh were not looking to replicate the medical model. To do so, they noted in the 1971 planning grant application, "would create a physician substitute and lose a nurse."[101] They needed to develop the infrastructure for the next step—to educate nurse practitioners and the teachers of nurse practitioners.

The program was also unique because of the way the participants developed more formalized perceptions of nurse-physician interaction, inference and decision making, and teaching and learning methods. There was more to the program than clinical experience and on-the-job training. All involved understood that although the particular skills and knowledge were important, their application to patient care would not happen if both nurses and physicians failed to realize their potential to work together. In other words, Bates and Lynaugh proposed a paradigmatic change in the way primary care should be practiced and taught. This involved the education of both nurse and physician in higher-level interaction skills, a detailed sequential approach to physical assessment and clinical thinking, and development and testing of models of teaching and learning that could be integrated into graduate education that focused on advanced clinical practice. Based on their experience with the planning grant, they began to envision how their curriculum and teaching methods could be integrated into both undergraduate and graduate education, and how the competence of their program graduates could be measured.

In 1972, Bates and Lynaugh received funding from the National Institutes of Health, made possible by the 1971 NTA, for a three-year training grant. Its purpose was to develop a medical nurse practitioner program in an ambulatory setting, initially as a continuing education offering, and to develop strategies to more effectively implement the role in the community. Inherent in the program was the training of nurse practitioner faculty.[102] As Lynaugh noted, "The most serious problem we had all the time I did this at Rochester was that we didn't have anybody who knew how to teach this stuff. It was tiring; you had to get somebody else there."[103] Because they could not recruit enough educators who had these skills, they developed an intensive summer course, similar to the original medical nurse practitioner program, to develop a pool of faculty who could work as part of a collaborative teaching team with a physician colleague.

The faculty problem also contributed to logistical issues for implementing their program on a larger scale. For Bates and Lynaugh the program was incredibly time intensive as they felt compelled to closely monitor the nurse-physician pairs. As Lynaugh noted:

> The whole style of practice and how patients would be seen in various practices, all that had to be improvised, and tried out, and so it was quite a strain on the people who were doing it for the first time. . . . The style that we devised for those first several years was kind of devised under the premise that you could give a block of experience in practice and education to the learners and then set up a fairly intensive support system to follow them as they went back to their practices and began to work with the physicians. So we did a lot of circuit riding, basically. And they came back. The nurses came back every week for a day. Then, [we] would go visit the practices. Because we could never get the physicians to come back. Even if we fed them they wouldn't come.[104]

In the 1972 grant, Bates and Lynaugh included time to develop evaluation tools to see if their program worked. This was, perhaps, one of the most important and controversial pieces of the program. Measurement in general was not a problem for nurse educators because quantification of nurses' work was part of its history, from Isabel Stewart's time-and-motion studies to intricate appraisals of education-program outcomes required by the programs funded by the 1964 and 1971 NTAs. This type of assessment differed from earlier efforts because it analyzed success based on patient responses rather than nurses' functional work. The parameters were meant to be patient-protective and to document the safety of the practitioner both to the public and medical and nursing bodies. As more people questioned whether nurse practitioners were safe, these types of data were invaluable in legitimizing them. The evaluation data toned down but never quite warded off criticisms that medical organizations raised about the quality of nurse practitioner patient care. Although the competence of physicians was rarely tested again after they passed their medical boards, the competence of nurse practitioners was constantly subjected to analysis.[105]

Another consideration was the selection of students. The program leaders chose them based on their involvement with an existing practice in an ambulatory setting, and the expectation that they would work there after completing the program. "They all had to have jobs," Lynaugh noted. "They had to have a written guarantee that they would be able to use the new knowledge and skills they had gained in practice. The physicians had to promise to participate. They never did, of course, but they had to promise."[106] This kind of agreement was fairly common around the country in the early 1970s for nurse practitioner and physician assistant programs.[107] The newly minted practitioners had to have a home base to practice the skills and knowledge gained in the program, and they needed initial supervision.[108] In an area such as Rochester, with a large academic health center and many physicians, there was no motivation from either the public or the medical profession for nurses to establish independent practices.

There were nurse-run practices in certain extremely poor rural locations across the country, usually supported by Public Health Service funding. Lucille Kinlein in Georgia was one of the more prominent examples, as were the nurses working with the frontier nursing services and the Alaska Public Health Service.[109] But unless they practiced in rural New York State, the nurse practitioners working in close proximity to the Rochester medical center and its affiliates were hard-pressed to gain independent access to admitting privileges or radiology and laboratory facilities, and it would have been antithetical to the collaborative model serving as the foundation for the programs. As Lynaugh noted, "It was problematic because you really couldn't expect a nurse to refine and develop her skills unless she could employ them on a regular basis with some kind of supervision and guidance from somebody who knew how to do this, and second, on a public policy level, it didn't make any sense to prepare a person to do something that she wouldn't be able to do."[110]

Another reason for physician sponsorship was to protect both the nurse and the physician. In 1971, New York reopened its Practice Act and over the next two years the New York State Nurses' Association, the New York State Medical Society, and the Hospital Association of New York contested the definition of nursing as a distinct and independent profession. Although this legislation (N.Y. State Senate Bill, No. 1918) addressed generalist nurses and not nurse practitioners, the underlying subtext of the debate was their emerging and challenging role. In any event, the program placed their students where physician sponsors could dispel challenges from colleagues that the students, and later graduates, were practicing medicine.[111] Challenges to nurses practicing in these roles were a reality.[112] But by relying on physician sponsors for supervision and protection, the program directors, as they soon discovered, lost a certain degree of control over the amount and quality of teaching offered to their students. This was the reality of early nurse practitioner programs.

Confrontations to nurse practitioner programs also came from within the nursing profession. Although by this time, the enormous federal funding for these programs through the 1971 NTA pressured many nursing education leaders to follow the money, occasional voices protested. Perhaps the most outspoken nurse leader was Martha Rogers, head of the division of nurse education at New York University, who saw the nurse practitioner role as one that discarded nurses' identity. Likening the growing nurse practitioner movement as akin to the "emperor's new clothes," Rogers believed nurses who took on enlarged roles that incorporated traditional medical skills became subsumed in a medical identity without the power and authority to wield it.[113] Responding to an article by Lynaugh and Bates describing the clinical practicum offered by their medical nurse practitioner program, Rogers's close colleague Mary Kohnke retorted, "it would be of great service if people in such programs would stop the euphemistic language and tell it like it is. These programs, purely and simply, prepare physicians' assistants."[114]

Nurse practitioners themselves sometimes seemed unclear about their purpose. Were they training to be the doctor's assistant, or were they supporting and enlarging a special set of skills and knowledge particular to nursing? Both approaches were validated in surveys and opinion pieces in journals.[115] The Rochester program was probably a mix of both: the medical nurse practitioner was clearly a hybrid who could practice medicine at a particular level but with a nursing perspective. This was true of many of the programs developing during this time and later. But lacking a particular language to describe their practices, the newly minted practitioners could only resort to typical terminology to explain themselves. They were either practicing nursing or medicine. There wasn't a word to describe that place in between. The Carnegie Commission's 1970 report, "Higher Education and the Nation's Health," supported alternate scenarios that could help standardize curricula, labels, and expectations, but these issues went unresolved.[116] Although many nursing leaders believed the movement of nurse practitioner education into graduate nursing programs and the integration of some of the same skills into the undergraduate curriculum might strengthen continuity and consistency of language and ideology, it did not clarify the issue of identity.

The medical nurse practitioner program supported by the NIH grant took the experiences from the 1971 planning program and formalized them into a two-session program, each twenty weeks long, including classroom instruction, highly supervised clinical experience, and guided laboratory practice. The program faithfully followed the text developed by Bates and included conferences on medical nursing problems organized by organ systems but centered on patient problems. By looking at the course outline, it might be difficult to discern differences from a medical curriculum, and it was consistent with that taught to medical students. In fact, Bates used her text and, later, videotapes to teach medical students the same skills. But there were differences: the highly supervised clinical experience provided to the nurses (in contrast to the typical medical education experience of "see one, do one, teach one"), the context in which nurse practitioners used the skills, and the performance evaluation conducted in the patient arena. Additionally, the nurse practitioner students were older, had a mean of over nine years' experience as clinicians upon entering the program, and were already placed in a practice before completing the program.[117]

Over the next two years, forty-eight students (with tuition covered by the federal grant) completed the program at Rochester, not including the seven students in the special summer session for faculty, at a cost of approximately $140,000 per year over three years.[118] Considering the amount of time and effort required of co-directors Lynaugh and Bates to manage the program, this was an extraordinarily good investment by the federal government via the division of nursing, which spent $19.5 million from 1972 to 1975 for special grants and contracts for nursing.[119] During this same time period, approximately three thousand nurse practitioner certificate and master's-prepared students graduated from DHEW-sponsored programs. By 1974, 131 programs for nurse practitioners existed, eighty-six certificate programs, and forty-five master's programs. The number of certificate programs grew substantially faster than master's programs at first, but with the infusion of federal money after the 1975 NTA, more than half were graduate programs by 1980.[120] An enormous amount of money was floating around for experimentation with curricula and development of new programs, and nursing school deans felt financial pressure to use the money as well as amazement over how much there was. These programs became lifelines for graduate and undergraduate programs at many schools, as the federal funding kept them solvent based on the support they received for their nurse practitioner programs.[121]

By the end of 1973, with Rochester undergoing a major curriculum overhaul at both the undergraduate and graduate level under new dean Loretta Ford, Lynaugh and Bates saw the opportunity to gradually convert the certificate program to a bona fide graduate-degree program. They developed plans to continue the nondegree for at least three more years, charge tuition once the grant ended, and aim for a student mix of half continuing education students and half graduate students; these students came primarily from the family health nurse clinician graduate program, which eventually became the graduate program in primary care.[122]

By 1974, Lynaugh quite accurately argued that local agencies customized their care delivery systems to incorporate nurse practitioners and relied heavily on them for patient care services. Spurred on by the success of existing programs and the opportunity for generous funding, the Rochester programs—as well

as those at SUNY Buffalo, SUNY Upstate Syracuse, and various programs in
New York City, such as the PRIMEX program at CUNY—were producing fairly
large numbers of nurse practitioners.[123] In fact, by 1977, New York had the largest
number of programs by state (seventeen), followed by California (sixteen), and
had the second largest number of practitioners after California.[124]

By 1977, private organizations such as the Robert Wood Johnson Foundation
closed the circle begun by the Kellogg Foundation by funding fellowship programs in primary care for both nursing faculty and students.[125] Rochester ben-
efited from both of these programs. And unlike the University of Florida, the
Rochester academic health center concept maintained its momentum even
when some of the major participants, such as Lynaugh and Bates, left for other
opportunities. Loretta Ford, first dean of the School of Nursing in 1972, kept the
ideal moving with the help of enlightened faculty, many of them trained
through the pediatric and adult medical nurse practitioner programs.

The University of Florida and the University of Rochester

The exemplars presented by these academic health centers, the University of
Florida, and the University of Rochester, are highly illustrative of the growing
focus on expert clinical practice in both medical and nursing education, and on
practice as something greater than on-the-job training. Experience and repetition no longer sufficed in a health care environment that demanded from
nurses broader and more intense decision making and critical thinking. Faculty
at both places believed in the need for clinicians who were able to think intellectually about their patients and their practice; these beliefs created the foundation for changes in clinical education from the baccalaureate to the graduate
level. These ideas were not limited to the two cases, but were in play in numerous places across the nation at both faster and slower paces. Many nursing education programs seemed to derive their influence from Smith's model at
Florida, and later the Rochester model, but each place claimed its own identity.

Both programs required ingredients similar to the early individually negotiated practices outside institutions of higher education—nurses and physicians of like mind, wanting to improve their practices and their patient
services, comfortable with themselves and in their roles. Money, however, is
thrown into the mix in the academic centers—foundation and federal research
funding for Smith, and even more abundant largesse through foundations and
the federal government for Bates and Lynaugh at Rochester. These programs,
and those developed by innovative nurses and physicians who knew how to
"follow the money," probably would have survived without it, but development
would have been slower and creativity less free reigning. Money equalized

many things, going to both small and large, private and public institutions. It created not only the practitioners themselves, but also the faculty to teach new recruits and the support to build curriculums and develop teaching models. It changed the course of graduate education for nursing from administration and education to clinical specialties, producing a growing cadre of expert practitioners, albeit with little experience and expertise as educators for future nurses.

The cases also highlight a growing revelation, something akin to Dorothy finding the Wizard of Oz to be a mortal man behind the curtain. Although the programs and the students required a great deal of effort by the pioneering nurses and doctors, teaching the skills and knowledge and practicing as a specialist in an expanded role really was not that hard to do. After the initial excitement of learning and practicing, most nurses understood what their physician colleagues always knew but rarely divulged—there wasn't any magic in the skills, and the knowledge was something nurses could take on and safely apply.

Chapter 4

Stealing the Spell Book

The Walt Disney animated movie *Fantasia* includes the tale of "The Sorcerer's Apprentice."[1] In the story the old sorcerer instructs his young apprentice to straighten up the laboratory while he rests. While the sorcerer is sleeping, the apprentice, who seems already to have a slight passing knowledge about magic, snatches the sorcerer's magic hat, and calls up an enchantment from the secret spell book to enable the willow broom to sweep and carry water for him while he performs his other work. But instead of one helper, he mistakenly conjures up scores of identical marching brooms with buckets that eventually create a massive flood that overwhelms the laboratory. The apprentice, perhaps because he cannot yet control the magical knowledge to counteract the spell, is carried away in a giant whirlpool. He is rescued by the sorcerer, who commands the water to recede and returns the broom to its inanimate state.[2]

This story has several parallels and some discontinuities with health care in the late 1960s and 1970s in the United States. The sorcerer, the controller and dispenser of magic, could be metaphoric of medicine or nursing organizations, as well as health care institutions, the federal government, or third-party insurers. And just as the napping sorcerer created an opportunity for the young apprentice to experiment, the failure of medicine and nursing organizations to strategically respond to changes in health care created opportunities for different practitioners to take on skills and knowledge traditionally controlled by the medical profession. And, unlike the apprentice who had to be rescued by the sorcerer, the new practitioners emerging in the 1960s and 1970s seized the moment in academic institutions and local practices and spread across the nation, changing public expectations of who was qualified to provide particular types of health care at specific times and places.

Different types of practitioners emerged during this period. Some, such as physician assistants, were in fact deliberately created de novo by physicians to support their work.[3] Others, such as nurse practitioners, arose from existing professions and realized an opportunity to expand their skills and carve out new practice boundaries with the help of some enlightened physicians, nurse educators, and public support. And, as in the tale, the newly minted practitioners sometimes looked the same and were not easily differentiated from one another. Yet all of these health care providers—nurse practitioners, physician assistants, and other types of associates—emerged in "whole sight" of the nursing and medical leadership, who may not have quite realized their potential or their emerging power. And like the folktale, the numbers of new providers grew, but in this case they could not be stifled or made to vanish, although many in the medical and nursing profession mightily tried. Both the nursing and medical professions then vociferously predicted that these emerging practitioners (depending upon which profession was predicting at a particular time) might cause patient care disasters, but they were wrong.

Although comparing health care in the 1960s and 1970s to this folktale is somewhat simplistic, it provides a way of thinking about the new providers that emerged during this time, how they took advantage of opportunities to "experiment with the spell book" to meet demands for health care and to cement their professional authority, and how, with limited success, they tried to differentiate themselves from others. In the story we never quite learn if the apprentice achieves his freedom and status as a sorcerer in his own right, or whether he always required the sorcerer's presence to use the spell book. But we do know that although newly emerging providers—including X-ray technicians, orthopedic and urologic assistants—initially warranted strict supervision, many soon practiced with minimal oversight or none at all once legislative and funding mechanisms caught up with practice realities.

Perhaps one of the clearest outcomes emerging from the creation of new practitioners during the 1960s and 1970s was the political divisiveness and overlapping of practice boundaries that occurred. These roles evolved before any type of strategic planning occurred in terms of how they were prepared, how many were needed, and what they would do. Although the motivation for new practice models was multifaceted, as seen in the previous chapters, most of these practitioners emerged in clear American entrepreneurial fashion: where the money and the opportunities were available. All were involved in the remapping of a particular social and political place already held by nursing or medicine and characterized by their concomitant power and authority. Many times the desired spaces—from the bedside to the exam room and into the home—overlapped and were contested, both between and within the medical and nursing professions themselves.

For medicine in particular, the debates that began in the 1940s over the role and authority of the general practitioner found their way to a larger forum in the 1960s.[4] The debates polarized the American Medical Association (AMA), the American Nurses' Association (ANA), specialty medical organizations, and groups of physicians and nurses in general during a time of growing demand and expectations for health services amid declining numbers of general practitioners. Clearly, the new providers, both deliberately and in an ad hoc way, took advantage of the opportunities presented by this debate and by professional medicine's inability to generate successful strategies for recruiting physicians into the vacuum of primary care. At the same time, the professions and organizations creating the new providers also failed to optimize opportunities. They neglected to effectively plan for incorporating them into the health care system at large and to establish guidelines for determining how many providers of this type were needed by physicians and the public. These difficulties generated a great deal of controversy over who controlled the new providers, the source of their authority, and when they would gain their voice to speak for themselves, all during a time when general practitioners were losing voice and authority.

In a sense, the medical profession was working at cross purposes. Its members created new assistants (e.g., physician assistants) who, on the surface, looked and worked quite similarly to general and family practitioners at a time when the professional authority of these groups was particularly vulnerable. For many reasons, physician assistants quickly gained public and medical acceptance, especially in underserved areas where the need for providers was so desperate. Family practitioners, on the other hand, found the going harder as they competed with higher-status specialties for medical student loyalty and professional influence. Over highly contested terrain, both the family practice physician and the physician assistant maneuvered for the authority to speak for themselves, perhaps like the apprentice trying to gain legitimate access to the spell book.

This chapter examines primarily the providers that physicians created—the physician assistants—and contrasts their stories with the conflict at play within medicine itself as it tried to reconcile the roles of the general and family practitioner and the specialist in health care.[5] The reconceptualization of general practice into family practice was one strategy the AMA and general practitioners used to solve some of the political dilemmas that the generalist-specialist rift created. But this strategy came too late. As general practice reframed itself yet again, physician assistants and nurse practitioners emerged on the health care scene as viable but also dangerously duplicate responses to some of the same problems.[6] The perceived similarity between them served to amplify the debates.

Translation Problems

From the mid-1960s on, numerous new categories of practitioners such as physician assistants, nurse practitioners, nurse associates, and various medical and surgical assistants emerged and contributed to the already complex dialogue surrounding health care professionals. There was indeed a translation problem as practitioners and the public alike tried to make sense of the different categories that appeared so quickly. What were the appropriate names for these providers? Should they reflect their creator—physician assistant or physician extender (somewhat akin to the nameless sorcerer's apprentice). Or should the names reflect their status as a familiar type of provider with larger responsibilities, like nurse practitioners? Were all physician extenders the same? The process of labeling was empowering to the newcomers and served notice to physicians, the normative group, that an entity existed that was important enough to have its own brand. Naming them specified relationships, setting certain groups apart while giving continuity to others. In other words, the name itself became as important as the function of the group.[7]

The labeling difficulties surrounding the new providers were part of the politics of nursing and medicine. As new programs emerged, names were independently devised to try to distinguish them from others. The MEDEX was one example contributing to the confusion.[8] The label derived from the French words "extension de medicine," meaning physician's extension, represented a new type of provider. The MEDEX was typically a discharged medical corpsman trained through a rigorous clinical preceptorship by a physician who agreed to employ him after graduation. The MEDEX seemed similar to the physician assistant, but was the MEDEX a physician assistant or a different type of provider? And what about the orthopedic assistants, who applied and removed casts and other devices and assisted in the operating room? How were they differentiated in practice, training, and authority?

The title "nurse practitioner" was confusing to many other health professionals as well. The term traditionally meant someone who practiced general duty nursing. As it began to be used in the mid-1960s, the term connoted specialized expertise. Its use generated another level of lexicon and cemented the hierarchy already emerging in nursing related to significantly different educational preparation; a diploma, associate degree, and baccalaureate degree all allowed the same entry into registered nursing, and the type of education placed the nurse in a particular status level. The technical-school-trained licensed practical nurse, an occupation that did not require high school education but was also called a nurse, created additional confusion for a public familiar with neither the terminology nor educational disarray of the nursing profession. Similarly, the term "nurse associate" as proposed by Henry Silver and the American Academy of Pediatrics in 1968 was also confusing.[9] "Associate of whom?" many critics countered. To the nurse—or to the physician, as Silver intended? The clinical nurse specialist was another type of practitioner who became part of the provider mix during this time period.[10]

Because the titles of new providers proliferated without oversight until the end of the 1970s, names were used interchangeably and created a confusing mélange of job descriptions and claims concerning outcomes. Many studies, both federally and privately funded, used the term "physician extender" to include physician assistants, nurse practitioners, nurse associates, nurse assistants, MEDEX, PRIMEX, and others.[11] Similarly, federal reports also combined the different types of providers into a general term of physician extender.[12] In a 1973 public health service manual, nurse practitioners are included under this umbrella, although they were separately defined and categorized by federal pay grade.[13] In a study funded by the regional medical program in a small New Mexico community and later published in 1971 in the *Journal of the American Medical Association*, the provider is labeled a "physician assistant." Two years later, in a book of conference papers on intermediate-level health providers, the same person in the same position is titled a "nurse practitioner."[14] In fact, many commentators, including nursing authors, tended to refer collectively to the nurse practitioner and physician assistant, although supporters and adherents of both types of programs believed they were explicit categories with specific ideologies and alliances.[15]

In addition to the confusion over labels, individual practitioners used different language to describe the process of negotiating clinical practice. Nurses discussed expanding or taking on new skills, and implicitly not "asking for permission."[16] This language implied the power to make choices or have agency to acquire a different skill or knowledge repertoire. In fact, this was an entirely active process; nurses had to agree to take on new knowledge and skills. They could have chosen to decline the opportunity, and some did, especially those who were reluctant to take on certain responsibilities that required knowledge or experience they did not have or were uncomfortable using without physician supervision.[17] Physicians, on the other hand, spoke of delegating skills to nurses and physician assistants.[18] To delegate something infers causation or volition, meaning that one group must decide, because of circumstances such as economics or politics, to deliver or assign actions, ideas, or objects to others, "entrusting of authority" to the "delegate."[19] A hierarchy is implicit—someone with power decides to allow others to do things usually reserved for those of higher rank. Agency remains with the delegating parties, while the receivers remain under their control or assume it only temporarily.

The idea of agency is important when thinking about how relationships developed in the 1960s and 1970s among nurse practitioners, physician assistants, and physicians, and how compatible practices emerged despite competing motivations and differential status. Nurse practitioners provide an interesting illustration. Both Loretta Ford and Henry Silver at the University of Colorado had similar aims of creating partnerships to provide better patient care, but they had different perceptions of the ideology behind their ideas. To Ford, the nurse practitioner was clearly a nursing model, a verification of what she was already doing and a way to expand and improve access to health care for underserved populations against the backdrop of a physician shortage.[20] In contrast, Henry Silver described the joint effort as a response to physician shortages and physicians' need to improve preventive health services for children. He even used a different name, nurse associate, in his writings on the subject.[21] From their parallel conversations emerged two models of patient care that were distinctly different in principle, agency, and name, but that met the needs of both practitioners and patients. To Ford, the nurse practitioner was a nurse practicing in an expanded role—not a new category of health professional. To this end, nurse practitioner education belonged in institutions of higher nursing education. To Silver, the nurse associate represented a new subset of medical worker who happened to have basic nursing education. Although the nurse practitioner worked collaboratively with the physician, Silver believed the physician still controlled the socialization, oversight, and most of the education, which could have occurred anywhere. From these diverse perspectives, Ford and Silver managed to work collaboratively and educate numerous nurse practitioners who went on to negotiate their own practices and formulate their own identities.[22]

The important question was whether the label mattered. Were the new providers really so different as to require different labels, classes of pay, and different legislative oversight? And how could they most effectively and efficiently fit into the health care system to improve access to primary care? Was the need for primary health care so great that there was room for all? Or, depending upon the political alliances they formed, would they disappear when the sorcerer awoke and saw them as interlopers, akin to the apprentice in the fairy tale?

The Disappearing General Practitioner

The future of practitioners such as physician assistants and nurse practitioners, no matter the ideology, depended in part on the general practitioner. After World War II, Americans were deluged with new scientific discoveries and applications of medical and surgical knowledge gained during the war. But perhaps their greatest need was for basic health care: well-baby and child care, immunizations, normal deliveries, care associated with aging, common and uncomplicated surgical procedures, and the management of the growing pool of people with chronic illnesses. Traditionally, the general practitioner provided this type of care as an all inclusive, all-knowing, familiar, and typically high-profile community figure. But the "Marcus Welby" model of the kindly family doctor was already obsolete before World War II, particularly in urban centers, although it long remained a nostalgic cultural icon.[23] In reality, most were not really generally focused. Many general practitioners limited their practice to pediatrics or adult care, although they also performed surgery and obstetrical deliveries as part of their general medical practice.

As medicine became more specialized, general practitioners and their organizations searched for ways to preserve their cultural authority. It was relatively easy to maintain their status with patients despite fleeting patient loyalty. General practitioners and their organizations had more difficulty maintaining their status within a medical system dominated by specialists, who by the 1940s were the most powerful voices in American medicine.[24] They continued to cling to power through their professional organization as AMA delegates (voting members of the AMA constituency), through state society leadership, and through the AMA committee on general practice until about the late 1950s. However, the specialists had strategic positioning on the AMA board of directors, the council on medical education, the advisory board for medical specialists (which determined the qualifications for certification), and through leadership of organizations such as the Association of American Medical Colleges (AAMC) and the Institute of Medicine (IOM). As such, they politically controlled the AMA and most organizations influencing health care policy and medical education.[25]

The general practitioners, it seems, had lost their place. What exactly was their contemporary role in health care? Were they gatekeepers and the managers of health and illness? Were they the foundation from which all other specialties emerged? Or were they an increasingly redundant form of practice? The public still demanded both medical services and personal attention from their doctor, but it was becoming more and more apparent that most people needed emotional support and reassurance, not medical services. The health care system was increasingly hostile to this type of patient and to physicians who practiced this way, and this was manifested by the structure of financial and system resources, hospital privileges, and access to useful knowledge and technology. It was increasingly difficult for general practitioners to make a living, although individual practitioners disputed the economic and workplace difficulties.[26]

To the emerging powerful specialists, general practitioners could not claim a concrete function. They did not provide an exclusive nor extraordinary scientifically based procedure or treatment, nor could they serve as gatekeepers. Since World War II, they lacked the numbers and professional power to control the flow of patients within the health care system. Perhaps most damning, many of those practicing failed to consistently upgrade their skills, and those that had were purloined by newly emerging specialties. Not only were the Marcus Welby–type general practitioners an anachronism, but their numbers in general were shrinking.

Even general practitioners themselves could not come to a consensus about their place and could not decide how to construct an identity the public understood. The lack of a clear purpose alone provided ample reason for diminishing student interest in the field, which led to a dwindling pool of active general practitioners. There were, of course, other important reasons for students' declining interest in general practice, such as the commonly acknowledged long work hours, low level of income compared to specialists, and the increasing prestige accorded the highly technical specialties. But perhaps the feuding that occurred within the general practice organizations themselves provided a significant backdrop for disinterest.

Part of the problem was that the general practitioner came to be identified by "what he lacked rather than what he had."[27] General practitioners traditionally performed deliveries and routine surgery such as appendectomies and tonsillectomies, procedures now claimed by the specialties of obstetrics, general, pediatric, and ear, nose, and throat surgery. These specialties already had well-developed residency and certification processes in place that excluded the general practitioners, and there was very little chance that modern certification boards of the 1950s and 1960s might certify general practitioners to perform these procedures. In fact, there was no certification for general practitioners, and many both in and outside of the profession pointed to this particular fact as a sign of declining authority and significance. To certify or not to certify was a great point of contention within the general practitioners community. Certification implied specialization, which was the antithesis of general practice. Many general practitioners sensed an inconsistency in creating a specialty to fight a specialty, and this philosophical dissonance reinforced the reluctant response to this course. On the other hand, specialty organizations quickly developed certification exams and staked out the functional if not cultural terrain for their roles, thereby locking out general practitioners from performing certain surgeries or using particular equipment.[28]

General practitioner training was scrutinized as well. General residencies were rare until the early 1950s when the AMA Council on Education and Hospitals formally established them, and even these programs were philosophically controversial and, at times, of questionable quality. Residency training was equated with specialization, something the general practice organizations could not reach consensus on until the late 1960s.[29] Instead, general practitioners were typically trained in rotating internships, usually one year in length, in an optional postmedical training program. In this type of curriculum the interns rotated through surgical, medical, obstetrical, orthopedic, psychiatric, laboratory, and radiology services, gaining general experience, but not expertise, in all areas.[30]

There were attempts to improve the image and quality of general practitioner residencies. The 1959 report on preparation for family practice, sponsored by the AMA with political weight from the American Academy of General Practice and the AAMC, proposed new two-year graduate medical pilot programs to create a mixed specialty practice of internal medicine and pediatrics, but excluding surgery. The programs attempted to address the functional concerns surrounding the quality, character, and declining numbers of general practitioners, but the controversy raised by the omission of surgical training kept the programs in medical limbo.[31]

These programs were attempts in the wrong direction as they did not address the basic problems of general practitioners. Without changes in the way patients accessed health care or some sort of regulatory control over the kind of provider the public first engaged, general practitioners could never gain a foothold as a necessary part of the system.[32] As the AMA appointed numerous task forces and committees to study the general practitioner issue, and as committee after committee from the early 1940s on recommended certification, designated residencies, and secure hospital privileges to entice students into the area, the solution to stop the declining numbers of general practitioners in the communities and the small general hospitals remained elusive. Residencies were created that never filled, and hospitals and communities still needed a workforce that never appeared.

General practice was becoming the waste bin of medicine. It could not claim an exclusive body of scientific knowledge or a specific procedure or technology that was clearly its domain, but consisted of a combination of knowledge provinces from other specialties considered less prestigious and important, such

as pediatrics, general surgery, and internal medicine. As such, it was a hori-
zontal specialty cutting across many others; this alone might have been better
presented by the general practitioners as a strength rather than a weakness.
Instead, there seemed to be a prevailing sense that any physician could provide
this type of care. Perhaps most damning was the fact that many patients could
take care of themselves—they could be their own general practitioners unless
they developed an acute serious illness.

Specialist physicians in general probably did not fully understand the
intricacies surrounding general practitioner practice. A lack of respect and
acknowledgment of the importance of the informal and low technological skills
general practitioners could claim as their area of expertise, such as communication and patient interaction skills, pervaded the medical profession. General
practice was caught in a quandary: many physicians believed they could provide
it without special training. After all, how difficult could it be to treat a sore throat
or an ear infection, or help a young mother with developmental child care problems? The whole area of general practice seemed to be one which was left behind,
classified as a social service more than a medical service.

These issues were complex and added to debates concerning who was the
best practitioner to care for patients at particular times. Although some specialists denigrated general practice skills, others found them valuable enough
to claim for themselves. In a bit of a reversal, the executive director of the
American College of Physicians claimed that the specialized knowledge gained
in internal medicine provided the perfect background for family practice. "A
man certified by the American Board of Internal Medicine," he noted in 1965,
"is the ideally trained man for adult family practice as currently defined."[33]
This was a reasonable and perhaps profitable declaration, considering that by
1965, 75 percent of the college's membership claimed to serve as the family
practitioner for many patients.[34] Rather than documenting the quality of the care
these specialists provided, the statement illustrates the college's perception of
the economic potential presented by public demand for basic preventive and
continuous services and their bid for this market share. Dwindling numbers of
general practitioners and public demand created the opportunity for other
physicians and other types of providers to claim this territory.

Physician Assistants: Extending the Physician's "Arms and Brains"

In 1961, Charles Hudson, a Cleveland, Ohio, physician and member of the AMA
Council on Medical Services, formally proposed creating one or two new groups
of assistants for doctors to help relieve a different kind of shortage—that of

interns and residents in the hospital. The new assistants, he believed, should be nonmedical, nonnursing personnel, without existing biases or loyalties. He used the term "extern" to describe an advanced medical assistant who handled technical procedures and had some degree of medical responsibility, and who served at the prerogative of the individual physician. This person, he suggested, might be given a bachelor of science in medicine or a bachelor of medicine.[35]

Hudson also predicted many of the issues that plagued early physician assistant programs and made the position unattractive to organized nursing but enticing to individual nurses. He recognized the growing use of more and more technical experts in the hospital (including laboratory, radiology, and venapuncture technicians) to relieve busy physicians and nurses. He also understood that the job, if not conceptualized properly, might prove unpopular because of the lack of potential for advancement. He forecasted the difficulties of an assistant interposed between medicine and nursing, the political dangers of asking nurses to take on these additional tasks, or of developing a half-nursing, half-medicine hybrid, especially without consulting the nursing leadership. Nor did he think this type of position meshed with the goals discussed in nursing education circles at that point.[36]

Using Hudson's proposal, discussions with colleagues, and personal experience, Eugene Stead, a physician in the department of medicine at Duke University, developed his idea of the physician assistant to help relieve overworked community hospital physicians.[37] Stead's physician assistant program is an informative one to examine beyond the fact that it was the first. Stead's position as a faculty member in the medical school of a southern university also opens up a broader perspective. His program was an example of academic medicine's attempts to help solve the problems of general practitioners in the community, and was one of the few medical initiatives that combined interests of the two, usually dissonant, parties.

Stead focused particularly on the plight of community physicians because they covered extensive terrain, from the patient's home to the hospital, and he heard many of their pleas for help through the university's medical education department. He particularized the type of assistant the community hospital physician needed. This career as physician assistant, he noted in 1964, would be "open to men with a high school or junior college degree, or to any person who was sponsored by a physician."[38] In his early conceptualization of the program, the students received a year of training in a physician-directed area in the medical center and one year of experience in a community hospital, and then moved on to employment positions with a sponsoring physician directly supervising the new assistant.[39] Stead believed that this "man" could be licensed with very little change in the state's medical practice act, although the AMA's tepid support of the physician assistant later on made this possibility more challenging.

The overworked community physician, usually a general practitioner, was not the only reason Stead developed the physician assistant concept. His philosophy of medical education somewhat paralleled the discussions occurring at the same time in nursing education: physicians needed to be freed from daily mundane tasks in order to practice safe, high-quality patient care. His program created "a new position in the health field . . . capable of extending the arms and brains of the physician, so he can care for more people."[40] He was also responding to a nursing shortage. He believed "there is a need for males to be committed to the health field to fill a gap between the physician and the nurse." This gap, he noted, "cannot be filled by additional training for nurses because nurses are already in very short supply."[41]

Stead had several reasons for starting the physician assistant program in 1965 as an avenue for men interested in a medical career but not in physician training. Although in the late 1950s he worked successfully with individual nurses such as Thelma Ingles, a professor of nursing at Duke University School of Nursing, to investigate an expanded role for nurses, he found working with the administrators, other faculty, and national nursing organizations—especially the National League for Nursing (NLN)—problematic and somewhat traumatic. Ingles spent a sabbatical year with Stead and his colleagues in the medical school in 1957, taking classes and attending hospital rounds with residents and physicians. She later took the clinical knowledge she gained from this experience and incorporated it into a clinical master's program she developed with Stead, with funding support from the Rockefeller Foundation, using a blend of physician and nursing instructors. The NLN declined to accredit this program in part because of the large amount of physician involvement. Stead was also keenly disappointed in the tepid response from the nursing faculty as a whole to his ideas. He wrote often of his frustration and disappointment that nursing education did not include physician instructors.[42]

In contrast, Henry Silver and Loretta Ford successfully collaborated and developed the nurse practitioner certificate program at the University of Colorado the same year Stead developed his program for men. This raises an interesting question: Why did Ford and Silver succeed in developing a workable collaborative model between nursing and medicine, but Stead did not? Part of the explanation lies in Stead's difficult experience with organized and academic nursing. Although his earlier work with Ingles convinced him nurses could safely perform traditional medical skills and understand medical knowledge, the less-than-eager reception to his ideas by the NLN and other Duke nursing faculty cemented his view of nursing as uninterested, difficult to work with, and antagonistic toward taking on the dependent role of physician assistant. He, in turn, may have been perceived by the faculty in the school as difficult to work with and transparent in his attempts to co-opt nursing education and practice, fairly popular views among some nurse educators and leaders. [43] Stead was also caught in the ongoing conflict among nursing faculty, between those like Ingles who wanted the freedom to practice nursing in the broadest sense possible, and those who were not quite ready for this type of practice. As such, personality, place, and politics played a key role in the character and success of the early programs.

Stead's difficulties went beyond his experiences with organized and academic nursing. They reflected his gendered perceptions of the kind of help his physician colleagues needed. As Ingles herself noted, "He [the physician assistant] is to the physician what the extremely capable secretary is to the top level executive."[44] In Ingles's highly gendered analogy the traditional female nurse would have been an apt fit, but it may have been too far a stretch for Stead to imagine women as physician assistants as he originally conceived the idea, out on rural roads late at night or putting in the same hours as the solo general practitioner. He clearly envisioned an assistant who kept the same schedule but did not command the same salary as the physician who employed him.

Stead worked well with individual nurses, as he and Ingles developed a fairly innovative clinical nurse master's program model. He also utilized nurses as instructors in the early physician assistant program, and included content common to nurse training programs in the curriculum. He credited a nurse, Kathleen G. Andreoli, as one of the reasons for the program's success.[45] But Stead firmly believed that men rather than women made better candidates for the physician assistant program, and there were few men in the nursing profession. Military corpsmen, one group of men he targeted early on, came ready trained with more advanced technical skills they had been applying in military hospitals and in battle situations in Vietnam. They were also acculturated to a strict hierarchical military chain of command and would be more comfortable in the assistant role Stead envisioned for them. "These men," Stead wrote to a Cleveland Clinic administrator, "work effectively for doctors. They do not work well with nurses, and they have the ability to do more than the nurse usually does."[46] As one patient explained in a letter to Stead: "As a hemodialysis patient . . . with an artificial kidney at home, I've been assisted by several military corpsmen moon-lighting their jobs at Walter Reed. I have found them to be uniformly dedicated, conscientious, and entirely professional. They are highly skilled in the machines and their use, more so actually than the MDs. . . . Moreover, they recognize clearly the line to be drawn between their area of competence and that of the fully qualified doctor."[47]

Stead was frustrated by the nursing shortage and the problems it created for physicians, and he looked to a new layer of health professionals to manage the daily work of medical care. Nurses were in such short supply, Stead believed, that "they have no time for learning."[48] Stead later realized that the community clinic and hospital were not the only places physicians needed additional help. The Duke University hospital also needed a worker to free up interns and residents for the important learning they needed, and nurses were in too short supply to provide that help. Calling the present arrangement in hospitals "somewhat chaotic," Stead envisioned a worker to serve as a consistent and stable assistant to physicians and remain with them long after interns and residents had rotated to new services, or trained nurses had left the labor market for marriage and family issues. The physician assistant, Stead believed, "could keep the shop in order so that the less career-dedicated persons, and people working more transiently in the health field, could feed in and out more easily. He would give stability to an area previously characterized by turnover."[49]

Even if nurses could be of assistance, Stead clearly saw them from a traditional gender, class, and race-specific perspective. They were, in his eyes, white, middle-class, temporary workers, and therefore their potential in the physician assistant role was limited. White nurses, in particular, tended to leave the labor force shortly after their training when they married or moved on to other professions or other workplaces.[50] The idea that nursing was a transient workforce was a fairly common perception even within the nursing profession itself. As Dorothy J. Novello, head of the Pennsylvania State Board of Nursing, noted, "the major problem is not what can we do to get more girls into nursing, but what can we do to keep the girls in nursing once we have them there. . . . We are losing them to other professions and their homes."[51]

Despite Stead's experience with career-oriented nurses such as Andreoli and Ingles, he still believed the new professionals would predominantly be male. "I do not believe that enough women in our society who wish to make a career in the health field their primary goal can be identified," he explained. "Most women still want home as the primary career and work in the health field as a secondary career."[52] Stead's views were particular to his program, as most others admitted women from the start who were both nurses and nonnurses. But his program was the most public one, setting the standards and the image for physician assistant programs for years. His graduates appeared on the pages of *Look* in 1966, one of the most popular magazines at the time.[53]

Stead's preference for men for the physician assistant program drew comments from educators and leaders who challenged his assumptions about nursing. Early on, Ruth B. Freeman, a professor in the Johns Hopkins University School of Hygiene and Public Health, noted that she was "very interested in knowing why you feel the physicians' assistant should be male. I can see certain advantages in terms of extending the work life of the individual recruited inasmuch as women do tend to take considerable time out for childbearing and rearing. However, it does conflict with your comment that this might be an upward channel for nurses."[54] She went on to remind Stead of a growing sentiment among practicing nurses, noting that those "who leave nursing and particularly hospital nursing do so because they do not feel free to do the things which they have been prepared to do. If they were, in fact, allowed to use their judgment to a greater extent and to share more fully in the care of the patient, I think many who leave 'for family reasons' would be right on the job."[55] Freeman understood the possible attraction and opportunities this position held for nurses, and saw expanded roles as a way to keep women in nursing rather than a reason for them to move out of nursing. If practicing nurses were given greater decision-making authority to reflect the skills and knowledge they already had, they might be able to help physicians, create a more stable workplace, and gain greater job satisfaction.

Stead replied to Freeman a week later, explaining that at that time his ideas were not firmly planted and based on a very limited series of pilot observations. But he did not distance himself from his earlier statements. He wrote, "I think the problem in nursing lies in the fact that we have not produced many professional nurses, nor do we seem likely to do so in the future. I would like to leave them an unobstruct[ed] line of development, but I would not like to be paralyzed by their inability to reproduce their kind in large quantities."[56] If nurses were available, and it seems there were available nurses, as Ingles exemplified, Stead preferred those who chose their profession as their primary interest, who were unencumbered by family and home responsibilities. These were the professional nurses Stead might consider for physician assistant training. And in a way, this reflected less a bias toward nurses (which he admitted) than a view of women that was based on particular assumptions layered by class, gender, and race. During this time, the proportion of women in the medical profession slowly grew. The influx of women interns and residents, and their particular needs for release time for childbearing and rearing, or perhaps certain schedule adjustments, when they felt empowered to ask for them, may have added to the chaos in community hospitals fed by increasing patient loads, and by physician and nursing shortages.[57] Medicine, traditionally white, upper-middle class, male-dominated, was not accustomed to providing accommodations.

Stead's idea for a new practitioner was in fact a formalization of the efforts that entrepreneurial and desperate physicians undertook for years: training assistants to help them in their busy offices and to provide coverage when they had to travel or were ill. Many physicians personally trained individual nurses, usually those working in their offices. But Stead's initial approach, and one taken by many other physicians, looked to individuals without any previous medical experience or those who were military medical corpsmen, and tailored their training to the particular physician's practice. Stead's program also provided a basic level of standardized education and expanded the idea to large numbers of overworked physicians.

One well-known example of a traditional assistant, probably because he was the focus of a published account in 1967, was medic Buddy Treadwell, who worked with physician Amos Johnson in his practice in Garland, North Carolina. Johnson was a powerful person in both his community and in the general practice profession. He earned profound patient loyalty, served as president of the American Academy of General Practice, was an active member of national AMA committees, and president of the North Carolina Medical Association. Johnson personally trained Treadwell and employed him for more than twenty-five years in his busy solo practice, probably starting in the early 1940s. This relationship worked for Johnson. As president of the academy and as an active board and committee member, he frequently traveled around the country, and Treadwell served as his backup in his absence. According to Johnson, Treadwell exercised medical judgment only when the doctor was in town. When the doctor was away, Treadwell handled problems by protocol.[58]

The common threads between traditional assistants such as Treadwell and Stead's more formally trained physician assistants were the individualistic and very local character of training, high patient acceptance, a dependent relationship with the physician, and attempts by physician employers to keep their assistants below the radar of local medical boards and licensing organizations that were responsible for assuring the basic qualifications of medical professionals. Using assistants in this way, no matter who they were or how they were trained, was illegal in all states as licensure boards defined this type of work as practicing medicine without a license.

The reluctance of medical boards was only one of the larger issues confronting Stead's ideas. As Hudson earlier predicted, the interjection of a middleman between the nurse and the physician, especially when done without consultation with the nurse leadership, proved incendiary. Not only would this new intermediary break the traditional line of communication between them, but it could, as one nursing leader wrote, lead to increased turnover and decreased recruitment of nurses. "There are already nurses who leave the profession," she noted, " . . . because the job roles and functions are too contained to allow creative nursing care. . . . Other nurses leave because there are too few ways to increase responsibility and salary in hospitals."[59] Nursing leaders were caught in a contradiction—many believed nurses could easily fill this role, but if they did, they lost these nurses from the bedside where the critical need existed. What the leaders really wanted was the ability to participate in the planning and decision making surrounding the physician assistant, a role that Stead was not prepared to offer or discuss. Nursing leaders saw Stead's new provider as more than a doctor's assistant, as a dangerous challenge to nursing's status in the health care environment. If a role of this sort was to be developed, nurses wanted to create it themselves in a way that was professionally substantive and advantageous.

The ANA and the Physician Assistant

The ANA was suspicious from the beginning about the physician assistant role, and not only those produced by the Duke program. Although by the late 1960s the ANA and AMA were immersed in a greater degree of dialogue at the conference and committee level, moves by both organizations generated suspicion. The ANA became even more defensive in 1970, when the AMA called for the development of a hospital nursing service as part of a dependent physician-led team, rather than the complementary, independent one (nursing supervised by nurses) existing in most hospitals. Part of the strategy was to have nurses provide more patient care services approved and supervised by physicians, although it is difficult to imagine how the AMA believed busy physicians might accomplish the additional work of team management.[60]

Walter Bornemeier, president of the AMA (1970–71), amplified the emotional temperature of the debate when he extended an invitation to the "285,000 inactive registered nurses . . . to come back into medicine with higher pay and status as that of a doctor's assistant."[61] Ernest B. Howard, executive director of the AMA, forecasted Bornemeier's offer earlier that year in an address to the Boston University School of Medicine, when he proposed recruiting 100,000 nurses to be trained as physician assistants.[62] Although both men probably thought they were giving nurses some special authority or gift, like Prometheus receiving fire from the gods, the ANA saw it as yet another attempt by medicine to control nursing. Dorothy Cornelius, then ANA president, replied publicly via the *American Journal of Nursing*. She "deplored the unilateral action by the AMA," noting that "it was not the prerogative of one profession to speak for another."[63]

But, as nursing leaders argued for a larger independent role for nurses rather than the dependent physician assistant they saw as an interloper between themselves and the physician, practicing nurses in clinics and at the bedside seemed to have settled into a more flexible reconciliation. In a 1971 study conducted by Duke University, nurses who had contact with university-trained physician assistants were asked to comment on their relationships with them and their work. Almost all of the comments were positive, and many illuminated the disconnect between the nursing leadership's position and that of practicing nurses. One nurse illustrated that both the physician and the nurse considered basic screening tasks and routine physical exams (both tasks nurse practitioners and physician assistants in general were taking on) to be onerous work: "He [the physician assistant] takes over many of the time consuming chores of both the physician and myself—i.e. emergency care of injuries—dressings and treatments I used to do—screening patients—doing physical exams. I feel that our patients get more personal attention since his arrival."[64] Another nurse exemplified the work she believed was important: "As we do have not a receptionist his [the physician assistant's] presence leaves me free to take care of the paper work and telephones—a job that used to get slighted."[65] Several of the comments spoke to the importance of personality in developing working relationships. "Our physician assistant is not only a well trained professional person, he is an exceptionally brilliant, well adjusted co-worker and a friend," one nurse wrote.[66] All in all, the nurses generally agreed the physician assistant was a welcome addition to the health care team.

Dorothy Mereness, dean of the School of Nursing at the University of Pennsylvania, also believed the physician assistant (although she interchanges the physician assistant and nurse practitioner) was a reasonable option that might help keep nurses in the profession. The ANA needed to keep communication channels open with the AMA so that nurses could take advantage of the new roles and participate in their development. "It is distressing," she noted, "when one realizes that the professional nursing organization had not already developed a position on this issue before the AMA issued its statement [on training nurses as physician assistants]. . . . If members of organized nursing continue to view with alarm this development, they may be relegated to the role of observer and lose an opportunity to shape the destiny of the profession."[67] The NLN established an ad hoc committee to study the physician assistant role in 1969 and prepared a report in April of that year, more than four years after Duke began its program. But they did not officially share the report with the ANA, with which it was engaged in a fierce battle for control of nursing education program accreditation. The political conflict between the ANA and the NLN prevented a broader and more organized response to the AMA, and directed their attention away from what was happening at the level of the practicing nurse.

To the ANA, this was yet another episode of the AMA missing an opportunity to develop a partnership that could facilitate better patient care and make nurses colleagues rather than dependent associates. Instead, the AMA proposed a traditional model built on physician supervision of nursing practice. Unlike the individual liberal-minded medical practitioners who worked closely with early nurse practitioners, Bornemeier and the AMA leadership were more culturally bound by their medical identity and unable to perceive nurses as anything more than physicians' helpers, no matter how much authority and decision making nurses took on, and many practicing nurses shared his belief. Ultimately, the ANA did not trust their constituency to recognize, as it did, the AMA's attempt to gather nurses under its jurisdiction. The AMA proposal was enticing to many practicing nurses, but as the ANA argued, it also had the potential to subsume them, creating even stronger dependent relationships in an assistant role. It was, as ANA president Hildegard Peplau noted during a board discussion, "an issue of control," perhaps, inadvertently explicating the point of contention for both organizations.[68]

The ANA clearly could not control all nurses, and in 1973 the National Board of Medical Examiners (NBME), which the AMA and various medical specialty organizations used to certify practitioners, invited nurses to participate in the physician's assistant certification exam. In fact, certification across all types of occupations was already becoming a powerful cultural tool that had salience in the marketplace.[69] At this time no nurse practitioner certification existed although the ANA and the American Academy of Pediatrics were developing one for pediatric nurse practitioners. Those working in expanded roles wanted and needed a way to legitimize their practice to their physician colleagues, a stand the ANA acutely understood but could not accept. Nurses practicing in expanded roles who passed this exam earned the credentials to practice as physician assistants, demonstrating a particular level of proficiency for a limited medical skill set, and became certified to practice dependently with a physician. The NBME invitation to nurse practitioners was attractive to them during a most uncertain period of role definition for expanded practice.

Horrified by the intrusion on its professional turf, the ANA quickly issued a reply to the NBME through the memo, "Nurses, in the Extended Role, Are Not Physician's Assistant." In it the ANA contrasted nurse practitioner strengths (including the state-approved process of evaluating basic nursing education, established state licensure, and the legal responsibility and authority for their own practice) with the nascent AMA action to accredit physician assistant programs, the lack of physician assistant licensure, and the dependent practice of physician assistants. The ANA reminded nurses that the certifying exam was not "a legal sanction to practice."[70] In other words, the ANA countered, nurses who passed the physician assistant exam and practiced as such lost their authority as practicing nurses. The physician assistant was not a nursing role, although the ANA could not adequately convince some nurses of the difference.

Defining Physician Assistants and the Name Game

The ANA was not alone in its difficulty with the physician assistant concept. The AMA, and in particular the powerful council on health manpower, was not altogether comfortable with the physician assistant, either. This council, according to AMA policy, was required to agree upon a definition, description, and need for the role before education standards could be developed, and it was taking its time deliberating.[71] The reticence stemmed in part from an informal moratorium in 1971 on the licensure of new health personnel.[72] So many overlapping and redundant types of new providers emerged during the late 1960s and 1970s that many organizations wanted more rigid categorization to allay confusion. The council believed there was really no reason to rush development of educational guidelines for a role that could not achieve licensure, albeit temporarily, although all organizations wanted to be positioned to their own advantage when the moratorium lifted.

Another reason may have been the ambivalence of the council members, and the AMA organization in general, to the idea of the physician assistant. Stead complained to the AMA in 1970 about a report in the *Journal of the American Medical Association* that praised the progress of the development of the physician assistant role. "Your authors have no sense of urgency," he argued. "They don't know that in spite of all the talk, very few persons [physician assistants] are being educated."[73] In his letter Stead emphasized the growing urgency for physician assistant services. In North Carolina, "we have systems that are collapsing. One of our physician assistant students is taking one of his clinical rotations with a doctor near the coast. The nearest doctor is thirty-four miles away. The preceptor has had an acute myocardial infarction. The doctor thirty-four miles away urges us to leave the physician assistant student there and supervise him by telephone. . . . We cannot even find a graduate physician assistant to send, they are too few and too much in demand."[74]

Overoptimistic reports were dangerous, Stead believed, because they could not generate the public pressure needed to galvanize the AMA and government and private funding agencies into action to support physician assistant programs. Stead wanted the AMA to rapidly develop well-defined educational and accreditation standards for physician assistant programs, similar to those devised for schools of medicine by the AAMC. He understood that in order for the physician assistant concept to succeed, the programs had to develop a consistent level of quality because their graduates were certain to be highly scrutinized by their physician employers, perhaps even more so than a newly trained physician. Stead could guarantee the quality of his own graduates, but not those from other programs. He wanted the programs to fall into some sort of defined order before they reverted back to the highly individualized traditional model of each physician training his own assistant.

Stead's concerns about proliferation were not unfounded. Both nurse practitioner and physician assistant programs grew fairly rapidly and without consistent guidelines. By 1970 the DHEW listed 67 programs for physician support personnel (both nurse practitioner and physician assistant), and in the next year, 112. They operated in at least twenty-five states, and all were different in name and in requirements for admission. The length of training also fit the highly individual model and ranged from fourteen weeks to five years. The programs were emerging in all sorts of places, such as medical schools, medical centers, two- and four-year colleges, clinics, and public and private hospitals.[75]

MEDEX, first developed by Richard A. Smith at the University of Washington in 1969, was a prominent example of the new physician assistant programs emerging during this time. Smith, a Howard University–trained physician, had a long history of national and international medical service.[76] Smith also worked in the surgeon general's office in the mid-1960s, and became familiar with the reentry difficulties military corpsmen experienced as they returned to civilian life after working independently on military bases or on Vietnam battlefields. Carl Toney, an army medic in Vietnam, was one example. Toney came home from the war and went back to his old job as a general medical orderly at Columbia Presbyterian Hospital in New York City. He felt quite frustrated in this job after his dynamic war experiences, and began a long period of short-term medical positions before he heard about physician assistant programs and the value they placed on his military experience. Although he did not become a MEDEX (he graduated from Duke's physician assistant course), his story is fairly typical of the men who entered these programs.[77]

The MEDEX program was specifically designed to place students into underserved areas before they graduated and included an innovative matching strategy pairing students with practicing physicians who urgently needed help. Most of the physician sponsors were solo practitioners who could not afford or were unable to attract additional physicians to join their practices, and worked in small communities in Washington, Alaska, Montana, Idaho, and Oregon. Sponsors accepted personal and financial responsibility for teaching and utilizing the MEDEX within their own practice, in essence creating the role and providing socialization as the student learned to master a particular skill set. There was no formal hospital-based experience unless the particular physician sponsor held hospital privileges and the training the student received was individualized to a particular practice.

The funding sources for these programs were quite diverse and fragmented, with little communication or standardization between agencies. Some of the earlier physician assistant programs obtained funds from private sources and government agencies. Smith's program received federal funding in 1969 from the Health Service and Mental Health Administration (HSMHA) as a demonstration project.[78] Other funding agencies within HSMHA took responsibility for physician assistant programs supported by the regional medical programs and the Indian health service. Still other funding came from the bureau of health manpower education, the NIH, the office of education, the office of economic opportunity, and the manpower administration of the Department of Labor.[79] More centralized federal funding for physician assistant programs came with the 1971 Comprehensive Health Manpower Training Act.

The MEDEX programs, similar to the Duke program, were highly successful. After five years, nine programs existed and several more were in development.[80] Unlike Stead's program, the MEDEX programs admitted women. Although few entered early on, by 1978 24 percent of the students were women, and 18 percent of this group were registered nurses.[81] At this early point both the MEDEX and the physician assistant exhibited better records of working in underserved rural areas with individual physicians than nurse practitioners, and also had better recruitment results for blacks and for practices in traditionally black areas than nursing in general.[82] The MEDEX programs were also more successful than the physician assistant programs in general in meeting the needs of underserved rural and urban communities. About 60 percent of graduates of one particular MEDEX program worked in communities of 50,000 people or less, compared with 48 percent of all physician assistants.[83] Other studies, including one from the congressional budget office, confirmed that MEDEX graduates were more likely than physician assistants, nurse practitioners, and physicians to work in communities of this size or smaller. MEDEX graduates also tended to work in primary care and family practices, probably due to the placement system used by the programs.[84]

Despite the success and acceptance of certain signature programs, the AMA continued to move slowly, and perhaps deliberately so, on physician assistant standards and education. They did, however, adopt guidelines for developing new occupations in 1969 and, in 1970, a definition of the physician assistant. But the AMA could not agree on what this new person would do or what they would be called.[85] Physicians debated the label and, indirectly, its symbolic implications, to a greater extent than other groups because they had the most to gain or lose. These new providers, physicians believed, could never be true associates because they lacked their knowledge and professional standing. They also assumed physician assistants could only provide substandard care and worried that patients might not have the ability to distinguish the important subtleties between the different levels of services. The right title helped to make the differentiation clearer.

Stead believed the label "associate" should not be problematic. He acknowledged that "names in the health professions . . . do get us in trouble. People look on a physician with an MD as a kind of uniform product, when actually you know MDs are no longer interchangeable."[86] Nurses, he added, "are even in worse trouble. . . . If you use the word 'nurse' it gives a fairly uniform picture to the physician and to many consumers of health care. But, interestingly enough, this picture is quite different from the picture the word 'nurse' means to the nursing educator."[87] And, indeed, all kinds of titles, most of them referring to famous historical figures in medicine, were examined at the time, including "Osler," "Flexner," and "Pinel," among many others.[88] Physicians at the AMA council and committee level strongly agreed the label mattered, going as far as submitting a recommendation to the house of delegates in 1971 that the term "associate" could be used only to refer to another physician.[89]

Clearly the differentiation was important to the AMA, illustrating an undercurrent of discomfort with the physician assistant role. But, as the AMA debated, the Duke program already called itself a "physician associate" program and started a registry with the same title in 1971. Graduates began the American Academy of Physicians' Associates and issued a journal, *The Physician's Associate*.[90] Many other programs changed their names to "physician associate" just as the AMA solidified its opposition to the term. As D. Robert Howard, director of the Duke physician's associate program in 1971, noted, "The timing of their [AMA] move lends itself to no other interpretation than one of reaction, rather than one of action. In any event, it is certainly a good example of locking the barn after the horses have gone."[91]

"Analysis Paralysis" and Specialization

Stead was impatient with the AMA, and when Walter Bornemeier, the AMA president, suggested that Stead and his colleagues formulate the educational standards themselves based on the program at Duke, they quickly agreed.[92] Bornemeier then forwarded the standards to C. H. William Ruhe, secretary of the Council on Medical Education, possibly to stimulate some action by the committee. But Ruhe took offense to the tone of the letter that accompanied Stead's proposal, especially "your comment that 'the council must appreciate this and not drag its feet indefinitely.' This implication is disturbing and unwarranted. To put it bluntly, this is simply untrue."[93]

The council held responsibility for standards, but not for defining the occupation. Thus Stead's proposal was premature because the responsible council (health manpower) had not yet defined the specific role, nor had it determined if the role was needed or should be reproduced even as programs continued to proliferate. The Council on Health Manpower was, indeed, working on this question and approached the issue in step with medical specialization: it requested each specialty organization, rather than each type of physician assistant program, to define the particular types of assistants it needed. Over the last two years, many specialty organizations surveyed their membership to document the need for this new type of assistant on their team and to develop detailed job descriptions. By 1971, the American Academy of Orthopedic Surgeons and the American Urological Association already completed the process and were invited to develop, in conjunction with the Council on Medical Education, criteria for accreditation of educational programs for assistants.[94]

By treating the physician assistant as an appendage to specialties, the Council on Health Manpower assured inconsistency in the role. The functional approach—focusing on specific bodies of knowledge and skills rather than a paradigmatic shift in the health care system—was similar to the way the AMA responded to the concurrent dilemma of general and family practice. Physician assistant education paralleled medical education, with specialization politically and culturally overtaking the generalist. This was not Stead's original intent. His program was a local response and institutionally based rather than organization affiliated. Stead developed standards for the AMA that were out of sync with the way it conceptualized the physician assistant, and he found himself and his program mired in organizational politics.[95]

Stead accepted none of the cautionary explanations offered by Ruhe and deplored the AMA's "analysis paralysis."[96] He had direct evidence of the critical need local physicians had for physician assistants, and the situation seemed to be worsening, as requests for his students and his graduates poured in. Some progress, of course, had been made, and by March 1971 the Veterans Administration counted fifty-four graduates of physician assistant programs of all types, with at least 350 students enrolled in various stages of training. The programs were reporting up to 150 applications per week. About a quarter of the graduates worked in small towns or small cities, primarily in the northeastern part of the country. The remaining graduates worked in urban, industrial, prison, or group clinics such as Kaiser Permanante.[97] Of the thirty-six Duke graduates listed in the Veterans Administration's report in 1971, about half worked in a university clinic, primarily at Duke. Thus Duke not only educated but also hired its own graduates, thus somewhat limiting the program's impact in rural areas.

Despite this, Stead was still alarmed by the AMA's failure to progress on the accreditation front because there were no standards to assure the quality of the new programs. His response to Ruhe captured his frustration in one short sentence: "If the AMA were doing anything, you could say it in less than three pages of single-spaced type."[98] In a companion letter to Bornemeier, Stead replied, "Enclosed is a typical AMA staff letter and my reply. There is nothing in this communication which makes me optimistic."[99]

In contrast to Stead's impatience and discontent, Ruhe believed that the committee was not intentionally slow or recalcitrant but genuinely concerned that they "should not plunge ahead and do something inappropriate which will only lead to grief later on."[100] In essence, Ruhe believed the AMA was right to try to plan for and control the development of all new types of health providers emerging during this time. And his position made sense as the ad hoc, rapid proliferation and unevenness of physician assistant programs illustrated. But he also used language that indicated he believed the physician assistant was a temporary solution to manpower shortages. "I can think of nothing which would be more disastrous," he noted, "than to set about the production of large numbers of persons to perform certain tasks and then to learn later on that there was no market for their services."[101]

Ruhe was in a unique position to be deliberate. He was deeply involved in the efforts by the American Academy of General Practice and the AMA section on general practice to develop a family practice specialty board, and served as an ex officio member of the liaison committee for specialty boards, where the crux of these discussions took place. Fully aware of the newly approved family medicine board in 1969, Ruhe may have believed that this was finally a viable solution to stop the declining number of practitioners in this field. If so, physician assistants might not be needed and were thus a temporary solution to a problem already solved by the medical profession.

The AMA's stand on the physician assistant, and accreditation in particular, changed abruptly with the prospect of large-scale targeted federal funding for physician assistant education through the 1971 Comprehensive Manpower Training Act. To obtain funds through this mechanism, programs were required to generate and apply specific education standards.[102] The AMA quickly adopted new guidelines for physician assistant program accreditation around the time of Stead's frantic appeal and the beginning of federal largesse.[103] By 1972, the AMA announced the first programs receiving accreditation. They were based in institutions of various types—hospitals, academic medical centers, and medical schools—and three of the four were in the South.[104]

As federal money became more available, physician assistants subspecialized, probably for some of the same reasons driving physicians and nurse practitioners to do the same—the salaries and the prestige were higher, and the supervision needed by physician assistants and nurse practitioners to practice in many states could be found in these areas.[105] Except for the MEDEX graduates, physician assistants began to gravitate toward tertiary care institutions, specialty groups, hospitals, and industry clinics, and not necessarily high-need rural or generalist areas. Yet demand for training in family practice or primary care remained high and represented the largest practice area even into the late 1990s in some states such as California.[106] In 1974, almost 44 percent of physician assistants worked in family practice with only about 7 percent in the surgical subspecialties. By 1993, the national distribution mirrored medical specialization in general: surgical subspecialties represented the second largest type of physician assistant practice (21 percent), with about 35 percent of physician assistants still engaged in family practice.[107]

Gaining Access to the Spell Book

Physician assistants were influenced by more than economics and status. They were shaped by practice realities, to be sure, but they also mapped their professional identity to that of the physician, working closely with their medical sponsors. This arrangement provided a certain knowledge and skill level. But it also provided socialization, rhetoric, and acceptance into a practice model built on a decaying but still formative tradition of the old family doctor, suggesting a measure of the relationship between "performance and identity."[108]

Although much was made by the early founders of the physician assistant's dependent identity, this was somewhat of a smokescreen almost from the beginning, as a means to an end and as a negotiating point. It soon became quite clear that physician assistants had to use some level of independent clinical judgment to provide the kind of services physicians and patients needed. Dependency was logically incompatible with the need to "do something," and to assist the physician. Not surprisingly, physician assistants became quite excellent practitioners, creating an identity and voice all their own from the perspective of their numbers and organizations. Many researchers in the 1970s and 1980s tried to show differences between the various types of emerging providers (nurse practitioners, physician assistants, MEDEX) and physicians, typically in primary care or in particular types of clinical settings with defined populations. But study after study showed little or no difference in quality of care.[109]

Perhaps because of their proficiency and their relationships with physicians, physician assistants ran into boundary issues with other professions, particularly in the legislative area. Early on, Stead predicted physician assistants would have a fairly easy march through the state practice act process. But the path was more difficult as both the boards of nursing, and in some places the boards controlling podiatry and pharmacy, took issue with physician assistant licensure attempts. In 1977, podiatry organizations in Pennsylvania complained to the state Board of Medical Examiners and Licensure that physician assistants were taking over traditional podiatry functions.[110] Nursing boards were sometimes particularly contentious. In many states, nurse practice acts prohibited nurses from taking orders from the physician assistant. If nurses could not legally do this, physicians had to be present, somewhat negating the assistant function so important to them.

Overall, the physician assistant gained access to the spell book, if indeed the spell book can be defined as the metaphoric tool encompassing not only the skills and knowledge to care for a particularly defined population group, but also providing the language, rhetoric, and image needed to gain legitimacy in the medical system. The spell book provided access to both the marketplace and a cultural space that superseded clinical authority at the bedside. Physician assistants succeeded because the public and the medical profession needed them, and because they astutely developed a clinical identity both supported by and differentiated from their physician creators. The physician assistants did this in a more effective way than physicians themselves, as the family practice specialty still failed to gain broad medical student interest and physician popularity, even with the approval of the American Board of Family Practice. Of course, the numbers of family practitioners grew rapidly at first after the specialty board came into existence, but the growth generally slowed and never reached the proportions envisioned by the AMA. Not so the growth of physician assistants, which doubled in number from 1974 to 1993.[111] In fact, family practitioners began to see the physician assistant as a threat. Even though the board of directors of the American Academy of Family Physicians officially supported the physician assistant in 1974, not all its members were as embracing. An Oklahoma delegate keenly stated his position when he asked his colleagues, "Do you want to endorse this monster, the physician's assistant."[112]

It may be that the physician assistants learned how to access and appreciate different publics—the poor, rural, underserved populations—while medical organizations focused inward, seeing themselves as their public. General practitioners and eventually family practitioners kept regenerating themselves and their spaces, incorporating new technology and procedures, and battling other specialties such as pediatrics and internal medicine to keep themselves culturally relevant and financially viable.[113] In any case, medicine across the board continued its specialization and segmentation, providing both the entry and the foundation for new practitioners such as physician assistants—the ultimate regeneration of medical practice—to gain access to the spell book.

Chapter 5

The AMA and ANA under Siege

As individual practitioners and nurse educators reshaped practice, public and private interests at the national level focused on a different sort of practice politics for the right to define the kind of practitioner they believed Americans wanted and needed. By the end of the 1960s, issues surrounding clinical practice for both the American Nurses Association (ANA) and American Medical Association (AMA) became more a matter of crowd control than the altruistic notion of linking disciplinary knowledge with social concerns as new providers and professional organizations maneuvered for recognition and power. Nurse practitioners and other emerging types of providers and the specialty organizations supporting them provided the underpinning, both directly and tangentially, to politically charged issues that ran the gamut from national health insurance to access to care.

Both the AMA and the ANA were private special interest groups with responsibilities to both the public and to their dues-paying constituents. The organizations, active in health care causes across multiple levels from their inception, maintained their dual public outlook of service and altruism mixed with a fair dose of self-interest. Enormous political, social, and economic power was embedded in these organizations, and they were, by nature, both "inward and outward looking."[1] Both the ANA and the AMA had power over their members to some extent—the AMA in terms of its ability through the state medical societies to censure members and control licensure (through the incestuous and mostly unacknowledged relationship of the state societies and the state licensure boards), and the ANA through its support of the state associations and their general welfare programs. Both groups controlled matters affecting the larger community, such as entry into practice and workplace standards, and thus indirectly, the practice domain. They also, along with other organizations such as the American Hospital Association, influenced national health care legislation and funding for professional education to a very large extent. Their power shaped clinical practice in a way that was economically rewarding and socially influential for their membership, and beneficial to the community at large.[2]

These private organizations thrashed out public and private health policy issues, both among themselves and others, all the while manufacturing and selling popular opinion, with variable success, to support their stands on the new health providers.[3] Unfortunately, these negotiations sometimes lacked any sort of strategic alliance or planning that might have fueled a policy engine to improve access to care for the growing pool of uninsured citizens, or to stem escalating health care costs. These issues, of course, were at the rhetorical forefront of each organization, but no consensus existed between the two organizations on how to turn the rhetoric into reality without losing authority and economic power.

The American Nurses Association and Nurse Practitioners

At best, the ANA was ambivalent about nurse practitioners during much of the last half of the twentieth century. Certainly, the organization tried to protect and maintain the role as part of the nursing profession. There are numerous examples during this time period of the ANA and its representatives working with various medical specialty groups and federal agencies to illustrate the importance of this type of nursing care provider (chapter 7). The ANA supported nurse practitioners as strategies to respond to increased demand in the health care system for primary care practitioners. But, the ANA was unable to create a space in the organization that met the educational and affiliation needs of this growing group of nurses.[4] This ambivalence stemmed from its mission to serve the public, but also from a prolonged inability to agree on a philosophic position for practicing nurses with advanced education and those in expanded roles. Where exactly did these nurses fit, and what would they do? Until the mid-1980s, most of the ANA's general population were less educated than nurse practitioners and were more concerned with workplace issues such as salaries and job security than professional advancement. How would recognizing these specialized, diverse, and independent nurses reflect upon the larger, less-educated ANA constituency?

There was, however, something more transcendent about the ANA's indecisive stand on specialization. Nursing had a tradition of denying the presence of "differentiation" or hierarchy, except through the paths of education or leadership.[5] The idea of sameness for the generalist nurse was a historically contingent and highly useful concept, at least until the 1950s. Cyclical shortages, education ideologies, and command structures demanded that colloquially, "a nurse is a nurse is a nurse" in both spirit and concrete economic rewards. This consistency, more in theory than reality, implied both students and graduates were functionally interchangeable; that is, they could be placed, rotated, or moved according to institutional needs without hiring additional workers. Specialization, either through expertise, focus, or advanced education, implied that someone else was "nonspecial," practicing at a lower level and perhaps even earning less money.[6] For the ANA to embrace specialization, which included the notion of expert and expanded practice, the idea of sameness had to be demystified and its constituency made comfortable with an inherent sense of collective inequity.

In fact, multiple layers of specialization were already embedded in the profession. Nurses with advanced education typically served as public health nurses, educators, and administrators. After World War II, as the complexity of patient care increased, more and more nurses searched for specialized and advanced clinical education not provided in their basic programs. This movement was spearheaded in part by nurses working in areas such as psychiatry and public health, and, later, in dialysis and critical care.[7] But, at the time of a major reorganization of nursing professional organizations in 1952 that set the foundation for how the ANA responded to nurse practitioners, over 40 percent of nurses practiced as private duty nurses, and most of them were diploma trained.[8] The most widely subscribed nursing journal was the *Trained Nurse*. This journal approached nursing from a traditional sense of duty and devotion to the patient and resisted efforts to differentiate nurses by their educational status.[9]

Organization leaders such as Hildegard Peplau (who was an ANA president and executive director) strongly believed in advanced education and expert clinical practice for nurses, but they were small voices in an enormous and inflexible organization based on a grassroots house-of-delegates structure similar to that of the AMA. Until the mid-1970s, Peplau and her primarily academic colleagues could convince neither their fellow board members nor the larger organizational delegate structure, to agree on where these nurses might practice, or how they might be prepared.[10] And by then, many nurses were finding educational energy and support from physician organizations or on their own, leaving the ANA to fight hard and long to try to regain their loyalty and trust over the next few decades.

While the organization grappled with basic and graduate education issues, clinical practice at the grassroots level rapidly changed. Many of the ANA leaders themselves responded and developed clinical programs at their own institutions, as Peplau did in 1964, preparing clinical specialists through a federally funded graduate program in psychiatric nursing at Rutgers University. But in general, the organization failed to keep pace with the changes and lacked a language, mechanism, and vision to embrace the possibilities advanced clinical practice offered. The organization spent money and time on workplace and economic security issues, on problems and strategies that bolstered their membership numbers, and on cooperation with the state nursing associations, but left clinical concerns adrift. Clinical practice did not become the highest priority issue at the ANA until 1968, when it finally usurped economics and general welfare.[11]

In fact, the ANA's uncertainty with respect to both the place and purpose of nurses with clinically focused graduate education spilled over into other arenas. This confusion created an uncertain foundation for dialogue among multiple parties about educational preparation for entry-level nurses in general. The ANA's ambivalence showed in its inconsistent language and action on practice and education issues and colored the later ANA response to expanded clinical practice and advanced education, and, in particular, to nurse practitioners.

Establishing Goals

Soon after the restructuring of the existing nursing organizations in 1952, the ANA leadership slowly embraced expanded and expert nursing practice and clinical education as both a political and practical strategy. To address these issues, the ANA's House of Delegates created the Committee on Current and Long-term Goals in 1954. Out of this committee came strategies to address clinical practice and its relationship to education. In 1956, goal 1 targeted efforts to continuously improve the standards of nursing practice, including enlargement of the scientific principles of nursing, and support of nursing research to apply these principles. By 1958 this goal was elaborated and tied practice to standards of education.[12]

Explosive growth in technology and knowledge marked this time period, and nurses and physicians typically incorporated these changes into their practices through self-education and reallocation of professional responsibilities. But the ANA rightly understood that informal methods such as self-education were no longer enough, especially when nurses' roles were rapidly changing. A report from the 1960 convention noted the increased need for "a practitioner [generalist nurse] who could perform critical, independent therapeutic functions for patients. Effective performance of these functions requires the ability to independently assess, evaluate, and interpret health needs and to follow these judgments with appropriate actions."[13] Although the ANA leadership seemed to understand and could articulate these changes through the use of language such as "independently assess" and "interpret health needs," it could not yet convert these ideas into clinical practice and education strategies.

The ANA's approach to practice interests in particular was further complicated and explicated by its frequently changing language and by where it placed practice within its organizational structure. Practice interests initially resided in functional occupation sections in 1952 during the reorganization. The following year the occupational and clinical groups jostled, and the ANA appointed a committee to define the terms "functional" and "clinical" to head off disagreements. This ad hoc committee determined that clinical interests might be best served in conference groups across functional sections rather than in specific clinical interest groups.[14]

Three conference groups emerged from the 1956 convention and reflected the confusion surrounding the conceptualization of practice by both leadership and constituents. The operating-room nursing and psychiatric nursing conference groups represented clinical interests, while the research conference group corresponded to more functional interests. Two more clinically focused conference groups, geriatric nursing and maternal child health nursing, formed later in 1960.[15] Then in 1966, the conferences became divisions of practice to set standards and develop certification boards, and in 1968, a Congress for Nursing Practice was added to coordinate the work and provide a unified approach to division work. Starting in 1972, separate councils for nurse practitioners (also nurse educators and researchers) were added and operated under the divisions of practice.[16] The formulations were the ANA's attempts to maintain relevance, preserve its place as a spokesperson for all nurses, and to respond more quickly to a changing practice milieu, including the rise of separate specialty organizations. But in doing so, the ANA created multiple layers of authority that diluted its efforts and that of its constituents, and cost a great deal of money.

The ANA organized somewhat more coherently around nursing education. Regrouping after its lobbying defeat to prioritize funding for collegiate programs through the 1964 Nurse Training Act (NTA), and inspired by the 1963 surgeon general's report, "Toward Quality in Nursing," the ANA formed a commission to develop a decisive position paper to more effectively influence the public and policy makers about the ANA's position on nursing education.[17] The result, *Educational Preparation for Nurse Practitioners and Assistants to Nurses*, was published in 1965.[18] This was the first definitive public statement on nursing education by the ANA that endorsed baccalaureate nursing education as the entry level for generalist practice, and it was rather bold considering most of the ANA's constituents were still graduates of diploma programs.[19] Despite its constituency, the ANA leadership wanted to be more definitive in shaping the appropriations debate next time by heading off construction and capitation funds for the diploma schools, even as it continued to support recruitment of women and men to them.[20] To control the debate and prepare for future skirmishes, the ANA wanted to have in place sound guidelines defining nursing practice and nursing education that reflected relevant contemporary standards.

The ANA report on educational preparation itself was outdated, however, and far behind the changes already occurring in practice. Moreover, instead of strategically focusing on the graduate level, developing new innovative educational endpoints, and widening its vision of the practice arena, the ANA maintained its focus on the hospital nurse and kept revisiting old political issues, such as the education level required for practice as a professional nurse. Of course, the ANA was again—perhaps strategically—in the short term playing to its constituency. But by taking this approach the ANA failed to recognize advanced and expert practice when it mattered most—during its early period when the movement might have been captured and nurtured. Instead, it mired itself in the entry-level debate, which still remains unsolved.

The Second Goal

The second goal formulated by the ANA's committee on current and long-term goals indirectly addressed clinical practice and advanced education by directing the ANA's attention toward recognizing superior expert performance and personal achievement.[21] Although not yet forecasting the nurse practitioner movement in general, distinguishing the need for multiple knowledge layers to build skills and a mechanism for rewarding expertise were precursors, one could say, of expanded nursing practice. The idea of setting up standards of excellence, incorporated in goals 1 and 2, rather than basic competence, was an extraordinary social and political concept. To this point, basic competence was assumed when a nurse graduated from an accredited nursing program and was seen as an equalizing benchmark across the profession in terms of status and economic well-being. But this was only a fairly loose means of guaranteeing proficient and safe practice since an empowered education program accreditation process had been in effect for only a short time in the mid-1950s. The ANA only approved a legal definition of nursing practice in 1955. The purpose of this set of guidelines was to frame state practice acts by explicating the functions, standards, and qualifications of nursing practice.[22]

The new definition, the ANA believed, supported the group's call for mandatory state licensure of nurses. By 1958, only about twenty states passed mandatory licensure laws, each characteristic of the state. These laws, however, served only as the minimal standard of competency, and many in the organization, if not in nursing at large, believed the ANA should support much more stringent and higher practice competency levels, primarily through certification.[23] But the new definition was itself problematic because it prohibited "acts of diagnosis and prescription of therapeutic or corrective measures."[24] These were areas where nursing practice was already unofficially expanding in intensive care units, public health, and outpatient clinics. The language used in the definition was based on recommendations by the ANA occupational groups. It may be that these groups supported the traditional concept of equity, and they were unable to envision or acknowledge the changes occurring in practice both inside and outside hospitals. An admittedly admirable mission to bring about some sort of standardization for legislative and consumer protection purposes, the definition quickly became quite limiting and restrictive, although many states adopted it over the next decade.

Achievement of clinical practice excellence, as presented in goal 2, was a separate and more refined concept than existing legislative standards mandating basic competence. Measurement and evaluation of clinical excellence was eventually manifested through certification processes and as an entry requirement in the proposed American Academy of Nursing.[25] The benchmark set up an eventual ideological confrontation between supporters of standards of basic competence and those who saw clinical excellence as the true yardstick. It was also one of the issues most strongly contested a few years later by numerous specialty organizations, in particular the National Association of Pediatric Nurse Associates and Practitioners (NAPNAP), which found the standard too restrictive, hierarchical, and symbolically tied to the entry-into-practice debate (see chapter 7).

To compound the problem, the ANA had a hard time deciding what excellence meant, who defined it, how it was achieved, and the organization's role supporting and building it while maintaining consensus and equity within the organization. After the ANA assumed responsibility for the development and implementation of practice standards from the National League of Nursing (NLN) in 1958, it appointed the Intersection Committee on Recognition of Superior Performance to implement goal 2. From the start the committee reflected the ambivalence of the organization surrounding clinical specialization as the members were drawn from the eight occupational sections of the association. These were role-based groups such as general duty nurses, private duty nurses, and educational administrators, consultants, and teachers, groups typically representative of a very traditional model of nursing education and practice.[26] Perhaps recognizing this discontinuity, in 1962 the intersection committee itself recommended reorganization, with the clinical groups rather than occupational sections constituting membership to more readily lend themselves to the identification of excellence. Despite reformulation, the committee members recommended establishment of baseline competencies or common cores of functions and standards that same year, rather than providing guidance for defining excellence.[27]

This was a key time for the organization to be thinking about clinical expertise. By the early 1960s, both an increasingly vocal constituency group and some members of the leadership recognized the need for different and more advanced clinical knowledge. In a memo to the conference groups in July 1960, Hazel Gill, the interim chair of the Maternal and Child Health Nursing (MCHN) conference group, recommended that the officers respond to a motion by the Oregon Nurses Association to plan a joint clinical and scientific conference. The Oregon association challenged the ANA to accept responsibility for supporting continuing clinical education, declaring that "the planning of programs designed to improve nursing practice [is] the proper activity of the ANA and the SNA."[28] That the Oregon constituent group members believed they had to remind the ANA board of directors of their responsibility to improve patient care through clinical educational programs seems somewhat extraordinary but substantiates the organization's dilemma of reconciling functional and professional, economic and clinical issues. Up to this point even the ANA conventions were focused mostly on workplace issues, economic welfare, bylaws, and policy changes of the organization, not on clinical practice.

Slowly the voices of the clinicians and those who supported clinical excellence were being heard. By 1962, the ANA held its first clinical sessions at its convention, and Mildred Scheuer noted in her 1962 presidential address the many requests for regional clinical conferences.[29] Some state nursing associations began their own clinical conference groups in 1964, and by 1966 seven states successfully formed these groups and were able to channel information to the practitioners who needed it. As nurse educator Frances Reiter noted, these clinical initiatives marked "a departure as the old order changeth and maketh way for the new."[30]

Demands for Clinical Information

By the early 1960s, individual nurses deluged the conference groups with demands for clinical information and recommendations for clinical, graduate, and short-term programs. The Maternal and Child Health Nursing conference began publishing clinical and educational information via memos sent to its members in August 1963. More than two hundred nurses requested the first memo, and almost six hundred the second.[31] By the fifth newsletter, there were more than eight thousand requests. Nurses sent letters and postcards with remarkably similar appeals, pleading for "any information you might have on . . . [area of clinical interest]."[32] Teachers requesting help with teaching materials, students requesting materials for school assignments, practitioners looking for help—all were desperate in their appeals for help to care for their patients and to prepare them for their enlarging responsibilities.

Without the initiatives of the clinical conferences, the ANA in general would have had little to offer its constituents. As it stood, the ANA tried to meet their needs for clinical information, but there were at least two issues restricting its efforts. First, the ANA, after a ten-year program of reinventing itself, was again going through a major reorganization that would not be completed until 1966, and many of its resources were tied up in this process. Many initiatives on the clinical agenda, including creating certification programs and defining practice standards, were put on hold. The second issue was specified by ANA president Mildred Scheuer in 1962. "Finances," she noted, "were hampering ANA opportunities and responses. . . . Staff are periodically faced with the necessity to cut, to go slow, to limit programs and services and even to suspend important activities."[33] Clinical education programs were some of the services cut due to lack of money.

Financial problems followed the ANA through the decade of the 1960s, eventually limiting the organization's aim to act upon certification and standard setting until the early 1970s. By then it faced competition from newly formed nursing groups and various established medical specialty groups. ANA membership was always tenuous, and due to difficulties and underestimation of the cost of a central billing system initiated in the mid-1960s, a great deal of dues payments and renewals went uncollected for several years.[34]

By the end of the 1960s, membership in the ANA dropped to less than a fifth of the registered nursing population, and by November 1969 the ANA was more than $1.2 million in debt.[35] In the meantime, increasing numbers of nurses formed specialty organizations and their memberships were sharply rising at the expense of the ANA. As one MCHN board member predicted earlier, "We promised our membership that given an increase in dues that one of our considerations would be giving more help to the nurse, the individual nurse in her clinical practice. . . . I think they are looking to us, I believe that our planning has to have a note of urgency about it or we won't be in so many [members' thoughts] shortly."[36]

Growing Specialty Organizations

While the ANA remained essentially paralyzed with financial struggles and competing ideologies, practicing nurses continued to move into new and innovative clinical areas that tested and writ large the shortcomings of their own knowledge and skills. The boundaries defining professional skills and knowledge were inherently porous. As early minutes of the MCHN division note, much of the discussion centered on correspondence from obstetric and pediatric nurses reporting they lacked the knowledge to use equipment being introduced into the practice setting, and were being asked "to practice beyond their knowledge and abilities."[37] Nurses, the MCHN board remarked, were feeling "a lot of pressure from physicians to do things traditionally considered to be medical tasks, like starting Pitocin drips and performing vaginal exams."[38] The MCHN division was not the only group receiving pleas for help from nurses who experienced increased practice responsibilities. Just prior to the founding of the American Association of Critical Care Nurses (AACN) in 1969, cardiac nurse Norma Shephard sent out hundreds of postcards to nurses working in this clinical area to find out the kind of information they needed to improve patient care. She received over four hundred responses from nurses. "Send me all the information you can" was a frequent reply and not dissimilar to correspondence received by the MCHN conference.[39]

In contrast to the ANA's response, physician specialty groups reacted quickly to nurses' requests for training and programming, and actively reached out to the ANA for help with clinical issues. Both the American Academy of Pediatrics (AAP) and the American College of Obstetricians and Gynecologists (ACOG) requested input from the MCHN division during revisions of their clinical standards.[40] The AAP even offered programs to their members in the late 1960s on how to organize nurse associate training programs because nurses' demands for these programs was so great.[41]

Like-minded nurses who gravitated to various specialty areas keenly felt the ANA's slow pace and began to seek out fellow nurse pioneers to develop and share experiences and knowledge. These meetings at first happened haphazardly between groups of nurses, perhaps at physicians' meetings where they went to learn about the latest medical innovations. This was true of the AACN, the American Nephrology Nurses' Association, and NAPNAP.[42] Medical specialty organizations began to hold nursing sections at their annual conferences. The American College of Obstetricians and Gynecologists sponsored nursing conferences at its national meetings as early as 1959.

The ANA felt increasingly threatened by the rapid formation of "splinter groups" of nursing specialists and by nursing sessions in other organizations over which they had little or no control and tried to counter them whenever they could.[43] In response to the attempts of the American Association for Maternal and Infant Health (AAMIH) to organize a local nursing group in Pennsylvania in 1964, Margaret McDermott, chair of the MCHN division and a Pennsylvania resident, was encouraged by the ANA to start a state-level conference group to counteract it. The division officers also believed that a strong MCHN clinical program was needed at the national level "because of the efforts of other organizations to plan programs for nurses in this area of practice."[44]

This issue did not disappear. In 1972, the Indiana State Nurses' Association demanded the ANA undertake efforts to "halt the proliferation and promote unification" of all emerging groups.[45] "Organizations," one report noted, are "forming at an alarming rate."[46] These groups could possibly have emerged under the aegis of the ANA through the council and division of practice structure, as there was nothing in the ANA bylaws or governance structure that precluded this. Indeed, the ANA board believed they could squelch the new groups if they publicized their current activities at a persistent and desirable level. The immediate problem with this approach was the lack of financial resources.[47]

Large, influential organizations such as the American Heart Association and the American Psychiatric Association organized nursing sessions that functioned as organizational special interest groups. At first, the ANA participated via official representation at meetings and conferences, many times paying dues for the privilege. But ANA representation was always politically situated—on one hand trying to keep control of the decision-making process on nursing issues, while also keeping a close watch for professional intrusion. Many times the decisions and policies of the various organizations ran counter to those of the ANA, and ultimately it decided the funds and the time required to monitor a growing number of organizations was not well spent. Eventually the ANA took a stand on this type of membership, and in 1967 it passed a resolution that withdrew official ANA representation from committees on nursing and/or nursing education under the aegis of other organizations. The resolution stipulated that "future requests to the ANA for such representation be refused, but that the response state ANA's willingness to discuss matters of mutual concern about patient care with appropriate groups within the respective organization."[48] While the ANA feared losing the ability to define professional nursing issues, it also worried about isolation from other organizations. The ANA needed to know what was happening outside its prevue and to keep its organizational prerogatives as secure as possible.

The ANA certainly had reason to be cautious and suspicious. During this period of the mid-1960s, the ANA encountered infringement from many different directions, including the establishment of new nursing organizations. In 1965, the ANA learned that ACOG proposed a national organization of obstetric, gynecological, and neonatal nurses. Judith Whitaker, the ANA executive director, and Jo Eleanor Elliott, the ANA president, wrote to Frank Lock, president of the college, and Robert Kimbrough, medical director, expressing their concerns over the formation of yet another national nursing organization. Whitaker and Elliott tactfully suggested to the college that the organizations could affect patient care in a larger way if they both worked together. "We appreciate the fact that ACOG is as vitally concerned with patient care as we are," Whitaker and Elliott wrote. "But, we believe the professional organization of nurses has the responsibility to help its members improve their practice. . . . Would this be an appropriate time for us to explore ways in which both organizations could work together to achieve our mutual goal—better care of the patient?"[49]

The officers of the ANA conference groups had fewer political constraints and weighed in more strongly and pointedly to their constituents. "In view of the already existing conference group on maternal child health nursing at the national level and the development of several state and district levels," the officers reminded their members, "it would seem most inappropriate for ACOG to continue its efforts to form another nursing organization."[50] The officers also urged their members to consider already available resources for improving their practice, noting, "It would be equally unfortunate if nurses failed to make use of the resources available within ANA to further their clinical interests and improve nursing care."[51]

In other words, the ANA, through its various mechanisms, wanted to derail a potentially threatening and admittedly politically disruptive organization that was attractive to its membership. The college astutely understood the appeal its programs and professional support held for specialty nurses. Even so, Kimbrough replied almost a month later with this disclaimer: "Please be assured that ACOG has done nothing more than suggest the possibility of a nurses' national organization."[52] Lock himself replied to Elliott, assuring her that "no definite plan exists that I am aware."[53]

Their replies, however sincere, were considered somewhat duplicitous by Elliott, who had in hand an article published in December 1964 by ACOG board member Willis E. Brown calling for a national organization for obstetrical nurses.[54] She also had obtained a copy of a survey dated two weeks before Lock's reply to her that was sent to all nurses who had registered for ACOG regional conferences in the last year. The survey included questions about the need for a national organization of obstetric, gynecological, and neonatal nurses, the purpose of said organization, the appropriate amount of dues, and timing of regional and national meetings.[55] Whitaker, also aware of the survey, noted the ANA felt betrayed by the college's action. The ANA offered full partnership to the college by publishing notices of ACOG meetings in its journals and newsletters, and provided editorial and content input for the *Manual of Standards in OB-GYN Practice* as requested and published by the college.[56]

In fact, both the ANA and ACOG may have been at cross-purposes. The ANA clearly saw itself as the ultimate professional nursing organization that, adequately or not, addressed the clinical needs of its constituents through mobilization of its clinical conference groups at the state level. And in many ways, this ideal was absolutely necessary for the ANA to achieve its other purposes, particularly to influence federal legislation and to further its workplace and economic security strategies through its numerical strength. Professional nursing, in fact, needed a strong voice to counter the better-funded and more visible AMA and the American Hospital Association. To achieve this, the ANA had to work fairly rapidly to put in place an organizational structure that was flexible and reactive, and utilize a group of leaders who were facile negotiators. As the story of the NAPNAP will show in chapter 7, the ANA could not accomplish these goals.

The college, along with support from practicing obstetrical nurses, believed that the ANA could not move fast enough to organize its own groups, and it was right. Only seven state conference groups formed in the next year. Indeed, ACOG wanted to counteract the slowness of the ANA because of several vital, albeit self-interested, concerns. The college feared commercial groups, a code word for specialty organizations sponsored by various industry sources and over which they had little control, might step into the breach, as had happened with the Association of Operating Room Nurses (AORN). At least, so ACOG believed, they had a fairly stable history with the ANA and could negotiate with them. From another perspective, the college and its nurse supporters also disliked the ANA conference group title of MCHN because it included pediatric nurses. The college had little interest in pediatric nurses and even less appetite for challenging a fellow specialty organization, the American Academy of Pediatrics, for control over potential nursing constituents. The obstetric and gynecological nurses interested in ACOG affiliation also did not want pediatric nurses diluting their sphere of influence.[57]

Finances also played a part in the discussion as nursing sessions were growing expensive for ACOG. The college, like most other medical specialty organizations, financially supported the nursing special interest sections through its entire conference structure, from waiving meeting-room fees to underwriting program brochures. It wanted to offset this expense with a nominal dues structure and designed the national nursing organization as a way to achieve this. They did not, as an ACOG staff member noted to Margaret McDermott, chair of the MCHN conference group, "want to antagonize the ANA and did not view their attempt [to organize the nurses] as a splinter group."[58]

The college recognized, even if only marginally, the necessity and importance of maintaining a fairly amenable relationship with the ANA, but it needed, in fact, its own nursing organization. Perhaps the priority was the issue of control over practice during a time of inherent instability in the clinical specialty itself. But more likely, ACOG recognized that its members wanted control over how their nursing colleagues were trained and socialized. Although the educational meetings were but a small attempt to develop their "educated allies," they were, nonetheless, highly influential, loyalty-enhancing services that went beyond monetary value. For most nurses in this specialty, the ACOG meetings were the only substantial opportunities they had to keep up with changes in clinical practice.[59]

The conflict between the college and the ANA illustrates only briefly the larger dilemma facing the organization at the national level and its practicing constituents at the grassroots level. Both groups fought different but parallel political battles. Nurse practitioners fought for the immediate knowledge to safely care for patients and the ability to chart their own future: they had to be able to do something for their patients, and they wanted to define their own roles rather than wait for a remote and unwieldy ANA to issue standards for them. Practice was changing too fast. These nurses also waged a structural battle—they wanted organizational arrangements they controlled to facilitate collaboration with medical colleagues, receive recognition for their clinical expertise, and share common concerns with other nurses.

The ANA was not organized, despite exhortations to the contrary from various committees, to respond to these needs, and both practitioners and the ANA itself recognized this as a weakness. "These groups [specialty organizations] formed outside the professional organization," one ANA report noted, "because they saw no place in the ANA where they could pursue their specific interest, no place where they would be free to speak to their special concerns, no place where they could emerge as recognized specialists, no place in ANA where they could collaborate with medical colleagues."[60] The ANA had similar issues with the American Association of Nurse Anesthetists, the American College of Nurse Midwives, and the AHA-based Society of Nursing Service Administrators. The arrangement of ANA occupational sections did not allow for development of specialty groups within the organizational structure with these privileges, and nurses subsequently formed their own organizations.

The ANA fought ideological battles on many fronts, which stemmed from the one-organization philosophy. The conflict waged with the NLN surrounding the power to set educational standards for practice only abated in 1966. The debate rekindled in 1974 when the ANA launched its program to accredit short-term continuing education programs for pediatric nurse practitioners.[61] The ANA was also trying to maintain its traditional position as the voice of nursing politics and workforce issues. It was trying hard to be both "professional leader and professional representative."[62] These tasks were singularly difficult enough, but much more complicated to say the least as a total package. And to complicate matters, there were always the ideological confrontations with its medical counterpart, the AMA.

The episode with the college also illustrates the power of the medical specialties and their efforts to circumscribe the terrain of nursing without involving the AMA.[63] The college, indeed, shared some of the same core values as the AMA when it came to expanded clinical-practice roles for nurses. American Medical Association support for ACOG and other specialty organizations came from a generalized recognition of them as distinct and fairly strong professional groups. Concerned more closely with specific practice boundary issues, ACOG and other specialty groups could more effectively and independently address these issues according to their own jurisdictional politics. By doing so, the specialty medical groups created similar issues for the AMA surrounding consistency and continuity as the equally independently minded nursing specialty groups created for the ANA.

Controlling Nursing

On another front, the ANA and the AMA skirmished over the status and power of nursing. In 1958, the ANA established its first official liaison committee with the AMA. Almost all of the issues brought to the ANA-AMA liaison committee centered on national and general institutional issues such as the role of physicians in nursing education, the growing shortage of nurses in hospitals, and the changing patterns of nursing practice. Decades earlier, the AMA created its own committee on nursing, as had most other specialty medical organizations. The AMA nursing committee met annually throughout the 1960s with its counterpart at the American Hospital Association to discuss problems of shared interest that usually centered on the survival of diploma school programs and maintaining the supply of a cheap nursing workforce. Nurses were active participants in this group, attending and speaking at several of the general sessions at the annual AMA convention in San Francisco in 1968.[64]

Leaders of the ANA and AMA realized they needed broader dialogue at the national level to address their issues, and after a two-year negotiation process, the first national conference for professional nurses and physicians convened in Williamsburg, Virginia, in February 1964.[65] This gathering was exploratory in nature, "providing an opportunity for representative nurses and physicians to meet informally and away from the pressure of their usual responsibilities, to search for increased understandings,"[66] or as one physician later noted, to "break the ice, so to speak."[67] Unsure of what to expect, and perhaps reflecting the pressing issues each group brought to the meeting, the AMA requested the meeting be closed to the press in order "to create an atmosphere for free exchange without discussions being unfavorably reflected on either group."[68]

The group of eighty-eight (composed equally of representatives from medicine and nursing) primarily academic and organizational representatives tentatively made their way through the proceedings on their best professional behavior. They tried to curtail unintended insults and misunderstandings, although as participant Hildegard Peplau noted, neither group could distance itself from familiar, patronizing language. Peplau remembered that physicians referred to nurses as "the girls," and nurses to physicians as "the docs," as if each group had a singular identity.[69] The language was, indeed, symbolic of the general approach each organization took in communicating and working with another, and coupled with the substantial history of agitated discourse among the groups, monolithic language was possibly all that could be mustered. There was no effort, nor opportunity for the organizational leaders and academicians to adopt the language developed locally in individual collegial clinical practices. For the most part, active clinicians were not part of the group, and the leaders and academicians did not share their experiences.[70]

The primary discussion topics at the conference centered on nurses' roles and the ethical and legal status of their enlarging practice boundaries.[71] As in many other venues before and after, neither the physician's changing role nor the need for physicians to adapt their practices to changes in the public's health care needs was the focus of discussion. Everyone wanted to talk about nurses, especially hospital nurses, and it was this focus that stymied discussions. Although participants generally agreed on the pressing need for better communication models for doctors and nurses, they couldn't agree on the level of education that nurses needed for the expanded roles, nor who might supervise them.[72] None of the discussions broke new ground, and by 1967 the ANA board of directors declined to plan for the 1968 meeting, noting that although much more needed to be done in the area of nurse-doctor relationships, the meetings "were no longer meaningful."[73]

At this point, the AMA was also in the midst of ideological battles on several fronts, and nurses' expanded roles were perhaps one of the least threatening, although still worrisome, intrusions into the medical practice domain. Indeed, Robert Throckmorton, who initially led the Iowa Medical Society assault on chiropractors in the early 1960s and who was appointed general counsel of the AMA in 1963, was silent at the conference about nurses' expanded roles.[74] The AMA considered other issues to be more pressing problems—namely, intrusions by chiropractors and osteopaths into traditional medical arenas, growing group practice structures at the expense of the traditional solo private practitioners, and the ongoing attempts by Congress to pass some type of socialized medical insurance program.

One such example was the 1966 Comprehensive Area-Wide Health Planning Act (PL 89–749) that supported the development of ambulatory neighborhood health centers through the Office of Economic Opportunity.[75] Nurse practitioners were already employed in federally funded ambulatory clinics in urban areas, and money was appropriated through the office to fund nurse practitioner training. The AMA and its local state associations were more concerned and suspicious of the idea of clinics in general and their associated appropriations as state medicine. They wondered who employed the physician— the patient or the clinic board?

Underlying the suspicions was the AMA's traditional support for fee-for-service, private-practice arrangements in contrast to group practices. Instead of public clinics, the AMA argued that private offices should be developed within the traditional fee-for-service arrangement. The AMA's position was problematic as Medicaid capitated clinic visits at twenty dollars while the usual routine private clinic fee was eighty dollars. "Is it too much to expect," wrote one physician, "that the Comprehensive Health Planning Act will not interfere with existing patterns of private professional practices?"[76] The AMA similarly opposed the Neighborhood Health Centers Act of 1969, which used federal funds to establish outpatient clinics in areas of low physician accessibility, a proposed 1969 revision of the Hill Burton Act that would channel money to health facilities, including community health centers, and the 1973 Health Maintenance Organization bill. The issue for the AMA, among other things, was that the new centers and organizations were not physician controlled.[77]

The AMA was slowly losing its battle for traditional practice models on several fronts. In the late 1960s, chiropractors gained access to payment systems through state Medicaid programs. In September 1968, the Pennsylvania Medical Society's House of Delegates learned that chiropractic services were to be included in Pennsycare—the state Medicaid program—and that the governor already signed this legislation into effect in July 1968. The resulting house of delegates resolution on unsafe practices mirrored the AMA sentiment as it noted delegates' outrage at the use of already "insufficient funds to be wasted on payments for which nothing of medical value whatsoever will be rendered."[78]

Throughout the 1960s, the AMA used the campaign against chiropractors as its own rhetorical force multiplier, as a way of mobilizing member support that spilled into other issues, namely, the battle against Medicare and Medicaid. In fact, the AMA invested heavily in financial resources and professional prestige to defeat both antitrust lawsuits brought by chiropractors and Medicare and Medicaid legislation. By the end of the 1960s, the AMA was badly defeated on the entitlement issues, and in 1972 chiropractors gained access to the Medicare payment system.[79] By the end of the 1960s and into the 1970s, the AMA was working to refurbish the organization's reputation through various media presentations, and like many other instances in its past, it had an uncanny way of eventually supporting the various policies it once tried to defeat.[80]

The AMA faced problems similar to those of the ANA. The AMA, too, tried to be both professional leader and representative, but with diminishing returns and the loss of its traditional role as arbiter of medical education and economic workplace issues.[81] The growing number of medical specialty groups, their internecine conflicts, and their threat to a unified overarching AMA political mission also kept the AMA from focusing on nursing in a stronger way. Indeed, one of the greatest nursing concerns for the AMA at the time was the demise of diploma programs, the growth of baccalaureate programs, and unionization by nurses, and these concerns partially stemmed from the national nursing shortage rather than changing practice parameters.[82] These concerns were diametrically opposite those of the ANA and provided material for episodic skirmishes.

The AMA eventually developed smoother relationships with medical specialty organizations, establishing the Department of Specialty Society Relations in 1970. The purpose of this department was to coordinate the efforts of the various medical groups to respond more consistently to federal and state policy initiatives.[83] Although a reasonable aim, improved relationships between the AMA and medical specialty groups continued to require resources and effort on both sides. A slowly percolating grass roots resistance to the AMA itself also required attention. Physicians such as Caldwell B. Esselstyn, who joined forces with organized labor to support Medicare, and Samuel Standard, who testified in support of Medicare before the U.S. Senate Committee on Finance, were part of a growing vocal movement primarily based in academic institutions that challenged AMA authority and hierarchy, and its commitment to patients.[84]

Empowering the Specialties

As nurse practitioners developed a place in health care in the late 1960s and subsequent decades, they played a useful role for the AMA as well: nurse practitioners provided a new common cause that united factions within organized medicine to protect its position in health care. The AMA used the same tactics against nurse practitioners and the ANA that the Committee on Investigations and the Committee on Ethics (known as the committee on quackery) used earlier against a growing chiropractic movement. Common strategies included efforts to exclude nurse practitioner services in health insurance and workman's compensation payment programs; censure for physicians in collaborative practice arrangements; campaigns against nurses holding hospital privileges; lobbying against education funding; building ethical complaints; resisting efforts for practice enlargement through legislation; and encouraging disunity within groups.[85]

In fact, the nurse practitioner specialties in particular played nicely, although perhaps not intentionally, into the strategy of disunity within groups. The AMA, because of the efforts of medical specialty organizations to develop their own nursing organizations and the inability of the ANA to mount an effective response to the growing demand for clinical programs, had little to do but watch and wait. In the meantime, the ANA continued to focus on study after study that documented retrospective changes. Indeed, clinical practice was changing, and the best ANA could offer was documentation that the changes occurred.

Not only were other organizations—such as the medical and nursing specialty organizations, system-focused organizations such as the American Heart Association or institutionally focused groups such as the American Hospital Association—challenging the ANA and the AMA for political control of nursing practice and education, but they were confronting them at a critical time of relative weakness for both organizations. Changing constituencies, economic difficulties, and a distancing of the organizations' leadership from the sensitivities of the daily needs of patients created historically specific opportunities and supplied the opening for other groups to challenge these dominant organizations. These issues forced the ANA and AMA to turn their gaze inward, focusing their efforts on self-protection rather than reacting and responding with their best intentions and resources.

These challenges could have constituted an important watershed in American health care if each organization—or at least a collection of these organizations—had put aside traditional differences and worked toward a common goal of enhancing access and improving the quality of patient care across all levels. This, of course, was the rhetoric of the organizations. They indeed initiated policies that improved health care, but they did so episodically and through efforts aimed at maintaining traditional positioning by disempowering other groups. Combined, the groups would have had substantial political clout in sheer number of members, which they could have used to garner a substantial amount of public and private resources.

But this was not to be the dominant narrative of the time. Each organization, because of its particular history, ideology, cultural power, and economic reality, responded to the challenges in its own way, achieving different levels of political success in harnessing the growing power of medical and nursing clinical specialists and practitioners. Even when they appeared to be working together, they were practicing "subclinical" efforts to maintain their political hegemony.

Chapter 6

Coming Together, Breaking Apart

The National Joint Practice Commission
and the Politics of Practice

As the larger professional organizations navigated the contours of national politics, individual practitioners and those working in larger academic institutions developed new educational programs and redrew practice boundaries into the 1970s through the crucible of experience. The context of national health care framed these changes and kept individuals and organizations occupied in practice politics. As the Medicare and state-based Medicaid systems took full effect after their implementation in the 1960s, health care expenditures climbed. Despite this, there was unabashed optimism surrounding these health care reforms, which pumped huge quantities of money into the system and opened up services to large population groups such as the elderly and the poor. Demands for more providers to care for these population groups followed. But inadequate control over cost, a continued focus on acute care institutions and medical specialization, and a lack of national interest for planning facilities and technology supported unencumbered growth and increasing redundancy of institutions and services, especially in hospitals. These forces created the most expensive health care system in the world, but one that could not meet the public's needs for access to basic primary care services.

The expansion of nurse practitioner practice and education was closely tied to the national context as more and more money was pumped into nursing, medical, and physician assistant education programs through manpower funding initiatives in 1971 and 1975. In particular, the increasing number and popularity of nurse practitioners, both to the public they served and to the physicians they worked with, created opportunities. It indeed fueled improved patient access to services, but it also created competition over professional autonomy and for public trust.[1] Health care was big business, both in the currency of cultural authority and dollars, with physicians in control of most of these resources. But this was highly dependent on the patient, the particular health problem, and the location of services. In other words, individual needs and preferences combined with community characteristics to determine the kind of care the public sought and could access. Individual nurse practitioners increasingly gained power in rural and urban clinics, and in specialty areas such as pediatrics and general medicine when the public had access to them and physicians could not mount strength in numbers.

One of the issues determining the success of nurse practitioners was the tension between individual need and community tendencies. Clearly, nurses could take on certain knowledge and skills traditionally in the physician's realm and safely use them in practice. And, growing numbers of patients trusted and chose them as their providers either alone or as part of a physician-nurse team. While individual patients highly valued the care they received from nurse practitioners, however, the community at large still granted higher cultural authority to physicians, which helped maintain their hold on health policy issues such as public funding for new practice models, legislation surrounding practice privileges, and reimbursement issues. All of these shaped the implementation of the nurse practitioner role and the professional relationships between nurses and physicians in general as progress achieved on an individual basis was difficult to replicate at the national level. Individually negotiated practice relationships did indeed influence clinical care, but the process was painstakingly slow, locally situated, and idiosyncratic. Despite the efforts of nurse-physicians pairs to successfully come together to support clinical care, doctors and nurses still experienced contentious and awkward interactions that deflected attention away from patients. Practitioners needed a mechanism to facilitate better relationships in general to support the early momentum of the nurse practitioner movement or it was unsustainable.

The National Joint Practice Commission (NJPC) is an example of attempts to pull nurses, physicians, and their organizations together to both develop strategies for getting along and to model the behavior that made nurse-physician collaboration so effective at the practice level. The commission grew out of the recommendations of the 1970 report of the National Commission for the Study of Nursing and Nursing Education (NCSNNE) and was supported in its short ten-year life by the ANA, AMA, and foundation funding. As the details of its activities illustrate, its existence depended upon savvy commissioners who brought successful experiences as individual practitioners in collaborative relationships and then extrapolated them to the national arena. When their efforts failed to satisfy the agendas of their sponsoring organizations in the late

1970s, and their confidence grew beyond their political abilities, the commission broke apart. The AMA and the ANA retreated to their traditional communication pathways through various politically appointed task forces and committees, while individual practitioners continued to rely on personality and perseverance to maintain practice relationships.

Coming Together

The 1970 NCSNNE report (the Lysaught Report) recognized the potential impact of expanded nursing practices and the strained reality of doctor-nurse relationships. In addition to making sweeping recommendations for nursing education, the report also critiqued the political disagreements between the major professional organizations. It reminded them of their obligation to both patients and their membership to develop more cohesive and congruent understandings of the public's health care needs. The report particularly faulted the failure of the ANA and the AMA to develop a national approach to collaborative patient care, a key component of expanded nursing practice and one that required sound relationships between nurses and doctors.[2] Essentially, the commission chastised the national organizations for failing to support the momentum driven by innovative practitioners and educators.

One of the recommendations of the NCSNNE report was the establishment of a national joint practice organization as a leadership and policy-formulating body guiding state organizations on a more local level. Its purpose was "to discuss and make recommendations concerning the congruent roles of the physician and the nurse in providing quality health care with particular attention to the rise of the nurse clinician; the physician assistant; the increased activity of other professions and skills in areas long assumed to be the concern solely of the physician and/or the nurse."[3] This was congruent to proposals put forward by the 1971 report from the secretary of health, education, and welfare, *Extending the Scope of Nursing Practice*.[4] Jerome Lysaught, the director of the NCSNNE, believed the joint practice concept was one of the most important parts of the commission's recommendations, "because medicine and nursing continued to be largely separate and often times antagonistic and belligerent towards each other, and the impact on health care was shortchanged."[5]

For their part, the AMA and the ANA gave the request fairly serious consideration. Both organizations publicly supported the NCSNNE report and specifically the concept of a NJPC.[6] Their failure to participate in the development of the commission would have raised concerns of integrity and reliability and questioned their own intent. Both organizations already engaged in episodic activities such as joint conferences, and had interagency and state liaison committees, but nothing concrete had come of them. The NCSNNE proposal was different. The NJPC would be a more independent and thus more legitimate forum for taking the lead on important patient care issues, making recommendations, conducting research, and serving as a sort of clearinghouse from which their findings could be more easily disseminated to the states and the public. Both organizations realized that the commission was probably going to occur in some form and that they had a stake in planning and, perhaps more important, monitoring its activities. If the commission was going to exist, both organizations wanted to be informed of its deliberations, especially if they were going to provide substantial funding, and neither wanted to be the reason the commission failed to develop or succeed.[7] By November 1971, the ANA and the AMA issued a joint memorandum of agreement broadly supportive of studying the roles and functions of both professions with the understanding that it was basic to the "concept of change that adjustments be made by all parties."[8]

The organizations then formulated the guidelines for membership to facilitate an equal distribution of power and oversight: commission membership included an equal number of both physicians and nurses (eight each), a majority of whom were active practitioners and all of whom were members of the ANA or AMA. Each organization was also represented directly by a nonvoting staff person, drawn from their own liaison committees, who reported meeting details back to the AMA or ANA. The organizations appointed commissioners each believed would be organizationally loyal, and this was probably to be expected given the parent organizations' financial commitment and overt suspicion of the commission.[9] On the other hand, the AMA and the ANA gained little by obviously stacking the commission, as it was quite important for the public and other organizations to perceive it as an independent body, not obviously politically influenced by either group.

For an organization with a major focus on quality patient care, one important constituency was missing. The NJPC never had an at-large public member, even though this was a time of heavy public advocacy, with activist Ralph Nadar highly visible in the mainstream media. The commissioners discussed the idea from time to time but never came to a consensus, and there was never support from the parent organizations to involve the public in NJPC activities. Yet the work the NJPC envisioned undertaking required a public buy-in to move the agenda forward. Upcoming initiatives such as changes in state practice acts provided the opportunity in many states for public dialogue. Sidney H. Willig, a lawyer and consultant to the commission on the legal aspects of medical and nursing practice, noted astutely, "Don't propose something, see the backbiters kill it, and then say, 'Well, this didn't go to the public.' If you bring the public in from the beginning, you have credibility in the eyes of the public and of legislators."[10] The AMA certainly understood the need to court public support and capitalized on it. They initiated several advertising campaigns in popular magazines and mailings that pointed out the practice liabilities of practitioners other than physicians. The ANA, on the other hand, was less effective in this area, perhaps because it did not have the money or it did not trust the public to embrace expanded practice even though study after study showed the public supported it. Part of the mistrust came from the ANA's basic uncertainty of the concept itself, and its failure to harness the energy from a growing, vocal group of nurses.

The appointed commissioners worked in different specialties in different parts of the country, and were probably unfamiliar with one another; they knew each other by reputation rather than personal relationships.[11] All were appointed by their respective professional or specialty organizations and were considered strong leaders in their fields. Two doctorally prepared nurses (Shirley Smoyak and Virginia Stone) were part of the nursing appointees. All of the nurses practiced in expanded roles. Smoyak noted the irony of these nurses representing the ANA, which was still primarily focused on workplace issues and a majority constituency of diploma nurses. "When the joint practice commission was starting," she remembered, "the constituency for nursing was still not up to speed ['training school people']. So the minority who were nurse practitioners or beyond were speaking for the association."[12]

The commission and its parent organizations were precariously positioned. The AMA and the ANA provided the initial funding for the commission ($10,000 each), and could withdraw support if their particular positions were not supported.[13] On the other hand, the organizations agreed to cooperate in this very visible venture and had to accept a certain degree of liability, obligation, and movement on sensitive issues such as clinical supervision and practice authority. For its money, the ANA expected its board to have the opportunity to deliberate on NJPC recommendations before they became public, presumably capitalizing on the work of the commission through a melding of the ANA's own strategies. The AMA requirements were slightly more opaque—it "accepted a fair amount of independence for the NJPC," but more subtly based its continuing support on the "effectiveness of the group."[14]

New Bottles, New Wine

The first meeting of the NJPC took place on January 21, 1972, in St. Louis, Missouri. This was a critical meeting as most participants were unfamiliar with the NCSNNE report; they agreed in principle with the general ideas but were unaware of particular details. And, despite the commissioners' individual familiarity and support for collaborative practice, this national forum was an unfamiliar proving ground, as no one was quite sure what was expected of them.

These uncertainties were reflected in simple, symbolic actions at this first meeting. The layout of the meeting space, for example, seemed counterproductive to the perceived mission of talking to one another as nurses and physicians each met in a separate room. Perhaps Lysaught believed they needed to move slowly and that placing everyone together from the beginning invited the typical nurse-physician interaction. Smoyak remembered, "And I said, 'This is stupid. This is very dumb,' and I was not alone. . . . The nurses joined in. And we as a group went into the other room and said, 'You're going to have to help us bring the chairs in here, because we're supposed to be talking to each other, we can't talk through a wall.' "[15]

The commissioners determined the character and the mission of the group, but no one was quite sure where and how to begin. The exception was pediatrician A. Alan Fischer, who came prepared to accomplish something substantial. He suggested the group use a new group process model to generate discussion, and, encouraged by Smoyak, the psychiatric nurse, the group agreed. "Alan Fischer had figured out that he knew what to do," Smoyak recounted. "And we assigned four nurses, four physicians to each of these two big tables, and we went through the process to decide who we were and how we would proceed. . . . What should this group be? What should the mission be? So the outcome was we should develop mechanisms for scanning the environment to find out who's already working in collegial ways. Who's already doing stuff in a cooperative way between nurses and physicians? We didn't even use collegial. It was cooperative."[16]

From the beginning the commissioners were quite blunt and at times their discussion more closely mirrored traditional nurse-physician conflict than attempts at better dialogue. At the first meeting, Smoyak, an avowed public advocate and feminist, spoke to the idea of physician dominance. She noted, "The idea that the physician is always right, always the leader, always the decision maker, and the one who *permits* the nurse to advise, must go!" Her fellow commissioner, physician James Walker, responded, "The physician is the front man for nurses' actions. . . . If the RN wants to function in a larger role, then she must also accept the responsibility and liability for that role. Many nurses are reluctant to assume such responsibility."[17] If the NJPC was to survive and develop into an effective body for generating strategies for better patient care, nurses and physicians had to develop a new language and manner for engaging each other. In fact, in the closeness and intensity of the commission meetings, they became quite effective translators and negotiators despite the political nature of their appointments. The developing alliances of the commissioners in time reflected the negotiations going on at the more local level, and they seemed to be able to take control of the dialogue and, after receiving some independent funding, their own actions. They quickly moved beyond the influence of the NCSNNE, although the ANA and AMA tethers proved shorter and less easy to break.

The original objective developed at the first meeting by the commissioners seemed fairly simple: "The NJPC and its state counterpart committees should be established to discuss, study, and make recommendations concerning the roles for the physician and nurse in providing quality health care to our nation's people."[18] However, the subobjectives developed by the commissioners prior to their second meeting in April 1972 were, from the start, farther reaching than perhaps expected by the parent organizations and indicative of the commissioners' growing facility for dialogue and alliances, and of the social movements of the time period. They touched on access-to-care, the need to revamp delivery systems, examination of the authority and responsibility of the professions, changes needed in education systems to enhance new role functions of nurses and physicians, and examination of the gender and class context that formed traditional relationships. By defining these issues as part of the functional structure, the commission set forth a fairly liberal agenda. It represented, as the NCSNNE suggested in its own publications, "new bottles, new wine," in its approach to clinical and professional relationship issues.[19] But, this liberal flavor was tempered by its lack of diversity. Although President Lyndon Johnson signed the Civil Rights Act in 1968, and the Supreme Court ruled that busing was a legitimate method of integration in 1971, race is not mentioned in NJPC documents. All the commissioners and their staff were white and reflected the power structures defining medicine and nursing during this time. Race, along with gender equity, was not to be a focus of the commission.

Once the commission began to function, the states rapidly began to look to the NJPC for leadership across all sorts of issues, including guidance for setting up their own state joint practice commissions and developing state practice legislation that more clearly fit the changes occurring in practice.[20] The work load quickly overwhelmed the volunteer group. The commission lacked a staff and a permanent office. None of the commissioners received compensation for their work (early on they were meeting on a monthly basis), and all of them had other clinical and academic responsibilities. Money became a critical issue, and by the second year the commission still had few prospects for income beyond the parent organization contributions.

The commissioners wrote grants to various foundations and made several visits to the W. K. Kellogg Foundation to propose a funding structure for their activities. The foundation partially funded the NJPC in July 1973, providing $326,620 over a three-year period, to 1976. This money was channeled through the AMA's Economic Research Foundation (ERF) because the commission and its sponsors could not agree on incorporation terms.[21] With these funds, the commission gained a measure of independence, hired William Schaffrath as director, and established an office in Chicago, leasing space from the AMA.[22]

Getting Along

While the national organizations followed their own agendas, the commissioners individually crafted alliances and positions that were not always politically congruent with the larger parent organizations. This was also true at the state level, where the opportune combination of interested nurses and physicians created momentum but few resources and little support from the local organizations. Each state commission characteristically developed in its own way and time, and, in fact, some states were working on joint practice issues and statements a few years before the NJPC began. These early declarations addressed physician delegation of authority for very specific procedures and technical skills to nurses rather than nurse-physician collaboration in patient care, but they represented the growing dialogue and negotiations occurring in the practice arena at the local level between nurses and physicians, and the introduction of new technologies into the hospital environment.[23]

The joint practice activities in each state were a product of the people involved, the time, and place. In North Carolina, the joint practice commission began in October 1971, with eight nurses and eight physicians, one medical and nursing student, and both presidents of the professional organization as ex officio members, which indicated a high level of organizational support. Unlike the activities in most states, physician attendance at meetings was reported as better than nurse attendance, although the nursing organization initiated the dialogue. The Illinois joint practice commission organized in 1972. Similar to other states, physician participation was at first somewhat marginal, but the medical association removed its original appointees and replaced them with "concerned and interested practitioners."[24] West Virginia medical and nursing organizations also convened a liaison committee prior to the formation of the NJPC. Although the committee undertook the important job of reopening the Nurse Practice Act, one physician noted that "probably the only real accomplishment was that we learned to talk to each other."[25]

Not all states were equally successful. In Wyoming, nurses began the process of developing a state joint practice commission (JPC) but had a great deal of difficulty making physicians interested in the concept. Respondents to a NCSNNE survey of the Wyoming committee noted that "physician participation has been a real problem for this committee. . . . Physicians saw no need."[26] In Maryland, the state nurses' association wrote to the NJPC appealing for help: "We're having difficulty in the State of Maryland getting physicians to work with us. Specifically, our state's medical society has consistently refused to establish a State Joint Practice Commission."[27]

Although the NJPC clearly relished the rising activities of state commissions, it was obviously cautious for two reasons. First, a 1964 AMA-ANA sponsored initiative similar to the NJPC failed four short years after initiation. Part of the intent of the AMA-ANA group was to facilitate dialogue between leaders at the national level and practitioners at the state level, but the initiative became organization directed almost from the beginning. Although ambitious in scope, it never generated a larger movement, and the NJPC needed to learn from this experience.[28]

Second, the commissioners believed the early state commissions were "reactionary bodies, and sorely needed a positive platform of projects."[29] Although the North Carolina state practice commission seemed to be moving in a general direction of conversation and communication between the professions, there was still a great deal of controversy between the local medical and nursing organizations. "It would be far better for the North Carolina commission to address themselves to the accomplishment of positive goals rather than merely react to local issues," the commission noted.[30] These antagonistic bodies were unlikely to facilitate the type of change envisioned by the NJPC and could really only provoke polemic local reactions. The national commission believed the best way to manage these groups was to expand its joint practice concept to the regional, county, and city levels through outreach by its commissioners. It is here, the commission noted, "where change, if it is to happen, will happen."[31]

But first, the NJPC had to create a model for the states to emulate. The activities of the commissioners, while nationally situated, represented the most local and individual level of collaboration and cooperation. Their meetings were generously attended, with most of the sixteen commissioners (with similar physician and nurse attendance records) attending each one- to two-day meeting. Those who did not attend were quickly replaced by other interested people.[32] Smoyak noted, "As we got to know each other better and developed camaraderie and the rest, at the end of the meeting the guys [physicians] would say, 'So what should we tell them [the AMA]?' Because they always had to report back. The ANA couldn't care less."[33]

The AMA more closely monitored the NJPC activities although it had many other important and crucial issues to face, such as physician assistant standards, incursions into reimbursement systems by various other professionals such as optometrists, chiropractors, osteopaths, and nurse practitioners, and trying to uphold the AMA's ebbing influence in medical education. The nurse-physician relationship, although important, was not its top priority. But it was becoming a highly visible and public issue, and the AMA could little afford to ignore it. Besides, the ANA soon discovered that its interests were generally well taken care of by the nurse commissioners, who, although not always in agreement during discussions, tended to vote similarly. The AMA appointed men like Robert Hoekelman, Alan Fischer, and Otto Page, who because of their own practice experience and personality allied themselves and comfortably collaborated with the nurse commissioners, creating a powerful political voting block. These men understood the concept of nurses in expanded roles and were quite comfortable with their own work relationships. But perhaps most important for the success of the commission but problematic for the AMA, the physician participants were not readily loyal to the typical ideological "captain of the ship" role.

Those who were not as familiar with the joint practice concept were, as Smoyak noted, "easily co-opted" into believing in the goodness and utility of the idea.[34] Smoyak remembered her physician colleagues "paid" for their independent thinking and were reproached by the AMA when they reported back to the organization: "What they were supposed to be doing was to get these uppity nurses back in their place. . . . And people went off, and people came on. And whoever came on, we would co-opt. In one or two meetings they were talking joint practice. They'd go back to AMA, and AMA would get mad. . . . James Sammons [executive director of AMA] saw it as a personal affront to him that these physicians . . . were selling out the mission of AMA. So he would berate them when they would go back and report that colleagueship was a good idea."[35]

Individually, the nurse and physician commissioners modeled the joint practice concept to each other and extended this practice in visits by pairs of commissioners, a nurse and a physician, to the state associations and committees. They spoke to the believers, the skeptics, and the curious alike, to anyone who wanted to learn about the idea of joint practice. The best encounters came when practitioners of all sorts wanted to learn how to communicate and work better with their counterparts in other professions. The most difficult scenarios were in front of hostile audiences. Smoyak remembered a visit to the Delaware Medical Society as one of the worst experiences and told the following story:

> Bob [Hoekelman] was with me. We would say, "What do nurses do, what do physicians do, separately, today? And when you put it together, what does it look like?" And just saying, "When you put it together," you

could see nervousness in the audience. . . . The put-together thing we orchestrated where I would say something about physicians and he would say something about nurses. And then we would have a mock debate about how to do something. Here's how it goes in a joint practice. . . . We would have an argument about pediatrics, and an immunization program—what's normal, what's not normal, how do you teach it, who should be in charge of well-babies. Are pediatricians ready to let go of well-babies? And we'd have this debate in front of them so that they could see. . . . Well, that was an unheard-of conversation. They thought we'd lost our minds. So what I remember is that when I was speaking alone, and it was only for five or ten minutes, men (they were all men except for a couple of ladies) they were smoking cigars in the audience and reading the newspapers. And when Bob was speaking alone they listened to him attentively. And when we did our little mock joint practice thing, they couldn't wait to speak, and they berated Bob for putting up with this. . . . It was ugly. It was disrespectful, it was rude, it was awful. And they invited us to a late dinner in the basement. The president or somebody apologized for the treatment. One of the women . . . told me that I should get a grip and understand what womanhood was.[36]

Most of the time, their audience courteously listened and responded to their ideas. There was incredible national interest from nurses and physicians about joint practice in general and about the nurse practitioner role in particular, and both professionals needed better understanding of each other's various positions. Most physicians, Robert Hoekelman noted, "do not know what is meant by the 'expanded role of the nurse' because they don't know of the restricted role, except that traditionally nurses have performed as physician's helpers."[37] Many nurses, on the other hand, could not conceptualize how expanded practice influenced the physician's role in the health care system, or how one might complement the other. Each had a great deal to learn about a group they already thought they knew, and this was essential if nurses and physicians were going to get along.

Renegotiating State Practice Acts

In addition to its various other roles, the NJPC also responded to numerous requests for assistance from state commissions exploring their practice acts to address nurses' enlarging practice roles and physician delegation rights and responsibilities. Nurses questioning their legal practice boundaries, along with physicians either trying to protect collaborative practices or accusing nurses of

practicing medicine, were turning to state regulatory boards of medicine, nursing, and state joint practice commissions for consultations.

Many groups besides the NJPC were examining this issue, as there was a
growing number of court decisions and pressure from both the medical and nursing professions to examine the legality of nurses' expanded practice. The commission funded Virginia Hall, one of their legal consultants, to investigate these
issues. She published her report, *Statutory Regulation of the Scope of Nursing
Practice—A Critical Survey*, in 1974 with NJPC support.[38] The Institute of
Medicine issued a major position paper on the legal liability of primary care
manpower in 1977, and various federal government departments and services
and numerous academicians wrote extensively on the issue.[39]

Practice was changing faster than the regulations, and a great deal of legislative and state board activity was happening on both the medical and nursing sides
as these groups realized the opportunity for change, for gaining new powers, and
for tightening control.[40] Most of the medical practice acts were decades old, as
medicine never had to justify its claim to practice under the acts and therefore had
no reason to change them.[41] In Michigan, for example, the act had not been
updated since 1899.[42] Numerous state nurse practice acts were unopened since
the 1950s, when many states responded to the ANA's model nursing practice act,
and even so, practice changed quite a bit in the last ten years as nursing, unlike
medicine, constantly realigned and justified its practice boundaries.[43]

A lot of movement was occurring in the states over practice acts in the 1970s.
In 1973, an ANA survey of state nurses' associations found that 54 percent anticipated legislation amending current nurse practice acts in that year alone, attest-
ing to the high level of interest and activity. Forty-eight percent of the fifty state
associations surveyed anticipated legislation amending the medical practice
act—46 percent of these changes were to enlarge the physician's delegatory
powers, and 50 percent were intended to extend the authority of the medical
board to regulate other health personnel such as physician assistants and nurse
practitioners through joint promulgation.[44] The NJPC issued a formal statement
on medical and nursing practice acts in 1974, but this was somewhat after the
fact, as the state organizations that predated the NJPC moved faster.[45] By 1972
Massachusetts alone had several bills before the legislature that addressed
expanded roles for various types of health care workers, and other states, such
as Florida and Oklahoma, already had specific statutes defining physician
delegations.[46]

Opening practice acts was a fairly labile process, as the outcome was never
guaranteed. Revising statutes helped to protect the public and nurses working
in expanded roles. But if the new language was overly specific and detailed, it

also had the potential to circumscribe and restrict nurses' ability to respond to changes in clinical care and discourage innovation and flexibility. For example, some practice acts that seemed to support nurses' independent prescriptive privileges were rewritten to block them from prescribing except under specific conditions, such as direct physician supervision. Many nurse practitioners worked in areas of low physician supply, and this type of change required doctors to be present. Patients were affected because access to services decreased when nurses lacked the mandated supervision, but had the knowledge, to prescribe. In some states, medical boards held nurse practice act revisions hostage until physician assistants gained prescriptive rights.[47]

The NJPC actively tried to harness the energy generated in the states and to help support a more orderly regulatory process, but few states, even those asking for help, wanted to wait for the NJPC to create guidelines. Timing, and the need to develop a consistent framework for change while allowing each state its fundamental right to legislate, were some of the reasons the NJPC began to generate positions on this issue. Their 1974 statement on medical and nurse practice acts, although late to the debates going on at the state and local levels, was one of the few nationally situated unifying voices emerging to guide physicians, nurse practitioners, and state boards.[48] Although there was much dialogue at the federal, state, and organizational levels, very little was aimed at the grassroots, where local practice negotiations almost daily reformulated clinical boundaries, for the most part out of sight of legislators and state boards.

The Casebook, Together

Almost from the first meeting, the commissioners realized they needed to offer successful exemplars of nurse-physician teams to help frame the debates on joint practice going on in the organizations and in the states. They already knew about hundreds of anecdotal cases, and they proposed enlarging and bringing these stories together in a published book. Through ads in various professional journals, they called for nurses and physicians in primary care settings to send their stories and case materials to the NJPC for consideration. Establishing no format except for the setting (the cases had to be set in outpatient areas), the commission received more than 250 responses from practitioners in all sorts of specialties and diverse locations. From these, they chose twenty-four to include in a book funded by the R. W. Johnson Foundation, published in 1977.

The book, *Together*, was fairly radical for the time.[49] Although stories describing nurse-physician teams had been published since the 1960s, this book was an emphatic concentration of nurse-physician collaboration and evidence of its ability to increase access, provide high-quality patient care, and improve patient satisfaction. The stories ranged from those of nurse Jean E. Steel (who later became an NJPC commissioner) and physician Robert Funkhouser describing their private practice in Cambridge, Massachusetts, for mostly upper middle class and some Medicare patients, to that of nurse Susan Schweer, who practiced at the remote People's Health Center in the Appalachian community of Briceville, Tennessee. Her two surgeon colleagues, David Stanley and Robert Dunlap, were twenty miles away in Oak Ridge but available by telephone for consultation and referrals.[50]

Both Steel and Schweer were nurse practitioners. Steel completed the certificate program in 1974 at the Peter Bent Brigham Hospital in Boston, and Schweer finished the Vanderbilt University nurse practitioner program and her master's degree in 1972. Both had significant previous experience in independent nursing practices. Steel worked with the Boston Visiting Nurse Association and the Harvard Community Health Plan, and Schweer practiced in a clinic in an East Nashville housing project. She also started the medical nurse practitioner program at the School of Nursing at Meharry Medical College in Nashville. The physician collaborators were men who chose to work outside academic institutions and had volunteered their time in community clinics. Funkhouser took a two-year fellowship at the Harvard Divinity School after graduating from medical school, and spent half of his time (the other half in private practice) in neighborhood health centers in Boston's poor neighborhoods, clinics in nursing homes, and teaching hospitals. Both of the surgeons working with Schweer started out at the Briceville clinic on a volunteer basis, as did four other consultants who visited the clinic one afternoon a month.[51]

Although recommended by the commissioners at the first meeting, the casebook took almost five years to reach publication. Part of the reason was the incredible volume of submissions, and the sorting and selection process. The commissioners were also searching for funding for the publication, which delayed the process.[52] Another reason for moving cautiously may have been the response by the AMA to the cases selected for the casebook. The ANA offered little critique or dialogue because it provided opportune illustrations supporting its statements on expanded nursing practice. In contrast, the AMA voiced its objection through one of its physician appointees. "There are nurses [in the casebook]," he reported somewhat nostalgically, "who are practicing family medicine—there is no other way to describe it. They are on the telephone, they make decisions, they make referrals; the physician essentially acts as a consultant. These nurses say, 'Gee, this is the kind of nursing we always wanted.' Yet it comes close to the ideal of the physician's practice of social medicine."[53]

For the AMA, the cases provided evidence for continued vigilance to maintain physicians' traditional role in primary care, and for its participation in the NJPC in order to monitor its activities. The AMA even requested and was denied a prepublication disclaimer explaining that the cases did not necessarily represent the views of the AMA.[54] Yet, in his introduction to the book, Max Parrott, AMA president in 1976, graciously acknowledged the benefits that "accrue to the patient, nurse, and physician when the nurse and physician utilize to the fullest their talents and knowledge."[55] But he minimized and reduced collaborative practice to an "effective working relationship."[56] He reminded readers of the physicians' role as head of the health care team, a responsibility they could not legally or ethically evade. He pointed out that the benefits of nurses and doctors in effective working relationships had yet to be fully realized and understood beyond the local level.[57] It was too soon, in other words, for the AMA to give its unequivocal support to a concept that had not been scientifically tested and analyzed to its satisfaction.

Nevertheless, the casebook was quite well received by nursing specialty groups and individual nurses, selling 6,500 copies by 1980 and receiving reviews in at least one nursing journal. But none of the medical journals—not even the official AMA *Journal of the American Medical Association*—reviewed the casebook.[58] Smoyak spoke to other kinds of publicity. "I think it [*Together*] got a lot of good press too, because what happened is the ones that we didn't select for the book, they got into newsletters, they got into local things."[59] It was also used in numerous practitioner programs and found its way into legislative offices. Grassroots practitioners closely identified with the individually negotiated cases while the larger organizations either ignored it or accepted it according to the organizations' political expediency.

The AMA and the NJPC Statements on Clinical Practice

Just as the ANA suffered financial difficulties in the late 1960s and early 1970s, from which it was only beginning to emerge, so did the AMA. In late 1974, to balance its budget, the AMA board of trustees undertook cost-cutting measures. It eliminated two councils and sixteen committees, including the committee on nursing and council on health manpower.[60] The NJPC became the only formal interface between the AMA and the ANA on substantive clinical and health policy issues.[61]

The reorganization, along with the growing number of nurse practitioners and physician assistants, the increasingly public issues of program funding through the manpower and training acts, reimbursement concerns, and action in the states over the legal boundaries of practice refocused the attention of the

AMA on the NJPC. By December 1976 the AMA established a new ad hoc committee to compile information on practice boundaries, program and practice costs, and, perhaps most important, the potential for the new providers to gain reimbursement.[62] In other words, the ad hoc committee collected some of the same data already solicited by the NJPC in its various projects, as well as the IOM and several federal agencies. The committee was not only going to re-create the database, but craft its own master narrative to justify a platform for future action against new practitioners.

One of the early issues the AMA ad hoc committee addressed was the series of pamphlets (entitled statements) the NJPC issued between 1974 and 1977. The five publications were disseminated to members of the ANA, the AMA, policy makers, and various specialty groups. The first two, "Statement on Medical and Nurse Practice Acts" and "Statement on Certification of Nurses and Physicians," issued in February 1974, elicited little controversy from the larger professional groups. In fact, the ANA used the second statement, which spoke to the need for professional groups to develop their own certification processes, to justify its stand on ANA-sponsored certification for advanced nursing specialty practice (see chapter 7). But the more recent releases, "Statement on Nursing Staffs in Hospitals" (pamphlet 3), "Statement on the Definition of Joint Collaborative Practice in Hospitals" (4), and "Statement on Joint Practice in Primary Care: Definition and Guidelines" (5), were far more controversial.

The commission work to date was more focused on nurses' expanded practice and the realignment of roles in primary care. The problem with this approach was that most nurses and physicians were associated with hospitals and received their training there. Relationships within these institutions, however, shaped those in clinics and private offices. By changing the focus of their gaze to the point of clinical socialization, the NJPC challenged professional interactions in a space sacred to both professions. Authority structures inside hospitals were highly ordered and formalized, and there was less room for flexibility and applying innovative practice models. Perhaps most critical, physicians claimed their contemporary status and cultural power from their place within the hospital and organizational structures, which were formulated to prioritize physicians' decision making and authority. Developing position statements on joint practice on a broader state-level scale was tolerated and probably more easily contained by those groups who felt threatened by them, but when the NJPC took on, in a national forum, the political structures in hospitals by offering alternative organizational paradigms, many in the medical and nursing professions found this to be an assault on their basic sense of patient care.

In the statement on nursing staffs in hospitals, the NJPC took on the imbalance of power between nurses and physicians in hospitals as a priority.[63] The language was broad and unspecific, perhaps because the commission itself could not come to a consensus on the details and merely wanted to start a dialogue. Perhaps it wanted to avoid the controversy that detailed language would spark, but this approach actually stimulated enormous debate within professional organizations over the impact of the statement. Or, perhaps the NJPC used statements 3 to 5 more broadly as a test case to assert its independence from the AMA in particular, as the ANA approved them from the beginning. Whatever the case, the discussions over the statements, while highly provocative and enormously energizing, illuminated the basic problem with the NJPC concept—the commission was autonomous only as long as its work paralleled the ideology of both professional supporting groups.[64]

The NJPC discussed the first draft statement, "Nurse/Physician Relationships in Hospitals," the precursor to the third and forth statements, at its March 1975 meeting.[65] This fairly vague and lengthy draft (more than six pages) was based on the standard and traditional Joint Commission of the Associated Hospitals (JCAH) definitions of medical and nursing services found in its 1973 hospital accreditation manual.[66] The JCAH statements distinctly contrasted professional accountability between medicine and nursing: the medical service was accountable to a governing body, for example, the board of trustees, and the nursing service was accountable to the hospital administration. Medicine was a self-governing body, and nursing was not. The March 1975 version used the strong language of "equity": "Equity must be established in the relationships [between medicine and nursing]."[67] This phrase was removed from the September 1975 version, but it contained even stronger, comparative language like "parity," "same responsibility," and "same accountability," and gave nursing staffs of the hospital "overall responsibility for the quality of nursing care provided to patients."[68] The aim of the statement can be seen in the reporting structure changes. In the March draft, nursing is accountable to itself and the administration; and by September, responsibility for nursing care shifted from administration to the institutional governing body, thereby providing the nursing service with autonomy, accountability, and authority parallel with medicine within the institutional structure.

Another part of the statement explicitly directed at the realignment of power was a short but critical phrase, "organized nursing service." This language concerned many physicians on the commission and the AMA, although it was neither new nor original and already part of the original JCAH nursing service definition. The phrase seemed to be illuminated as it was positioned in the draft, and in this context it seemed profoundly more nuanced and challenging. In effect, the language indicated a separate but equal nursing staff with its own administration and accountability structure that was independent from the "first organized staff [the medical staff]" of medical providers.[69]

The AMA recognized the shift in authority and power and swiftly responded, asking the NJPC to reconsider and explain the impact on patient care if a "second organized staff were established within hospitals."[70] But the AMA was primarily interested in how the change might affect the authority of the medical staff, and declined to endorse the statement until the NJPC resolved these issues. On the other hand, the ANA Congress for Nursing Practice approved the statements without question.[71] It fit the publications the ANA itself issued on nursing practice.

The commissioners continued to revise the statement, tightening the language, and separating the draft into two distinct documents (statements 3 and 4). But the underlying meaning of the original draft remained—medical and nursing services should have parallel and equal autonomy and accountability. The AMA again withheld its approval of all the statements (3 to 5) in June 1977 without further comment. Commissioner A. Alan Fischer reminded the others that, as he predicted, "organized medicine would not look kindly upon our definition [of nursing and primary care] and guidelines documents."[72] Commissioner Otto Page noted that certain words in statement 3 "were unnecessarily abrasive and that physicians were not as autonomous as the statement was saying nurses should be."[73] The comments by Page and Fischer are particularly illuminating given that they were probably two of the most liberal and longest-serving physicians remaining on the commission. For them to have concerns indicates the tenor of some of the debates going on within the commission itself and the national organizations.

The fifth statement, "Joint Practice in Primary Care," had the greatest potential impact for nurse practitioners. Based on the description of primary care from the interim report of the IOM and remarkably consistent with the announcements issued by the ANA on expanded practice, statement 5 focused on comprehensive care across the health and illness spectrum and advocated active patient participation in their own care. Patient activism was not a new concept, as the American Hospital Association implicitly accepted this role in a new Patients' Bill of Rights in 1972. But it did not include the right to quality nursing care or to the same specific responsibilities that were expected from physicians, such as the right to know their physician's name and receive information.[74] This is where the NJPC statements charted new territory.

Statements 4 and 5 explicitly included nursing as an essential part of the patient's care both in the hospital and in the primary-care setting. "Neither the nurse or the physician alone," statement 5 proposed, "is prepared to address adequately the broad range of health, medical, and nursing concerns of patients encountered in a primary care setting."[75] The idea of shared responsibility was also transferable to the hospital, where "there is acceptance by nurses and physicians of each other's clinical judgment in their respective professional field. Both are subject to *clinical challenge* in the patient's interest."[76] The NJPC statements writ large in a national forum what was happening informally in clinical practice across many levels and in many settings.

The American Academy of Family Physicians (AAFP) particularly took issue with statement 5. The group's negative response should not have been unexpected, as its 1974 position statement on family nurse practitioners can be seen as the inverse of the fifth statement. The academy recognized expanded nursing practice only as it contributed to the medical care of the patient, and only as an indirect dependent service that occurred under the direct supervision of a physician.[77] In his response to statement 5, George T. Wolff, chairman of the academy commission on health care services, noted that the AAFP board could not accept the statement for many reasons. One problem was the use of the term "providers," as it linked all of them in one group without prioritizing physicians. Second, the board disagreed with the definition of primary care, noting that no one on the board was familiar with the language the NJPC chose (actually chosen by the IOM and cited as such in the pamphlet), and noted that the board stood by its earlier 1974 statement.[78]

The NJPC voted to publish the third, fourth, and fifth statements in June 1977. Considering the earlier lack of AMA and AAFP acceptance, approval by the NJPC commissioners seems extraordinary. Alliances within the commission offer a partial explanation. The physician commissioners, especially those who believed in the ideal of joint practice, held enormous power even if they were somewhat critical of the products. The bylaws required a simple majority (nine) of the commissioners to vote for approval, and absent members to be polled for their votes but without power to amend the statements. Only ten of the sixteen commissioners attended the June 17 meeting when the statements were put to a vote, and half of the physician contingent was absent (four members), as was the AMA liaison staff member. The minutes of the meeting do not reflect the vote tally, but one can speculate on the alliances. If all eight nurses voted to approve the statements (and they usually voted together), only one of the eight physician commissioners was needed to join their block. Given Fischer and Page's traditional support, only one of their votes was needed to successfully pass the statements for publication.[79]

The AMA ad hoc committee on the functions and reimbursement of new health practitioners issued its earlier-mentioned report, which included a response to the statements, five months later in December 1977, through the Council on Medical Service. In particular, the council took issue with the three most recently published statements. It was "concerned that the dimensions of expanded nursing roles recommended in these reports [statements] differ significantly, not only from those developed by physician-nurse dialogue in specific specialty areas, but from those concurred by the AMA house of delegates in previous AMA statements and reports."[80] Two areas in particular concerned the council: the independence of nursing staffs in hospitals, which held nursing service accountable to the governing body without accountability to medicine, and the absence of the requirement for direct physician supervision of other types of practitioners. The council, in fact, was quite within its purview to question the language, however after the fact it might be. At this point the AMA still contributed more than $25,000 per year to support the commission, and perhaps more importantly ensured the viability of continued private funding by allowing money to be channeled through its foundation.

Concerns about the commission from the membership supported the AMA's stand on the statements. As some of the more traditional members became aware of their organization's support for the commission, they began to write to the AMA and published their objections in journal articles. "It annoys me," one physician noted, "that a portion of my AMA dues is paying for the advancement of these ideas through the National Joint Practice Commission. . . . I went to their [NJPC] annual meeting and came away in a state of shock. I never knew the intensity of the contempt that nurses in high positions feel for physicians as a group."[81]

Essentially, the council believed the current physician commissioners were not supporting established AMA policy. At the least, the council recommended, it was in the best interests of the trustees to increase the number of appointees closely associated with the AMA as delegates or committee members.[82] This actually was not that different from the way the nurse commissioners were appointed, as almost all of them were members of ANA councils or committees, so the council was not recommending anything out of line with current NJPC practices. The physician commissioners tried to assure their nurse colleagues that appointment of AMA officers or delegates did not imply attempted "control of the commission by the AMA, but rather is seen by that body as a means of direct communication between the AMA and the NJPC."[83] In fact, new appointees with closer ties to the leadership probably did improve the level of contact between the AMA and the commission, but it also necessarily changed its character and the tone of the discussions. The AMA appointees essentially became as ideological and dogmatic as their nursing counterparts.

From 1977 on, the spirit of the commission shifted. As supportive and more liberal founding member physicians, such as Otto Page, Alan Fischer, and

Robert Hoekelman, left the commission in late 1977, the AMA appointed new, more closely aligned members. In 1977, half of the medical contingents were new appointees: John H. Budd, Charles M. Cole, Holier Rasmussen, and Hubert A. Ritter. Cole and Ritter were trustees of the AMA, and Budd was a past president. Ritter was the current president of the AMA ERF, and Rasmussen was a member of the American Academy of Family Physicians, one of the specialty organizations that actively confronted the nurse practitioner movement.[84] As Ritter noted during a September 1978 meeting, "The AMA was upset with the way things were going. That's why we're [the new appointees] here."[85] For the nursing contingent, the ANA appointed Jean E. Steel, a member of the Congress for Nursing Practice and a forceful advocate for nurse practitioner practice.

Breaking Apart

Joint practice in general and nurse practitioners in particular became quite common in clinics and private practices by the end of the 1970s, and there was a declining urgency of the commission's mission to focus on expanded nursing roles and nurse-physician collaboration. Enduring issues, such as changes in practice acts or nurse-physician communication, were somewhat stale and failed to arouse the same sense of indignation and resentment present at the commission's founding. These issues, to be sure, remained problematic, and episodic action flared over them. Interest at the state level was somewhat mixed. Regional joint practice conferences in Oregon and Washington were cancelled because they failed to draw sufficient numbers of participants—especially physicians—but those held in Michigan and Connecticut were well attended.[86]

By the late 1970s, the commissioners were still actively debating their autonomy from the professional organizations. "If the commission . . . polarizes itself into one representing medicine and another representing nursing, not able to address itself to the mission of this commission, then I think we will revert to organizational policies which are not reconcilable," one commissioner noted.[87] Another commissioner astutely responded: "It seems to me the commission can act autonomously in the sense that it can arrive at whatever conclusion and recommendations it wishes to make. However, I can not conceive of its trying to implement these [recommendations] regardless of the parent organizations' approval or disapproval. After we do our autonomous thinking, then we have to sell it."[88] Clearly the commissioners now grasped the political reality of their positioning with respect to the parent associations and realized their attempts to reshape the dialogue surrounding practice, however innovative and necessary, were politically naïve. They were not working from a position of power; they could generate ideas but had no organizational structure nor constituency to actively lobby for them on their behalf. They also underestimated the AMA's attention and overestimated the ANA's aim to protect them.

The AMA response to the statements provides an example of its growing concern, as well as that of other organizations, with the implications of nurse practitioners on clinical practice. While the American Academy of Pediatrics understood there was an obvious need to formalize the physician-nurse relationship, it believed the "three statements by the NJPC did not accurately define the current or the possible future for collaborative practice for physicians and nurses."[89] The academy responded primarily to the challenges to clinical judgment, noting that "one person must still be in charge. . . . Traditionally, as well as educationally, this is the physician."[90] The statements, the AAP suggested, "appear to have been written by nurses or for nurses rather than as a joint effort by nurses and physicians."[91] The academy demanded they be rewritten so that they were acceptable to patients, although at this point many studies, including their own, showed high patient satisfaction with nurse practitioners.

The commissioners, even those with strong AMA leadership affiliation, still believed their primary focus was the facilitation of collaboration through joint practice—this was an enduring issue.[92] But Sammons now argued that joint practice was a "poor phrase," as it "raised physicians' hackles" and triggered many negative responses.[93] By speaking against it, Sammons and the AMA were not dismissing collaboration; they just had a different hierarchical sense of who should be directing the process and the language to be used. To them, it was quite simple: collaboration was a good objective as long as the traditional power differential remained in place and physicians controlled clinical practice. Joint practice implied shared power, and there was very little the AMA was inclined to split with other providers, particularly nurses. From the AMA's perspective, joint practice was not a viable concept unless all involved remembered the traditional adage, "There can only be one captain."[94] Nurses were valuable in their role as assistants to the physician, he said, noting "the AMA choose the wrong name in naming PAs 'physician's assistant' . . . the nurse is the physician's assistant."[95] There were few examples that better illustrated the dissonance among the physicians actively working in joint clinical practices and the AMA leadership and many AMA members.

Somewhat after the fact and in an act of appeasement, the NJPC in 1979 requested written comments from the sponsoring bodies on the five statements.[96] The ANA again approved the statements except for slight editorial comments. The AMA response was different this time and was crafted along the lines of those suggested earlier by the Council on Medical Service. The AMA also demanded that the NJPC reissue the statements in revised form. The problem with this request, however, was that the statements, particularly statement 5, were popular. Distributed for free through announcements in professional journals—including the newsletter of the American Academy of Pediatrics— the statements were now frequently requested by medical and nursing practitioners and schools of nursing. "You should know," William Schaffrath reported in 1979, that "a large number of them have been circulated to individuals and groups in the U.S. and Canada, and some even abroad. They continue to be cited in the professional literature, and ordered individually and in bulk."[97] By May 1979, the first and second statements sold 1,500 copies each, statements 3 and 4 sold 3,300 copies, and statement 5 sold 5,500 copies.[98] The question confronting the NJPC was whether reissuing an edited version, in light of the large numbers of copies already in circulation, would make a difference, or if the "inflammatory" nature of the original documents and the debate surrounding them would only heighten interest in them.[99] In the end, the commission voted to keep the original text.

The commission continued on, but its funding situation was tenuous as the operational support the Kellogg Foundation began in 1976 lasted only until 1980, and no new sources were in place or even looked promising.[100] Finally, in June 1980, the AMA, without much advance notice, voted to terminate NJPC financial support, effectively closing it down.[101] Although the AMA acted first, the ANA supported its decision but held back on its own action until after the AMA declaration. Earlier, in May 1980, the AMA and the ANA met to decide if the NJPC remained their appropriate liaison mechanism and whether it should be limited to completing its current work.[102] By this point, Myrtle Ayedelotte and James Sammons had been meeting formally and informally for the last two years to discuss better relationships between the professional organizations, and both concluded that the commission was no longer an effective mechanism. They believed they might work better together if they and their various boards or committees met on a more formal basis in their own liaison committee, without the middleman or facilitation of the NJPC. Many other issues were confronting the professions, such as proposed changes in Medicare payment systems, and in particular, both organizations were concerned with the discussions surrounding the prospective payment system later initiated in 1983.[103] Both professional organizations believed they could more effectively respond to these issues if they developed a stronger alliance outside of the NJPC.

The commission officially dissolved on January 1, 1981. Chairman Richard Chamberlin, one of the longer-lasting physician commissioners, noted in his final report that he had just reread *Abstract for Action* and urged the commissioners to reexamine the section containing the original recommendations for establishing the NJPC. Although written in 1970, he believed that the section was still timely, as the "generic problem of role articulation in health practice remains with us in 1980."[104]

This historical episode illustrates the multiple levels of politics surrounding clinical care during the 1970s. In particular, it documents the possibilities and problems of a bipartisan national commission financially dependent on the largesse of professional organizations that are typically at odds. When it was successful, the NJPC mirrored some of the most innovative local individual efforts occurring in clinical practice, creating forward-thinking strategies for working together. But the commissioners never fully managed the differences between politics in the clinical setting and those needed to move national agendas. The NJPC was financially and ideologically beholden to its benefactors, the AMA and ANA, and at a critical time addressed health policy issues that both organizations saw as their prerogative. The NJPC was, in fact, in the way of direct communication between the groups. Even without its own constituency it did its job too well and too publicly, imploding, literally, coming apart in 1981 as it moved faster and more creatively than its parent organizations.

Chapter 7

Triangulating Specialty Practice

The ANA, NAPNAP, and the American Academy of Pediatrics

The 1970s can be characterized by the proliferation of specialty nurse practitioner organizations, as practice based on clinical focus became the norm. These groups, with ready-made constituencies, proved more durable and enduring than the National Joint Practice Commission (NJPC). In general they gained resiliency from their experiences in the practice arena, which served as a mechanism to bring together nurses and physicians with similar clinical interest. The members were active nurses across all levels of education, from diploma schools to graduate programs, whose common characteristics were an independent and curious spirit and completion of a typically free nurse practitioner training program. They came from all classes but remained for the most part differentiated by race, as long-standing disparities and discrimination remained in both nursing and medical education in general despite the civil rights movement.[1]

The specialty groups claimed legitimacy to exist through their growing numbers and power in the practice arena as patients gained familiarity and were comfortable with their services. Specialization inferred a level of expertise and authority, as it did in medicine, and these types of organizations used this power. They shaped American health care by maneuvering to control how much and what kind of education was needed to provide health care to particular populations, how many specialty practitioners were needed, and who controlled their practice.

The National Association of Pediatric Nurse Associates and Practitioners (NAPNAP) was one of the earliest nurse practitioner specialty organizations. The pediatric specialty was initially the most popular area for typically female nurse practitioners, and until the mid- to late 1970s, there were more pediatric programs than any other type. Gender was a factor as the mostly male physician assistants gravitated to family and general medical practices. A more substantive explanation is that the first program at the University of Colorado in 1965 created by nurse Loretta Ford and physician Henry Silver was pediatric focused, and the American Academy of Pediatrics (AAP, or the academy) and pediatricians in general grasped the idea of a nurse associate (Silver's term for the nurse working in an expanded role) earlier than most of the other medical specialty groups. Early federal funding through the Nurse Training Acts (NTA) of 1971 and 1975 also targeted education for expanded roles for nurses prepared in pediatrics in response to the growing need for children's health care providers stimulated by the entitlement programs of the 1960s.

The story of NAPNAP encapsulates the politics of creating space for the specialty organizations after the development of the nurse practitioner movement in the 1960s to their broad public acceptance by the end of the 1970s. The organization early on became enmeshed in a triangulated relationship between the academy and the ANA, as the practice changes occurring at local clinical

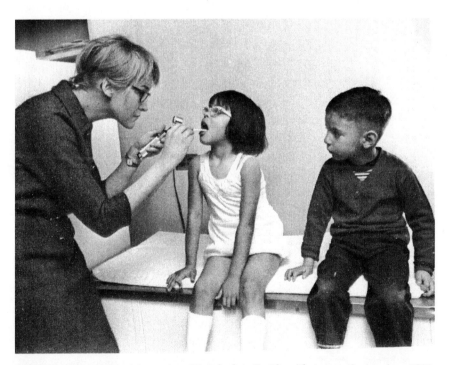

Photo 5. Nurse practitioner Ann Noordenbos Smith with two patients, circa 1965. Smith was a graduate of the University of Colorado nurse practitioner program. (Used with permission from Loretta Ford, personal collection.)

sites, "the bomb in the exam room," reverberated through the professional organizations, creating a grab for control.[2] These developments were the culmination of negotiations at the local levels in the context of individual practitioner and patient needs, federal funding for nurse practitioner and physician assistant programs before the development of national standards, and the professional organizations' efforts to manage their memberships and maintain their influence. This example explicates tensions both within professional groups and between medicine and nursing as they tried to dominate the process of defining the role (scope of practice), and establishing education and practice standards. All of these groups understood that those who controlled the standards controlled the practice arena.

Within the contextual fabric of NAPNAP, fast-moving, eager practitioners who negotiated the passageways of care for themselves and their patients provide a stark contrast to the more deliberate and slower professional nursing organization. The ANA, in the midst of the great financial, political, and philosophical instability of the 1970s, tried to be all things to all nurses, with neither the resources to do so nor a clear vision of the opportunities and hazards accompanying the complex reality of clinical practice. At the same time, the needs of individual pediatricians for educated allies were at odds with the sometimes duplicitous efforts of the academy as its leadership tried to reframe the rapidly changing health care environment and maintain control of pediatric practice.

The story of NAPNAP offers a counterpoint to the increasingly liberal and highly independent experiments nurses and doctors launched throughout the country at places such as the University of Colorado, University of Rochester, University of Florida at Gainesville, and University of Kentucky, to name a few, and in organizations such as the NJPC. These examples represent more localized arrangements with individual physician colleagues, and nurses in these places embraced their nursing roles in the context of expanded practice. They also appreciated their need for medical supervision, but did not require it for their legitimacy or power. Because the early NAPNAP leaders were developing a national organization that superseded local politics, they were dependent in their early years on physician groups that controlled greater resources and cultural authority.

The new nursing specialty groups learned early on to capitalize on the conflicting agendas of the medical and nursing organizations and to use the growing power embedded in expanded roles. Their emerging authority as increasingly skilled practitioners challenged the basic tenets of medical dominance and provided the evidence for policy makers that different models of patient care were viable. Study after study documented their safety, effectiveness, high patient satisfaction, and results comparable to physician care for particular groups of patients, such as the elderly, those in need of routine care, and the chronically ill.[3]

Fomenting Discontent

The academy was a clinical specialty organization as well as a professional and educational group, and could more easily imagine and develop different kinds of practice models than the ANA or the AMA. Academy members, especially Henry Silver of the University of Colorado, were part of a forceful vanguard of liberal-minded physicians who were early proponents of the pediatric nurse practitioner model. The organization's leaders chose to focus their efforts on harnessing the energy of this emerging group of providers by, first, trying to determine where they might fit within their constituents' practices, and second, how they might keep some sort of control over their growth. At this point, many individual academy members were curious about nurses' potential to formalize their expanded roles.[4]

In 1967, the academy surveyed its constituency to gain insight into their commitment to nurses' expanded role, gauge the extent of members' commitment to the idea of expending resources in this area, and to examine the distribution of task performances in private practice.[5] From the survey results, the academy determined that an "allied health worker" (a term that included all levels of nurses working in physician private practices) assuming an expanded patient care load only for health supervision could free up a minimum of 25 percent of the physician's time per week. If other aspects—including paper work, laboratory, technical tasks, and some illness care—were added to the allied health worker's responsibilities, at least 50 percent of a physician's time might be liberated.[6] The survey also revealed that less than half of pediatricians were utilizing nurses in expanded roles in their practices. Essentially, pediatricians realized the potential but were reluctant to delegate. Based on these results, the academy publicly issued the first of several policy statements supporting task delegation to the trained individual working under pediatrician supervision in 1969.[7]

At the same time, the academy published guidelines for training pediatric nurse associates. These principles were developed without formal nursing participation, an issue the ANA raised a few months later in January 1970 when it refused to endorse them.[8] Philosophically, the ANA believed it was inappropriate for a medical organization to be defining the scope of practice and educational requirements for a nursing role. At the least, the ANA wanted representation as part of a collaborative process.[9] It was a shaky start, resulting from naïve expectations on the part of the academy for ANA approval and a large dose of reality for the ANA when it grasped how rapidly the academy was moving with the pediatric nurse associate concept. But the two groups realized they had to work together, albeit cautiously, and agreed to form the joint ANA-AAP liaison committee, which met formally for the first time in February 1970.

Parallel Play and the Joint Guidelines

Perhaps the most important development resulting from the ANA-AAP liaison was the joint statement, "Guidelines on Short-Term Continuing Education Programs for Pediatric Nurse Associates," developed in 1970.[10] The guidelines stemmed from the original set the academy developed after its 1967 membership survey, and were re-presented to the newly formed joint ANA-AAP liaison committee at its February 1970 meeting. The ANA liaison nurses again strongly rejected the original academy statement, and reported their frustrations to the ANA board on the committee's progress. "It will be difficult to work through to a mutually acceptable statement," they reported, "and at the same time, move toward establishing the right of the nursing profession to determine its own scope of the practice of nursing."[11] But after much debate, posturing, and compromising on both sides, the liaison committee agreed on the joint guidelines eight months later and issued them in early 1971 in both association journals. They were widely distributed, with the ANA alone responding to over twenty thousand requests.[12]

Both organizations recognized the urgency to establish guidelines because numerous training programs for nurse practitioners and physician assistants were opening in rapid, entrepreneurial fashion in places as diverse as private physicians' offices and public health departments. The mechanism for most nurse practitioner education at the time was short-term continuing education or certificate programs, such as those offered initially at the University of Colorado and University of Rochester, rather than collegiate programs. And similar to the concerns of Eugene Stead of Duke University about physician assistant programs, both the academy and the ANA were worried about quality and control. No standards existed, and there were at least twenty-two training programs by 1968, and by 1972, more than thirty-five were in planning stages around the country.[13] Perhaps more important, both organizations wanted to have some say over the curricula and who controlled them.

Considering the ANA's long history of suspicion of medical organizations, its ability to collaborate with the academy on the guidelines is intriguing. In fact, one wonders how the two groups achieved consensus, except for the threat of each organization going it alone. Despite the disciplinary complexities flavoring the negotiations, the guidelines were quite progressive for the time. They also provided a point for much backsliding over the next few years. Both the ANA and the academy agreed that the "performance of these new technical skills . . . should be viewed as increasing the sources from which the nurse gathers data for making nursing assessment, as a basis for diagnoses and action, thus contributing directly to comprehensive nursing." "Nurses," the guidelines continued, "must have the opportunity to be engaged in independent as well as cooperative decision-making."[14] The guidelines addressed basic educational programs specifying that all, where possible, be developed jointly with nursing and medical collaboration, and supported in but not limited to placement in collegiate nursing programs.[15] These sentiments were in opposition to those issued by the AMA, which still advocated a dependent relationship with nursing and prioritized diploma training.[16]

The guidelines satisfied both groups because each held particular perceptions of their meaning and implications—a powerful sort of parallel-play exemplar. The language of the guidelines centered on provider quality and patient safety, but the underlying rhetoric and subtext focused on the issues of practice boundaries and control. They acknowledged the independent practice of nursing and nurses' ability to determine what was and wasn't nursing care, and did not oppose placement of nurse practitioner programs in collegiate nursing programs, the direction the ANA hoped nursing education in general might follow. The academy, on the other hand, gained a commitment from the ANA to include physicians in the education of nurses in expanded roles and had no requirement for pediatric nurse practitioner education to reside in academic programs.

In the next few years, however, the ANA, the academy, and later, NAPNAP reinterpreted portions of the guidelines, and each group felt betrayed by the others' misperception of the original intent. But in fact the guidelines, developed in good faith, fell victim to turf wars, miscommunication, and perhaps a plain lack of civility on all sides. The most contentious issues proved to be independent practice, the need for direct physician supervision of the pediatric nurse practitioner, and control over education. In any event, the guidelines were the first step toward standardizing the training of nurse practitioners. The practice and supervision issues continue to be the most controversial issues today.

Growing and Controlling NAPNAP

On May 2, 1973, pediatric nurses, physicians, and industry representatives came together in Columbus, Ohio, at a meeting called by Janet McCleery, a pediatric nurse associate.[17] Coincidentally, academy president Robert Heavenrich was also present. He later claimed, when confronted by the ANA leadership about attendance, that he "happened to be visiting Children's Hospital [in Columbus, Ohio] where the meeting took place and [he] spoke briefly to the group after lunch."[18] Actually the meeting took place at a hotel and Heavenrich had the location wrong, which compounded an already existing ANA furor over the meeting. It had been invited but declined to go.[19]

From this first preorganizational meeting came plans to create a nursing specialty group, NAPNAP, that focused on the primary health care needs of children.[20] Although the group discussed several affiliation options, the pediatric nurse practitioners from the beginning chose the academy rather than ANA.[21] They were not alone in seeking support from physicians for their organization as several other groups organized with their physician counterparts instead of the ANA.[22] Medical specialty organizations, sensing the economic and professional promise of "educated allies" and realizing an opportunity for larger numbers of conference registrants, increasingly held nursing sections at their annual meetings. And although one can speculate that the meetings served as ways to manipulate nursing, in fact, professional nursing itself was not rising to the challenge. Nurses seeking out new clinical knowledge had few other places to go.

Given the ANA's slow response to clinical issues and its history of hostility toward specialty groups, it is not surprising that Janet McCleery and her nursing colleagues looked to the academy and not the ANA for help when they created their organization. The early leaders attended academy meetings, saw the organizational support structure in action, and felt their nascent group could benefit from its organizational expertise. The AAP also offered a channel to industry contacts that already provided support for nursing clinical sections at academy meetings. Many health care companies used pediatric nurses as consultants, and it was these nurses, such as Ann McRedmond, the nursing consultant from Ross Laboratories, who opened communication with the pediatric nurse practitioners to start an organization.

All of the founding nurses were also familiar with the possibilities offered by collaboration with physicians. Working with the academy was similar to practicing with their individual physician colleagues—they were welcomed. Perhaps they were not equal partners, but pediatric nurse practitioners could learn and get along. As Robert Heavenrich noted to Janet McCleery after the Ohio meeting, "The AAP would welcome you [NAPNAP] if that is the desire of your organization, or perhaps your home will be with the Nursing Association. Or even still, you may stand on your own. At any rate, we look forward to a close affiliation with you."[23]

The formation of NAPNAP and its choice for affiliation and alliance occurred against the backdrop of the 1970 guidelines. Although the ANA and the academy could work together, the ANA mistrusted the physician group and felt it needed to remain vigilant to preserve nursing's practice prerogative. From the ANA perspective, the academy's production of education and practice guidelines without consulting nursing was just one example of continued attempts by medicine to control nursing practice. This theme pervaded relationships between the ANA and medical professional organizations in the 1960s and 1970s, and it was not tempered by NAPNAP's inclination toward the academy.

But from the perspective of many of the early founders of NAPNAP, the ANA was not to be trusted. Many diploma nurses felt betrayed by the ANA's policy statement in 1965 proposing the baccalaureate degree as the required entry level for nursing practice. Their distrust was compounded by the guidelines for short-term programs that supported collegiate education for nurse practitioners.[24] In this context, diploma training was an insignificant benchmark for practice and required that nurses trained in this way restart their nursing education. Most of the early leaders of NAPNAP and, in fact, most nurse practitioners were diploma graduates who received their advanced clinical training in short-term certificate programs rather than collegiate programs. As NAPNAP leader Sally Walsh noted, "Diploma nurses may not have felt acknowledged by the ANA." She went on, noting the "ANA made a major mistake by invalidating [their] hard work."[25]

The entry into practice issue was only one, perhaps rhetorical, issue. NAP-NAP founders also believed the ANA saw their small group as a threat, and their perceptions were not far off the mark. In fact, the ANA was quite concerned about emerging specialty organizations (chapter 5), even before NAPNAP. President Hildegard Peplau highlighted her concerns over the "emergence of splinter groups" in 1972.[26] Around the same time, Pearl Dunkley, chair of the ANA Nursing Practice Department, sought clarification about discouraging or encouraging the formation of specialty groups. How, she asked, can the ANA deal effectively with those that are formed under the aegis of other organizations?[27] These were critical issues for the ANA. How could it keep control of professional nursing if each special interest independently formed its own constituent group?

During this time, there were many ANA investigative meetings to obtain information about nurse practitioners and the growing specialty organizations they tended to join, and to see if they could develop better communication channels with them. In April 1972 the ANA board of directors met with the executive directors of nurse practitioner and other specialty groups to generate ideas for organizational structures they might find agreeable.[28] At the 1972 national convention, the ANA held a "rap session" for pediatric nurse practitioners, with both nurses and pediatricians present, and discussed their ideas for an internal mechanism to meet pediatric nurse practitioner education and affiliation requests. Hildegard Peplau even addressed expanded nursing practice in her address to the ANA house of delegates. "All of us know that registered nurses can do more than many situations permit," she noted. "Nurses in schools, industry, clinics, and health centers, in ghettos, Indian reservations, rural areas, nursing homes, military installations and the like have illustrated this fact for many years—long before Medicare, Medicaid and the Physician Assistant."[29]

The ANA also met with independent practitioners on September 18, 1972, to discuss the definition of roles, legal problems associated with expanded practice, the need to purchase malpractice insurance, and the possibility of third-party payments.[30] The first formal meeting of the ANA and nurse practitioner specialty groups occurred in Kansas City, Missouri, in November 1972, before NAPNAP was founded, and the groups identified common interests such as certification, accreditation of education programs, and defining the expanding nursing role.[31] Clearly the ANA was paying attention to nurse practitioners and was trying to gain a strategic position with these groups, not only for control, but because there were obvious critical issues associated with their practice roles for which the ANA could offer support.

As the academy proposed affiliated membership and before the ANA met with specialty nursing leaders, the American Association of Critical Care Nurses invited nineteen national specialty nursing organizations to develop strategies to communicate and work better with the ANA. The groups were demoralized by their antagonistic relationships, and were also fearful the lack of unity in nursing might encourage unionization efforts percolating during this time in various states.[32] In January 1973, thirteen of the nineteen invited specialty organizations met together with the ANA for the first time in San Clemente, California, a gathering that was designated the first national congress (and later, National Federation of Specialty Nursing Organizations).[33] For many years the ANA viewed the federation alternatively as a threat and as a way to keep in touch with the workings of other nursing organizations, but eventually it came to value its work and efforts to bring together disparate nursing organizations into a powerful organizing and political body. The overwhelming issue discussed at the ensuing meetings over the next ten years was certification for practice, what it meant, and how the organizations and the ANA could develop a meaningful and mutually beneficial process. This was one of the most critical concerns for NAPNAP leaders in their affiliation negotiations with the ANA and the academy.

Between Nursing and Medicine

Despite its misgivings about the ANA, the NAPNAP organizing group met with both ANA and academy representatives in Denver, Colorado, in August 1973 to consider affiliation direction. There the group learned the ANA had already created a council of nurse practitioners in pediatric nursing under the new Maternal-Child Health Nursing (MCHN) division in February 1973, and this council was scheduled to meet at the ANA convention in September that year.[34] It was here that the ANA saw NAPNAP fitting into its organizational structure, and this should not have surprised NAPNAP founders. At least eight pediatric nurse practitioner special interest groups already existed within state nursing organizations, anticipating ANA's formation of a council.[35] Janet McCleery, the first NAP-NAP president, knew the ANA was planning to implement this structure as early as March 1973, when she learned about it from fellow pediatric nurse practitioner Patricia Stewart. The ANA discussed its plans in November 1972 with the ANA-AAP liaison committee, of which Stewart was a member.[36] This knowledge probably stimulated the May 1973 Ohio meeting from which NAPNAP emerged.

NAPNAP saw the council structure as a direct challenge to its existence as a new organization, and indirectly, worried it would compete with NAPNAP's claims to speak for pediatric nurse practitioner practice. But NAPNAP did not have much to fear at this point, as the ANA designed an arrangement that offered the councils little voice within the organization. The ANA refused to assure NAPNAP of pediatric nurse practitioner membership on the larger and powerful division of maternal child health executive council where policy making occurred, nor would NAPNAP as an organization have a representative on the board of directors.[37] Within this new structure of divisions, the pediatric nurse practitioner council was somewhat powerless. It could only communicate with other organizations, such as the academy, through the ANA-AAP liaison committee (consisting of division chairs and organization executive committees and staff), rather than directly, as was the norm in the practice arena and in earlier academy correspondence. Furthermore, NAPNAP could be part of the ANA structure only through its individual members rather than as an independent group. Finally, the pediatric nurse practitioner council would not have its own newsletter. Its announcements would be subsumed into practice section newsletters.[38]

For its part, the academy offered viability to NAPNAP because it allowed affiliation as an organization. NAPNAP could, if it remained independent, establish a liaison with the academy, its members could attend academy workshops, joint regional and local conferences could be initiated, and NAPNAP officers could be appointed to academy committees as organization representatives. But unlike the ANA offer, NAPNAP members could never gain the full rights and privileges of the academy unless the organization changed its bylaws and allowed nonphysicians as members.[39]

At the first NAPNAP general meeting on October 23, 1973, the membership voted unanimously to form an independent organization with loose affiliation with the academy. The meeting took place in facilities provided in conjunction with the annual academy meeting, and Walter Campbell, director of the department of community services of the academy, was the keynote speaker.[40] Both the ANA and the academy presented affiliation options and participated fully in the meeting. Barbara Bishop, a pediatric nurse practitioner and a representative of the ANA pediatric nurse practitioner council, and academy representatives Henry Silver, Robert Hoekelman (also a NJPC member and University of Rochester pediatrician), and Walter Campbell were noted as discussants from the floor in the meeting minutes.[41] Although NAPNAP tried to work with the ANA, as pediatric nurse practitioner Sally Walsh noted, "No one wanted to wait for permission [from the ANA]," no one wanted to "start at the bottom of the organization and work up."[42] Pediatric nurse practitioner Margaret Hicks reflected on the perception of the ANA leadership and the pediatric nurse practitioner entrepreneurial spirit: "We were all very young and didn't want older people telling us what to do."[43]

Through the council structure, the ANA believed it was responding in part to its membership's clamor for help in clinical settings. But the explosion in the late 1960s and early 1970s of specialty nursing organizations formed by nurses who felt the ANA was too slow to meet their needs for clinical knowledge may have been the most important incentive. The ANA correctly believed that specialty groups would eventually siphon off membership at a critical time, when declining membership and a bleak financial situation put the organization in serious jeopardy. Patricia McAtee, a NAPNAP leader, noted later, "The ANA hold on nursing is weaker now than it has ever been. It represents only 21 percent of all nurses. That's a shaky position. No wonder they won't recognize other nurses [organizations]."[44]

Emerging specialty organizations represented a critical constituency, but it was the ANA core membership—the generalist nurses who joined the association primarily through the state associations—who really needed to be satisfied. There was a growing discontent within this group who believed the ANA was focusing too many resources on nurse practitioners.[45] For these core members generalist practice and work place issues were key. The ANA feared losing the specialty contingent, but it was even more concerned about its general constituency, its largest group. There was less inclination for the ANA to worry about offending the specialty groups as long as it could keep core membership satisfied, nor did the ANA have the punitive power to punish those who chose to leave. One of the only ways the ANA could fight back without alienating this constituency was to support the clinical special interest groups that broadly included staff nurses and nurse practitioners.

Though a young organization, NAPNAP founders realized early on that they were in a strong position with the ANA. They were part of a growing movement of nurse practitioners and specialty clinicians and could choose their professional affiliation because medical organizations were clearly enticing them with financial and organizational resources. The ANA's relative weakness at the time, due in part to finances and the sheer number of groups with whom it had to negotiate, prevented it from slowing the march of new specialty organizations that were developing important political currency to determine their own courses. Loyalty to nursing was important to the NAPNAP leaders, as they identified as nurses, but it did not extend to the ANA. Patricia McAtee observed at the 1974 annual ANA convention: "The most difficult thing to see in a national organization is how really powerful you are [NAPNAP] and then to wield that power wisely and sparingly to attain goals. Make no mistake about how really powerful the PNP organization could be [as] a spokeswoman for the health needs of children. I think the ANA is more responsive *because* of NAPNAP and that we can use that to gain the things needed in the future."[46]

There were indeed several major "future needs" that NAPNAP and other specialty organizations required for successful and fruitful survival: accreditation of nurse practitioner programs, generation of a scope of practice, and certification for practice. These issues led directly to the questions of who controlled and defined nursing practice and were illustrative of the debates going on between medicine and nursing and among nurses themselves across all specialties, beyond the scope of the larger professional organizations. Who controlled practice? Was it the larger professional organization, the specialty nursing organization, the individual practitioner, the state, or all of the above? And what did control mean in economic, cultural, and legal terms to individual nurses practicing in the field?

Ultimately, NAPNAP's decision to affiliate with the academy meant the ANA had to negotiate with yet another new nursing organization to continue advancing its aims of professional autonomy and higher qualifications for practice. These issues, although positioning nursing in general to control practice, put the organization in direct opposition to many of the specialty groups it was trying to pacify. Not only that, but the ANA had to move much more quickly to implement its programs before the specialty organizations siphoned off membership. The organization was not up to, nor skilled at, either of these tasks.

Certification Location

Many professional organizations ostensibly use certification mechanisms to protect the public by assuring a certain level of service quality, but it's also a way to control entry into a profession and to help define it. The American Association of Nurse Anesthetists began certifying in 1946 and the American College of Nurse-Midwives in 1971. Both of these programs were independent of the ANA. In the triangulation of the ANA, academy, and NAPNAP, the battle for control over certification was highly contentious and more reflective of the wider national conflict for control over nurse practitioner practice rather than issues of quality, although in this instance quality and control became rhetorically inseparable.

Although the ANA had been working on certification for over a decade, albeit in interrupted stages, it began to move quite rapidly to put a process in place in the early 1970s, stimulated by a number of factors. Part of the reason for this increased activity was the demand from nurses who had already completed short-term pediatric nurse practitioner courses. In June 1971, five hundred nurses and thirty-six physicians participated in a regional conference in Boston on pediatric nurse associate programs, jointly sponsored by the ANA and the academy. Most of their discussions centered on demands for some form of certification and recognition.[47] The ANA was also prompted by the National Board of Medical Examiners' invitation to nurses to take the physician assistant certification exam in July 1973. This occurred during a critical time for the ANA as it struggled to differentiate the nurse practitioner from the physician assistant and tried to stake out nursing's patient care territory (chapter 4). Its rapid response to the board's invitation was not only a strong rebuke, it was the first time the ANA forcefully and publicly took a stand on nurse practitioner practice. Nurse practitioners "have the responsibility and authority to delineate *their own* scope of practice," the ANA noted. "The law does not place the registered nurse under the direct supervision of any other health discipline."[48] This statement, later reflected and reinforced in the November 1973 draft "Scope of Practice for Pediatric Nurse Practitioners," was an early, if little noticed, foreshadowing of heightened discord between the ANA and the academy.[49]

The ANA also saw the national board's invitation as an untimely intrusion and in competition with its own initiatives. The ANA already had an exam in development, and in November 1973 it released new position papers and brochures introducing it, as well as a program accreditation process and scope of practice.[50] In fact, the ANA began to address the question of certification for clinical practice in 1958, when it developed ways to recognize superior achievement and clinical performance through goal 2 (chapter 5). In 1960, the ANA Intersection Committee on Recognition of Superior Performance established a twelve-year timetable to develop a recognition program that included certification for practice excellence. By December 1968, five interim certification boards were in place developing examinations coinciding with the newly formed practice divisions. At this point, certification was not linked to educational level or type of nursing practice, nor was it planned at first for advanced or "expanded" practice nurses. The exams were, however, intended to define excellence in specialty practice for practitioners of nursing, the language initially used by the interim certification boards to describe all practicing nurses, including nurse practitioners.[51]

But shortly after NAPNAP formed, the ANA converted the exam already in development by the interim certification board to certify nurse practitioners. After a year's delay due to financial problems and terrible infighting between the highly partisan staff and the ANA president, Hildegard Peplau, the ANA formally announced its pediatric nurse practitioner certification program in November 1973, to be administered by the Educational Testing Service of Princeton, New Jersey, and mailed guidelines for certification to the membership.[52]

The certification exam announcement immediately generated a great deal of controversy and animosity from both the academy and NAPNAP, which claimed they had not been consulted. In fact, the ANA had communicated since late 1971 with the academy on the certification process for pediatric nurses through the ANA-AAP liaison committee, even before the ANA formed the Council of Pediatric Nurse Practitioners. In November 1971, the liaison committee unanimously passed a resolution supporting the "ANA plan for certification for excellence in clinical nursing practice."[53] At the April 1972 liaison committee meeting, the ANA reported on its progress and "attention was called to the fact that a qualifying exam was to be prepared by ANA in consultation with academy, rather than prepared together with equal participation."[54] The committee members generally agreed that the ANA must take the initiative and major responsibility for certification.

The academy appointed pediatricians to participate in exam preparation via the Blueprint Committee (later renamed the Test Specifications Committee), focusing particularly on aspects of pediatric nurse practitioner practice traditionally considered the domain of the physician. The ANA Test Specifications Committee met in July and December 1973, and included an academy representative, two pediatric nurse practitioners in active practice, and two directors of pediatric nurse practitioner programs. This group, along with eighteen additional item writers (including four physicians), developed and refined the examination.[55]

As early as February 1973, the ANA reported to the liaison committee that the exam would be ready to be administered in the spring of 1974. The academy expressed some concern that it could not be represented on the certification board, an independent group that supported the process and had decision-making and policy-enforcing power. But the ANA pointed out that its bylaws only allowed association members to serve. In spite of the two-year collaboration process, the academy's request and the ANA's use of the bylaws to refuse it indicated the liaison was perhaps more fragile than the committee admitted.[56] Nevertheless, the ANA still believed it had the general support of the academy for its certification program. The liaison committee even began to develop pediatric nurse practitioner program accreditation standards so it could validate the nurse practitioners who would take the exam.[57]

There were additional, and in fact quite obvious, signs, however, that a disconnect existed between the liaison committee and the two larger parent organizations. Both had been circling the certification issue in their own ways, culminating in a great deal of activity that only slowly filtered down to the liaison structure. In June 1972, the academy announced plans for the "development of a national testing program as a minimal level of PNA certification."[58] In response, the ANA   which occurred
on Augus   its examination
proposal   rtification exam,
and reiter   ee meetings.[59]
   Despi   nsultation of the
joint liais   ification process
through a   P convention in
october 1   n, the members
learned a   fellows. Robert
Hoekelma   e academy leadership, an   ecided to certify
PNPs."[60]   e noted, "PNPs
[should]   member of the
National   nsistent with a
statement   February 1974.
NAPNAP's response to the academy's plan for certification was muted.[62]

The ANA and the academy were working at cross-purposes, and it is unclear if their efforts were the results of missed or misconstrued communication opportunities, deliberate attempts to control the certification process, or a combination of the two. It is clear, however, that both groups believed the certification process to be a highly symbolic and powerful issue. And each wanted to control the process.

Collapse of the Liaison

Unlike the earlier 1972 episode when the academy first announced its efforts to put a certification exam in place, the situation was not remediable. The pediatrician component of the liaison committee misunderstood its policy-making capacity and its power to commit the academy to a supportive role in the ANA certification process. Although the physician members communicated regularly with the executive and manpower committee of the academy, it was not always a two-way conversation. Perhaps the academy executive committee never saw the work of the liaison committee as anything more than a way of keeping track of rival ANA initiatives. Even more problematic, the academy was developing its own independent exam process without communicating with the liaison committee members or the ANA. Whatever the reasons, NAPNAP and the academy seemed to be genuinely surprised when the ANA announced its certification plans in November of 1973, shortly after NAPNAP's first meeting and Hoekelman's disclosure. McCleery noted, "All of us assumed the certification process was a *joint* effort between AAP and ANA; however, ANA did 'their own thing' without anyone's collaboration."[63] It is unclear why McCleery was misinformed as her academy counterparts on the liaison committee were actively engaged in the ANA exam process.

The ANA-AAP liason continued to erode. On January 16, 1974, in a move that surprised even the physician members of the liaison committee, the academy announced to its fellows and pediatric nurse associates that it was severing its connection with the ANA certification program for pediatric nurse practitioners. The announcement of the ANA certification program itself was not the only issue prompting the academy disassociation. It wanted a clearer delineation of its participation and influence in the certification process, and, in effect, the academy believed it was losing control. Shortly before the January 1974 letter, the academy again demanded representation on the interim certification board and on any similar committee working at the policy-making level toward accrediting pediatric nurse practitioner programs, but was again denied.[64] This was an important issue for the academy, not as a place for NAPNAP to have a voice, but for its own participation.

A more critical subtext in the letter was the academy's disgruntlement over the November 1973 draft of the ANA scope of practice for nurse practitioners, issued at the same time as the certification plans, that defined the boundaries of practice, including the level of education, what they could do, and who was responsible for their actions. Confusion and disagreement about the nurse practitioner concept in general writ large the issues fueling the conflicts between the ANA, academy, and NAPNAP from the beginning; the scope of practice was situated at the heart of the certification debate. In fact, each group defined a different practitioner—one that fit the needs and ideology of the particular professions and organizations.

In response to the ANA scope of practice document, the academy developed its own for pediatric nurse practitioners in early 1974, with input from NAPNAP, as a companion document to the disassociation letter. The AAP/NAPNAP scope, as it was later called, described the nurse practitioner as a nurse with other training in skills and knowledge traditionally in the medical realm, providing both medical and nursing services. Physicians were responsible for teaching and evaluating medical content. "Nursing," the academy reminded its membership, "should not be involved in either," nor should it define which group owned particular skills or where they could practice.[65] To NAPNAP, the nurse associate was "first a nurse," but because the associate took on medical tasks and services after the appropriate education, the provision of these services was no longer in the nurse's realm. They remained "the responsibility of the physician and must be performed under his direction, supervision and review."[66] In contrast, the ANA scope established the practitioner's independence: "The services offered by a PNP . . . reflects the nurse's ability to independently make and act on decisions related to health status. . . . She is accountable for her decisions and actions to the child, the family, herself, her peer group, and her colleagues."[67] There was no room or need in the ANA's definition for medical supervision.

Individual NAPNAP and academy members did not necessarily agree with the AAP/NAPNAP scope statements either. As one pediatric nurse associate wrote about the supervisory statement found in the AAP/NAPNAP scope of practice, "I feel this statement denies that the nursing profession has anything unique to offer to the role. . . . To me, harmony means collaboration between professions, not control of one profession by another, as has been described."[68] Another nurse practitioner added, "It seems to me that this statement from the academy, with NAPNAP support, serves once again to make nurses dependent on the medical profession."[69]

Members of the academy countered with their own criticisms. One physician wrote: "I feel that the only role that these people can play is in areas like Appalachia and in large cities where physicians are overwhelmed. . . . Most of the pediatricians with whom I have been associated who foster the philosophy of the PNP or pediatric nurse associate are those who really do not enjoy the general practice of pediatrics and like to delegate as much of the care as possible."[70] Another physician noted, "I cannot see continuing to call these people nurses. I feel they are a different kind of practitioner. If we continue to call them nurses, we accept a legacy from nursing which in the long run will interfere with their functioning."[71] If "these people" were called something else, the writer implied, the academy could develop a role with its own culture, standards, and responsibilities, and perhaps more control by pediatricians. Not all academy members felt this way, especially those who included pediatric nurse practitioners in their practice. A member of the Committee on Pediatric Manpower who worked with pediatric nurse practitioners, noted, "There is no better way to deliver quality health care."[72]

The academy used the certification exam as a cloaking device to shield its disapproval of the ANA's language in the scope recognizing nurse practitioner autonomy.[73] Couching its concerns in the rhetoric of patient safety, Robert Frazier, the academy executive director, wrote to the members, "It is now apparent that the academy's proposal of a pediatric nurse associate [PNA] to work under physician direction in performance of both nursing services and delegated medical tasks is not supported by the ANA. . . . The academy has the obligation to insure that the PNA is adequately trained in a program utilizing physician teaching or supervision for medical matters."[74] In fact, the academy was not the only physician organization that responded to the ANA scope documents. The American Academy of Family Physicians (AAFP) issued a position statement on family nurse practitioners in July 1974 in response to both the National Joint Practice Commission statements and the ANA scope document. The AAFP statement echoed, albeit even more forcefully, the language of the academy and was probably developed in conjunction with them. "Under no circumstances," the AAFP wrote, "should the family nurse practitioner examine and treat patients as an independent practitioner . . . and should not be employed . . . except under the direct supervision of a physician."[75]

In the disassociation letter, the AAP alerted its constituencies that it would develop its own certification process "with those agencies and organizations sharing a similar understanding of the role of the PNA," not necessarily naming NAPNAP as its partner, although its participation may have been assumed by both groups.[76] In fact, NAPNAP leaders only learned during a board meeting in mid-January 1974 that the academy dissolved its liaison committee with the ANA and that the ANA announced its pediatric nurse practitioner certification. Neither the ANA nor the academy communicated with them.[77] At the board meeting, NAPNAP leaders decided not to support the ANA process and met with the academy almost two weeks later, on January 31, 1974, to discuss certification, a process the academy had already begun.[78]

Now there were to be two different certification exams—one administered by nurses and one by physicians and nurses—and although NAPNAP was intimately involved in the exam, the academy for the most part controlled the tone and scope of the process. It had the resources—a central office, finances, and a flexible organizational structure—to support a rapid development process. By aligning itself with the academy on this issue, NAPNAP served, in a sense, as the academy proxy for control over pediatric nurse practitioner practice, at least for the first decade of its existence, and provided a great deal of legitimacy to the academy's efforts. In exchange, NAPNAP achieved representation on many academy committees at a level not promised by the ANA—indeed, the ANA did not want NAPNAP included in the liaison or other high-level policy-making committees—and obtained resources for organizational survival from both the academy and industry supporters on a magnitude the ANA could not match.

NAPNAP's alliance with the academy was critical in the battle for control of practice. Pediatric nurse practitioners were desperate for a certification exam as a way to formally document their competency and legitimacy, both to their patients and to their supervising pediatricians. Depending on the philosophy of the certifying organization, the credential indicated either a basic level of competency needed for practice, or the achievement of excellence, all providing different levels of patient safety assurances. The sponsoring agency also gained authority and power by controlling the gateways to practice through the development of the scope. One nurse practitioner succinctly noted, "If the pediatric nurse associate cannot be certified by the AAP I believe they [AAP] will establish training programs for non-nurses—as the physician assistant programs already in existence—whom they will be able to examine and certify—the pediatric nurse associate will be unable to find a job."[79] In fact, one percent of eligible nurse practitioners accepted the invitation of the National Board of Medical Examiners (NBME) to take the first physician assistant exam in December 1973, so the threat was real. The ANA proceeded with its own examination in May 1974, with fewer nurse practitioner participants than for the NBME exam. The ANA offered two certification examinations that year, one for geriatric nursing and one for pediatric nursing in ambulatory care. A total of ninety-nine nurses took the exams, and it is difficult to factor out the number of participants for each. Even if there was an equal split, the NBME was a more popular exam.[80]

Practicing pediatric nurse practitioners found themselves the focus of attention of several groups. The ANA mailed certification program brochures to its pediatric nurse practitioner council membership and members of the MCHN division. Practitioners also received the academy disassociation letter around the same time. Additionally, pediatric nurse practitioners and fellows of the academy received a memo from ANA executive director Eileen Jacobi about ten days later refuting the academy letter and outlining the ANA's collaborative efforts through the liaison committee to develop an exam process and its many consultations with the academy executive committee.[81]

Not surprisingly, pediatric nurse practitioners themselves found the actions of NAPNAP, the academy, and the ANA confusing and quite troubling, to say the least. Many found the ANA certification program itself confusing, unclear, and astutely understood that it was geared toward generalist nurses (those not working in expanded roles, such as traditional office nurses, hospital nurses, and the original targets of the exam) rather than pediatric nurse practitioners, although it was billed as a way to document expertise. Many also recognized a power play when they saw one, and the ANA, academy, and NAPNAP soon received letters from concerned pediatric nurse practitioners. A group from Jacobi Hospital in New York City declared to Janet McCleery:

> We have serious questions about the validity of the certification procedure produced by the ANA. . . . We are very interested in what position NAP-NAP is taking. . . . We are aware that there is some discrepancy between what the ANA-AAP liaison committee and what the academy executive board is saying. We feel strongly that as nurse practitioners we do not want to get caught in the middle of a political feud over who has jurisdiction over our practice. As you can tell . . . we are not impressed with the ANA's credentials in this area nor do we feel that the AAP has the sole right to govern our practice.[82]

A nurse from Pennsylvania wrote to Robert Frazier of the academy: "I cannot believe that the committees from our two organizations could not come to some agreement that is acceptable to both. None of us needs the confusion, uncertainty and expense that will come out of two programs of certification. I would greatly appreciate knowing more about the specific areas of disagreement. I realize there are two sides to this question and I am also asking the ANA to respond. . . . Surely the issue is important enough to warrant a second attempt at resolution."[83] A pediatric nurse practitioner student from Loma Linda University phrased the problem more succinctly: "Is your letter to be viewed as a struggle to see who will have the right to certify the PNP—the AAP or the ANA?"[84]

For a very young organization, NAPNAP quickly developed a loyal following, one that shared its concerns about ANA certification in particular and the organization in general. "For my part," a pediatric nurse associate noted, "I feel that ANA has lost to the organization an entire group now functioning as pediatric nurse associates or practitioners. I am ready for NAPNAP to work with the academy in preparing for certification."[85] Another appealed to the NAPNAP leadership for support: "It is my hope NAPNAP will make a stand and inform both organizations that we will not be a pawn in their game of chess or a whetstone on which they may grind their axes. Let's stand firm and together on this issue."[86] McCleery acknowledged the split from the ANA when she replied, "I agree that PNA's are caught in the middle of a feud between ANA and AAP; however, I am personally convinced that the AAP is most sincere in their interest in PNAs and not in exploitation."[87]

NAPNAP members were also confused about the quick loss of support for the ANA by the academy. Barbara Dunn, a well-regarded and highly active member of both NAPNAP and the ANA and later NAPNAP president from 1975 to 1978, wrote to Janet McCleery about her concerns, noting, "It is becoming increasingly evident to me that there is a general lack of communication within and between these organizations. . . . I feel that I am an active participant in both ANA and NAPNAP. Owing to my own feelings of confusion and frustration as a result of these recent events, I am wondering how the general memberships must feel."[88] McCleery replied shortly thereafter, pointing out the difficulties with the ANA, and strongly positioning her loyalties, "Several PNPs . . . have written to ANA seeking answers to specific questions about their certification program. To date, we haven't even received an acknowledgement of our inquiries. This is not only a lack of communication, but a lack of common courtesy."[89] Dunn ended her correspondence to McCleery with an appeal for reason: "Someone needs to proceed with a level head—it seems evident to me that thus far too much has been based on emotional reaction."[90]

The three organizations did not respond to "reason," as Dunn implored. All of them held different political agendas reflecting their core organization ideologies. The split between the ANA, academy, and NAPNAP revealed at least two "places" of nursing politics—NAPNAP's "grassroots" practice and ANA's broader policy-forming agenda—and a cleavage between the liberal ideals of nursing as an autonomous discipline and the daily realities of providing health care to clients while working intimately with other health care providers. The disjuncture between the three different groups—and the ANA was in conflict with several other specialty groups at the same time for some of the same reasons—reflected less a lack of common purpose than diverging historical and philosophical viewpoints and power issues. ANA leaders, perhaps because of their historical vantage point of nursing's contextual battles for recognition and autonomy, could not see NAPNAP's alliance with the academy as anything less than yet another paternalistic manipulation by medicine within the context of NAPNAP's inability to understand these larger ideological issues.

Although there was some truth to the ANA's views, its lack of self-awareness regarding its own conduct toward both the academy and NAPNAP was somewhat hypocritical. The ANA representatives were sometimes seen as being rude, condescending, and unprofessional. NAPNAP in particular complained of not receiving responses to requests for information, and of difficult, contentious meetings.[91] The ANA's behavior toward NAPNAP was flavored in part by the personalities of some of its representatives, and in part by the organization's inherent chauvinism. The ANA characterized the conflict as one between a major medical organization, the academy, and itself, with NAPNAP as an interloper, a splinter group. By situating NAPNAP in this manner, the ANA failed to recognize and respect the power NAPNAP held, how little support ANA had at this point from its nursing grassroots constituency for autonomous practice, and the importance of the emerging nurse practitioner movement. "I believe the ANA has really missed the boat," another PNA wrote to Janet McCleery. "The AAP offered a colleague association. The PNA is part of the pediatric team. The pediatrician is obviously the team leader. ANA by insisting on complete autonomy for nursing is negating or denying the team concept."[92] "I need the input of the physician," another nurse wrote. "I feel that I am indeed his associate, not his assistant; but I do not feel that I am or wish to be a solo practitioner. . . . If I did, I would have been a pediatrician."[93] All of these factors colored the ANA's relationship with NAPNAP.

Attempts to Salvage the Relationship

Shortly after the academy decision to disassociate itself from the ANA certification process and the liaison committee, the ANA tried to reengage. A negotiating meeting was set for November 1974. In the meantime, in March, the academy brought together NAPNAP, independent pediatric nurse practitioners, representatives of the U.S. Air Force (USAF), which also already had a certification process in place, and the American Board of Pediatrics to move its certification plans forward.[94] The participants agreed the consortium (the name given the group convened by the academy and renamed shortly thereafter as the National Board of Pediatric Nurse Practitioners and Associates) should ideally include the ANA, and it was invited to participate. This gesture, while politically astute, was unrealistic because the group proposed guidelines the ANA could not have accepted given its basic philosophy of rewarding excellence rather than basic competence and its stand on autonomous practice.[95]

When the ANA and the academy finally met in November, both organizations understood they needed to engage in creative and nondefensive dialogue to proceed in a unified and functioning relationship. After two difficult days, the much-anticipated negotiation meeting ended with a joint statement on the relationship between the pediatric nurse practitioner and the pediatrician that broke no new ground.[96] Although NAPNAP was not officially invited, its interests were indirectly represented. Mary Kaye Willian of the academy liaison staff was at the meeting. She was a pediatric nurse practitioner, NAPNAP member, and strong supporter. Willian kept NAPNAP's interests in the arena, although her loyalties were keenly tied to the academy. They employed her and she shared their philosophic views on the role of the pediatric nurse practitioner.[97]

In late November 1975, a joint meeting of NAPNAP, the academy, and the ANA was perhaps one of the last attempts to unfreeze the impasse on certification. The meeting was a contentious one, as the ANA and the academy were both losing their veneer of civility toward the other. One of the NAPNAP representatives, noted: "All in all, I thought the meeting today was frustrating and confusing. . . . I felt badly during the meeting that I could not offer more input for NAPNAP and the academy, but so much of the information and dynamics of the interaction were new and emotion laden. I felt [one of the ANA representatives] was baiting NAPNAP into taking a stand separate from the academy, or at least speaking up individually for the organization."[98] At this point, NAPNAP had much to gain from its alliance with the academy. It was its source of both financial and professional support and strength, and there were no guarantees from the ANA that it would negotiate with NAPNAP alone or offer support if it disassociated itself from the academy. NAPNAP's existence, at this point, depended on it, and the ANA keenly resented the alliance.

The ANA had more to lose at this point, as its exam had already been administered at least twice. Although the number of those sitting for certification was small, perhaps around one hundred nurses, the ANA believed its popularity would grow, and it fit their organizational strategies and their ideological stand on nursing practice. Essentially, the ANA's goal was to convince the academy and NAPNAP to halt their certification efforts, viewing the academy exam (as it is named in ANA documents) as an illegitimate incursion into nursing territory and an academy attempt to define and regulate nursing. This issue was the fulcrum for the ANA's inactivity on the consortium invitation and resistance to the entry-level examination.

Untangling NAPNAP from the Academy

The academy and NAPNAP continued their close alliance and formalized their affiliation in 1975.[99] And, in March 1977, 958 pediatric nurse practitioners took the first certification exam, and 823 passed, making it more popular than the ANA's offering. But the character of the relationship changed throughout the 1980s and 1990s, as NAPNAP became increasingly wary of the academy and its efforts to control the organization. The medical manpower shortage that seemed in part to fuel the expanded nursing role slowly abated, academy members increasingly viewed pediatric nurse practitioners as competition, and the academy executive board was highly sensitive to any perceived threats to its control over pediatric nurse practitioner practice. NAPNAP members themselves were changing. Early NAPNAP leader Sally Walsh noted, "We were coming out from under supervision of physicians to a more collegial relationship."[100]

Much of the subsequent conflict surrounded NAPNAP's increasing self-reliance and independent efforts to define practice and the academy's highly sensitive response and continued refusal to modify its position on the need for direct supervision. On August 18, 1981, the academy complained to NAPNAP about an article in a recent newsletter describing the plan by the Civilian Health and Medical Program of the Uniformed Services (CHAMPUS) to directly reimburse nurse practitioners (rather than paying them through their physician collaborators) for their services. The academy saw the inclusion of this item as an indication of NAPNAP's support for independent practice. In addition to the newsletter, the academy was also concerned about a new scope of practice draft that NAPNAP developed. In the context of these two items, the academy perceived a "change in NAPNAP's basic philosophy regarding independent PNP practice. . . . The AAP wants input [into the scope] as they feel the scope [as it was drafted] describes independent practice."[101]

These issues were important enough to warrant an academy emergency meeting on October 30, 1981. At this gathering, the academy developed a resolution that contained the following three points fortifying its traditional position on nurse practitioners: the academy must have input into the training of pediatric nurse practitioners and the certification process, and the health care of children must be supervised by a physician. The academy also demanded that the new scope of practice directly state pediatric nurse practitioners must work under the direction and supervision of the physician.[102] The academy threatened to withdraw from the AAP/NAPNAP affiliation if the scope draft did not include this language. In its own emergency session to respond to the academy, the NAPNAP executive board agreed. They delayed the publication of the new scope of practice and voted to reconvene the original task force that developed it. But they now also included other organizations in addition to the academy as members of the task force, such as the ANA Council of Primary Care Nurse Practitioners, the Association of Faculties of Pediatric Nurse Practitioner Programs, and the National Certification Board.[103] At the same time, as the board voted to affirm its belief in the team approach to health care, it also resolved that it did not support independent practice by nurse practitioners.[104]

Although the conflict was tempered for the moment, NAPNAP leaders began to sense a shift in the position of its constituents. NAPNAP published the scope draft in early 1982 and began to receive responses from the membership that indicated certain concerns. In particular, the members wanted a phrase inserted describing "our contributions to direct primary care," and questioned the contradiction of the clauses "collegial and collaborative" and "directed and supervised" [by the physician].[105] Ninety-nine percent of the membership felt their role was complementary rather than dependent, and believed the language had to reflect this difference. An astounding 93 percent supported direct reimbursement for nurse practitioners. The membership's strong position on these issues convinced the board to change its stance and revise the draft in March 1983.[106]

Over the next three months, the AAP executive board continued to threaten the affiliation if NAPNAP included phrases describing collaborative practice in the scope. This time, NAPNAP was at a different place. The academy was no longer essential for NAPNAP's existence: the organization had grown substantially, boasting 2,600 members by 1983. Although still small, the group was nonetheless very strong and well supported by its industry sponsors. NAPNAP held its own meetings, had a well-supported newsletter and journal, scholarship programs, and well-known consumer-advocate initiatives.[107] The membership had the support of physician colleagues at the grassroots practice level, many of whom wrote letters to the academy supporting collaborative practice rather than direct supervision.

By June 1983, the NAPNAP executive board noted a "change in thought and position by the AAP."[108] Several new academy board members who were more liberal in their ideas about nurse practitioners were elected, and they provided the voting block to maintain affiliation with NAPNAP despite the scope language. This was not a philosophical sea change, however. The board was still concerned about the substitution of "collaboration and third party payment" for "directed and supervised," but the reshaped academy board believed in and actively supported attempts to work out their differences rather than issue ultimatums.[109]

For NAPNAP, there was no turning back on the issues of collaboration versus supervision. This issue already more accurately reflected the daily realities of clinical practice. The board believed that membership responses obligated it to use broader statements "rather than a term [supervision] that could be interpreted as a physician having to be in the room with the NP. It was also important to use terms that describe what we [nurse practitioners] are actually doing, such as diagnosis."[110] The new scope of practice, with its focus on collaborative relationships with various other health professionals, was approved by the NAPNAP board in November 1983. At this meeting, the academy made one last effort requesting a statement against direct reimbursement, but this idea was not sustainable. NAPNAP already had in progress a position statement supporting third-party payment, and was encouraging its members to register as providers for the CHAMPUS program wherever state practice legislation might be supportive. In a final show of its increasingly independent stance, NAPNAP admonished the academy, noting the scope is "NAPNAP's document, not the AAP's."[111]

In the next decades, NAPNAP continued to mature as an independent nursing specialty organization, one with high name recognition and great constituency loyalty. It no longer has a formal affiliation with the academy, although it maintains a collegial relationship. The national board remains an independent certification organization.[112] By the late 1980s, the ANA, like the academy earlier in the decade, changed its approach to specialty organizations, in part because a new generation of leaders was more progressive, less removed from daily clinical realities, and, although still fighting for nurses' place in the health care system, no longer fighting for professional survival. And the new leaders realized the power they might wield if they worked with specialty organizations. Also, broader organizations such as the National Alliance of Nurse Practitioners and the American Academy of Nurse Practitioners emerged in the mid-1980s to take on the political and practice issues of nurse practitioners, and these organizations worked with the ANA.

In their recent scope of practice document in 2003, the academy responded to increased numbers and clinical practice expansion of nonphysician providers by upholding its decade-long position on supervision and independent practice. The academy continues to support supervision of nurse practitioners and all other nonphysician providers involved with child health care. Although now cloaked in the rhetoric of the pediatric health team and public safety, the academy continues to advocate for "a physician, preferably a pediatrician" to lead the team, delegate, and supervise care provided by nonphysician providers, and determine referrals. In other words, it still does not support independent nurse practitioner practice even in medically underserved areas, direct third-party payment, or prescriptive privileges for nonphysician providers.[113]

Chapter 8

Making Room in the Clinic

Throughout the 1980s and into the twenty-first century, nurse practitioner roles continued to reshape, expand, and formalize. By the late 1970s, more and more graduate programs began to offer clinical nursing degrees (which were required by the end of the 1980s by most states), creating a larger pool of nurses qualified to take active roles in the education and socialization of new nurse practitioners. At the same time, broadened feminist perspectives engaged consumers to take more active roles in their health care, while the economies brought about by the prospective payment system created a supportive environment for nurse practitioners to develop a professional character that was more proactive and independent of physicians. This more confident stance challenged professional medicine's control of the dialogue surrounding clinical practice, metaphorically making room in the clinic for nurse practitioners.

But even by the end of the 1970s, the successful model of care anchored by nurse practitioners and the features that were important in creating it were already in place to sustain it. This platform was one of collaborative practice and respectful negotiations to extend health care to more citizens. In turn, nurses broadened their skills and knowledge and practiced more closely to their fullest potential. Many factors, including the maturation of nursing, the needs of the public for health care, the local receptivity of physicians, the availability of federal and private funding, and policies to improve access all converged to support nurse practitioners by this time.

The 1980s and 1990s offer a different story, and can be seen as a period of both gained and lost opportunities. Attempts to control public and private health care spending, instead of strategies to increase access, were some of the key policy initiatives of the following decades. The temporary drop in spending seen in the early 1970s after wage and price controls (primarily through control of insurance premiums) rebounded until the late 1970s, when the health care industry organized voluntary efforts to control costs after President Carter threatened regulatory oversight. It increased again until the mid-1980s, when the prospective payment system resulted in shorter hospital stays, decreased payments to providers, and smaller medical and nursing staffs. This temporary drop was followed by another increase, which was then only slightly tempered by the managed care initiatives of the 1990s.[1] All of these factors in addition to the general economic trends of the country limited access to care for millions of uninsured poor and working-class families as hospital admission criteria tightened, insurance premiums continued to soar, community clinics closed, and outreach programs went unfunded.

These changes presented an opening for health policy strategists to devise a primary care ambulatory network based on the services of independent nurse practitioners or teams of nurses and physicians. But this did not happen as public and private support for large-scale changes never materialized, partially due to the lack of political will for planning, initial expense, low levels of interest in primary and ambulatory care, and the willpower to override the concerns of medical specialties and acute care hospitals. Instead, federal funding for health care targeted a different paradigm based on cost and competition, and nurse practitioners were seen as cheaper alternatives to physician care instead of a value-added model. Although this further opened up the health care market to nurse practitioners, and many health maintenance organizations began to hire them as gatekeepers and as participants on practice panels (lists of provider options for people in particular insurance programs), the connotations of the low-cost designation devalued their services. Many nursing organizations also touted nurse practitioners as providing low-cost and high-quality care, and this was true. But the typical American vernacular, "you get what you pay for," implied nurse practitioner services were not as good as those provided by physicians. Professional organizations spent a great deal of time highlighting an old, already documented issue, that nurse practitioners provided safe and high-value care.

Physicians and nurses still negotiate to define the borders of responsibility and authority for clinical care, and these contracts continue to be framed by the politics surrounding the professional groups and the larger policy landscape. In the 1970s and 1980s, organizations supporting nurse practitioners, such as the American Academy of Nurse Practitioners (AANP), provided broader convergence of awareness and coherence of nurse practitioners' general political and clinical interests. This organization and others in concert with the ANA became the moving force behind nurses' expanded clinical practice roles and responses to health policy proposals, although they could not convince the federal government to maintain funding for nurse practitioner education in the 1980s except for narrowly focused programs.

Negotiating practice remains an individually idiosyncratic process devoid of homogeneity, but these relationships sustain the nurse practitioner movement.[2] Clinical practice arrangements develop at their own pace depending on time, place, and personalities, and despite the particularities of state practice legislation or organization prerogatives. But their tone and focus are different than in the 1960s and 1970s because it is now complicated by political and economic competition that supports contingent practice barriers. Nurse practitioners in many states are not legally sanctioned to practice to their full capabilities because of restrictive state practice acts that mandate direct physician supervision and narrow prescriptive privileges. The reimbursement practices of public and private third-party payers that fail to cover or provide payment at lower rates for nurse practitioner services add additional impediments. In many states nurse practitioners must practice in more affluent urban and suburban areas with higher concentrations of physicians to obtain state-required supervision, adequate income, and support. And, nurse practitioners seek practices in more affluent areas for some of the same reasons as physicians—for the social and cultural opportunities. At the same time, the number of nurse practitioners increased exponentially and occurred during a period of physician surplus and a projected increase in physician supply.[3] Physicians, already under siege from shrinking reimbursements and oversight from health maintenance organizations, are now also faced with the effects of a movement set in process over four decades ago that began, in part, to help them with their busy practices.

When nurse practitioners are seen as competitors rather than complementary or collaborative providers, the politics of clinical practice change. Warnings concerning this potential dilemma were raised early on in the 1970s and 1980s by various manpower reports, including the 1981 report of the Graduate Medical Education National Advisory Committee (GMENAC), and the issue persists.[4] In a 1994 letter to the editor of the *New England Journal of Medicine*, one physician boldly wrote what many physicians only dared to speak about privately, "Now is the time for all physicians to support our profession and not the time to give away work to outside personnel."[5] Even more recently, a frustrated physician complained, "We have forces at work to deconstruct our profession of medicine, break it down into little pieces, and parcel it out for others to do."[6] Perhaps more telling is a satirical miniature toy duck developed by

Mattel, "the Quacktitioner," that elicited enthusiastic responses. "I'm ordering one for each of my physician colleagues," one physician wrote.[7]

Nurse practitioners are illustrative of the practice politics involved in delivering services to patients, the constantly shifting intellectual frame of knowledge domains, and the result these factors have on health policy. Because of changes in physicians' practice patterns, nursing practice and education, and the political maneuverings of professional organizations, physicians and nurses engaged in negotiations that met the needs and expectations of providers and patients in different ways. Patients found nurse practitioners to be reasonable, compelling, and sometimes the only way to access health care. Physicians traded pieces of their traditional power base, the components of clinical thinking, to nurses for the opportunity to focus on the more important, satisfying, and less boring aspects of medical practice. As nurses became more educated and competent in the care of clinically diverse populations, they engaged these patients without waiting for physician permission or approval. Other nurses new to the idea of broadened clinical practice willingly and even eagerly took on expanded nursing roles and claimed the process of clinical thinking as their own, shaping it according to their own ideology. Clinical thinking, even those parts physicians considered mundane, represented competency and political power to nurses. But it also meant something more—it gave them the framework to provide organized and meaningful care that patients needed.[8]

The AMA's Citizens' Petition on Physician-Nurse Collaboration is an example of this complicated practice terrain. Launched in 2000, the petition was a response to the 1997 Balanced Budget Act, which extended direct payments for Medicare Part B services provided by nurse practitioners by eliminating the qualification of geographic setting (payment was no longer determined by location). The AMA petitioned the Health Care Financing Administration (HCFA)—the agency responsible for establishing billing regulations for Medicare and Medicaid—to live up to its obligations to the program and the tax-paying public. In particular, the AMA wanted HCFA to develop strict regulations that ensured nurse practitioners collaborated with physicians, even in states that did not require collaborative arrangements, and prevent reimbursement for services that were not provided under "medical direction and appropriate supervision."[9]

The "citizen" in the petition consisted of the AMA and forty-nine other medical specialty organization supporters. It was not, as might first be imagined, the public at large, although the AMA and its constituencies do constitute a particular public. A media campaign followed its submission, and the language of the petition addressed the abuse and misappropriation of tax funds as

well as the possibility of substandard care if HCFA failed to establish collaboration requirements. The petition was couched in terms of patient safety and the
protection of the public's health, both traditional and long-held arguments reflecting physicians' claim to expertise through their exclusive scientific education.[10]

The action by the AMA and its partners was an effort to control who provides health care and, in particular, who receives reimbursement and in what
amount at the federal level for health services. But its efforts were too late and
had little influence over health care policy for two reasons. First, the public was
satisfied and approved of care by nurse practitioners either as independent
providers or as part of a team. Patients indeed chose care by nurse practitioners. Second, the AMA was proposing direct supervision and not collaboration.
This was a regressive stance unsupported by many individual physicians.
Although unacknowledged in the petition, and as history has demonstrated,
nurse practitioners and physicians collaborated in growing numbers over the
last four decades. They created extremely entrepreneurial, high-quality practice relationships that were not replicated, even if only in spirit, at the national
organizational level.

One-on-one negotiations between nurses and physicians in individual
practices illuminated each profession's source of power, be it the nurses' exquisite knowledge of their patients or physicians' knowledge of pathology and disease, and integrated them into a successful model that encompassed the
everyday realities of providing clinical care. In fact, in long-standing tradition,
individual nurse practitioners and physicians continue to push and reframe
practice without waiting for health policy or legislative changes. In many
instances, the only requirement for innovation is imagination and the compatible personalities of the providers.

Debates over boundary negotiations are illustrated more recently in the
AMA-sponsored scope of practice partnership announced in February 2006.
Although clothed in the typical rhetoric of patient safety, the main focus of the
partnership was to defeat the upcoming expansion of practice legislation in
several states for other health care providers.[11] In response, twenty-six other
health provider organizations—including those representing nurse practitioners, physical therapists, and psychologists—formed the coalition for patients'
rights. The coalition couched its purpose in the rhetoric of patients' right to
choose their health care provider, but it was also politically focused on preserving the practice boundary expansion of its supporters.[12] Episodes and
examples like these document a significant loss of historical perspective surrounding the consequences of a public debate geared to undermine each group's
professional authority and attempts to turn political disputes into moral issues.

This is the case when patient rights and safety become fodder for political positions that are based in both public trust and professional self-interest.[13]

Another contemporary example of boundary negotiation is the rising employment of nurse practitioners in hospitals as part of the larger clinical care system. In response to clinical errors by sleep-deprived medical and surgical residents, the Accreditation Council for Graduate Medical Education (ACGME) initiated common standards related to resident duty hours in July 2003. Similar to the function of nursing students in hospital diploma programs of the last century, medical residents typically provided much of the labor of clinical practice in hospitals as part of their training. The residents traditionally worked long rotations that many times extended over twenty-four to forty-eight hours or more, with little opportunity for rest under the premise that continuity in a case presented a superior learning experience. The new standards broke with tradition and specified maximum work hours over a particular time period and sent hospitals scrambling to devise new schemes for medical care coverage.[14]

The duty-hours policy raised questions somewhat consistent with those generated by physicians and nurses over the last forty years: How should the "work" of clinical care be organized to meet the needs of patients? Many hospitals responded to the ACGME policy by hiring nurse practitioners and physician assistants as part of the strategy. One urban Philadelphia academic institution of over 500 beds, hired thirty-six new practitioners in addition to more than forty already working with individual physicians in the institution. All but six of the practitioners are nurse practitioners, and they work in many different capacities depending upon the relationships they are able to negotiate with a particular set of attending physicians. The nurse practitioners make clinical rounds, write orders, prescribe treatments and medications, and plan and evaluate treatment based on laboratory and radiology studies they order. They work closely with the residents, and on some services report directly to attending physicians. They frequently provide patient education and outpatient care in clinics and during private office hours.[15] In each instance, the relationship and the clinical terrain remains individually situated even when most institutions have specific job descriptions. But the variety of services nurse practitioners provide indicates their reach. No matter how the practice relationships develop, nurse practitioners are now embedded in patient care in and outside of hospitals.

The range of settings that nurse practitioners now claim and services they offer present important developments in health care. In particular, they provide flexibility in a changing health care environment framed by new categories of chronic diseases and new standards of care. As advances in medicine made it possible for patients with chronic illnesses to live longer, new management problems came about as "unintended by-products of technologic change."[16] These problems, such as the long-term effects of chronic hypertension, hyperc-holesterolemia, and functional disabilities (for example, difficulty walking, dressing, or writing, and sexual dysfunction) caused by treatment complications and side effects represented quality-of-life issues for both patients and their families. Medical diagnostic categories did not easily capture these problems, but they were particularly responsive to care provided by nurse practitioners.[17]

The care chronically ill patients want and need helps exemplify why nurse practitioners are more than physician extenders or substitutes, and that they provide services that, while overlapping with medicine, are also different. Nurse practitioners cover the care continuum from health promotion and disease prevention to diagnosis and treatment to prevent or limit disability. These services are grounded by their nursing education and its particular ideology and professional identity. Nurse practitioners also learn how to work with teams of providers, which is perhaps one of the most important factors in the successful care of chronically ill patients. Using skills traditionally residing in medicine's realm does not make them "half-fledged" physicians: it makes them practitioners who integrate a range of skills from several disciplines—including social work, nutrition, and physical therapy—into their nursing practice.[18]

The health and illness profile of today's patients, along with the lack of access to basic health services, also supported the reemergence and demand for primary care physicians. But reasons similar to those contributing to a short supply of general and family practitioners in the 1960s and 1970s remain salient for modern medical students. Health policies that continue to reward acute care and medical specialists, and the nature and location of these types of practices, make recruitment into primary care and to roles as gatekeepers in health maintenance organizations difficult. Physicians cannot solve the access problem themselves. Although doctors provide much of the primary care today, a greater proportion of nurse practitioners work in rural and poor urban health clinics to serve these citizens.[19] These are some of the complexities that shape how the public decides who provides care at particular periods of time. In this case, supply of physicians and satisfaction with nurse practitioner care overrides medicine's cultural authority.

The intersection of professional cultures serves as the space where negotiations occur, and it is a vibrant place. The growth of the nurse practitioner movement itself, and its acceptance by patients, is the exemplar writ large. Models such as health maintenance organizations and the health systems of the armed forces incorporate nurse practitioners as primary care providers. Federal programs such as CHAMPUS directly reimburse nurse practitioners for their services. Many nursing schools support academic nursing practices using teams of providers led or supported by nurse practitioners for preventive and primary health care services.[20] Nurse practitioners are a key component of an innovative practice model—transitional care—that uses interdisciplinary teams to improve postdischarge outcomes of high-risk elders after hospitalization for chronic cardiovascular disease problems.[21]

At the broader organizational level, the National Joint Practice Commission is another example of the energizing effect of the nurse practitioner movement. Although lasting only ten years, the commission was in fact instrumental in supporting collaborative practice across many levels and activities to change state practice acts. These efforts helped sustain contemporary nurse practitioners. The commission's success was supported in part by other social movements of the 1970s. It existed during a time of turmoil and heightened social activism across the board—for consumers, women, antiwar demonstrators, civil rights marchers, and many others. For the nurse and physician commissioners, being part of the organization was, in fact, a form of activism at the national level, and it confirmed their agency and effectiveness while assuring a certain level of confrontation. Being embattled was energizing, eliciting strategic and intellectual creativity that helped both to actualize the commission's ideas and to lead to their downfall.

For both nurses and physicians at the individual and organizational level, agency to joust with or stir up the larger professional organizations was part of the reward of activism. Negotiation itself was a way to instigate political change, gaining individual nurses the power to exert some level of control over their practice. For physicians, it provided the opportunity to control, monitor, participate in, or benefit from a growing nursing movement that was only becoming more vocal, obvious, and effective. As Loretta Ford astutely noted, "I don't want less chaos ever, because chaos is opportunity. The nurse practitioner is not the end, it's the beginning."[22]

Nurse practitioners were commonplace across the country by the end of the 1970s, and the intensity of the struggles abated with the exchange of subject identities from the activist to the status quo. There were, of course, other battles coming up over issues such as reimbursement and prescriptive privileges, but these were almost finishing touches, rather than outcomes of a larger political struggle. In their early years, it was quite empowering for nurse practitioners to practice in a place beyond traditional boundaries. There were opportunities on the edges, and, in fact, nurse practitioners' work with patients many times depended on the exact premise of marginalization—out of the gaze of those who might have tried to limit their practices.[23] For nurse practitioners, becoming "normalized" to a certain degree carried both the power of legitimacy and the danger of "dulling of the critical edge that comes with being on the margin."[24]

The social movements of the 1960s and 1970s influenced expanded practice, but not always in positive ways. Nursing and medicine continued to be primarily white occupations. The number of underrepresented minority nurses and physicians grew slowly and did not keep pace with the proportion of these groups in the population. General practice nurses, no matter their race, never fully shared in the empowerment women gained from the feminist movement. Hospitals remained patriarchal institutions. As traditionally male fields such as medicine and corporate finance opened to women (although women and men from minority groups still found these areas difficult to access), fewer of them gravitated to the nursing profession. The growth in enrollments in undergraduate nursing programs slowed until the early twenty-first century, when a general nursing shortage supported higher salaries and better job opportunities than many other fields.[25] Nurse practitioner programs did not experience the same decline, and, in fact, their numbers continued to climb and were supported by men and women who were looking for more satisfying second careers.[26] The connection between the nurse practitioner movement and increased opportunities for women in medicine from 1960 onward is not clear, but nurse practitioner growth did not slow. More women admittedly entered the medical field during this time, but the numbers of nurse practitioners, fueled primarily by women, increased at a much faster rate.[27] Women had more choices, to be sure, and they chose medicine or nursing for particular reasons; nursing was not the fall-back choice.

The nursing and medical professions are undergoing an unusually high degree of internal scrutiny from individual practitioners, and externally from the public and health care policy strategists. Vociferous political arguments continue to encircle debates over the type of health care the American public needs and who should provide it, and the type and amount of education practitioners require and who should pay for it. The self-interests of professional organizations partially underlie these debates, and it is difficult to extract them from the public's interest. One example that melds historical contingency with contemporary issues is the debate over the level of nurse practitioner education. The lack of resolution in American nursing regarding entry level into general practice with diploma, associate, and baccalaureate degree entry points still recognized by state licensing boards complicates the issue. The general entry level inconsistency intrinsically influences graduate education for nurse practitioners because it means there can be no expectations for a student's consistent knowledge and skill level on admission or after nurse practitioner program completion.

The 2004 doctor of nursing practice (DNP) initiative from the American Association of Colleges of Nursing (AACN) is an important example that raises questions pertaining to the relationship between health care advocacy, practitioner education level, and negotiation of clinical practice. It also serves as a convenient contemporary exemplar examining the relationship between the interests of professional organizations and the health needs of the public. The AACN developed its initiative as a response to the growing complexity in health care. In the last decades, many schools expanded the number of clinical and didactic hours in their nurse practitioner programs to respond to the heightened level of patient care in hospitals and clinics. Many programs require credit loads greater than the traditional requirements for master's education in most other fields.

The doctor of nursing practice is one way to acknowledge the expanded course load and to add other advanced clinical courses and those of various other foci such as informatics. Supporters also point to the tradition of practice-focused doctorate degrees in other professions, such as medicine, pharmacy, dentistry, and psychology, with the doctor of nursing practice as part of this continuum. The AACN proposed the degree as the practice entry level for nurse practitioners by the year 2015, although each state, rather than the organization itself, holds the authority for enforcement. Nevertheless, the doctor of nursing practice concept increasingly resonates with some nurse educators; there are currently 46 programs in existence with over 140 more in various stages of discussion and development.[28]

While detractors agree that many programs should reevaluate their length, they do not believe the doctor of nursing practice is necessary for safe practice, or that it addresses any public need. The debate in nursing over this issue, they argue, will redirect attention and resources needed for other, more important initiatives such as health care reform, patient safety, and access to care. The practice doctorate could also negatively influence enrollments in research-based doctoral programs (Ph.D. programs) that are the source of badly needed nurse faculty and researchers.[29] They point to the 1986 Office of Technology Assessment (OTA) study that estimated nurse practitioners safely cared for more than 75 percent of patients typically seeking the services of primary care physicians, and to the hundreds of other studies since then that supported the OTA report and documented the safety, quality, and cost-effectiveness of care provided by nurse practitioners.[30] Detractors also use the 2002 Institute of

Medicine (IOM) study, "Health Professions: A Bridge to Quality," to support their position. This study questioned the need for the extensive science training found in medical education in view of the demographic changes in health and illness in the United States.[31] The AMA recently responded to the doctor of nursing practice initiative with a motion to monitor and publicize false claims by practice doctorate programs in terms of the clinical capabilities of their graduates. This issue is also creating a growing conflict between medical and nursing professional organizations during a time of relatively amicable relations.[32]

This story of nurse practitioners, then, as a whole, is not representational but emblematic of the tensions among individuals, groups, and organizations, and the difficulty of consensus. In reality it tells us how change is condensed into some sort of reasonable explanatory framework. The common thread is the influence of time, place, and person, contrasted with the mischievous forces of serendipity and idiosyncrasy that expose the fallacies of typical and reasonable explanations. The mission of the historian is to provide some sort of explanatory or perhaps alternative frame to ideas, experiences, and episodes that seem inherently unrelated or structurally intransient.[33] There are more ways to think about how a society decides who should provide health care and how these decisions are negotiated than deferring to the typical, seemingly monolithic characterization of medicine and its concurrent cultural authority without tearing down physicians' facility for what they do best—the intricate and painstaking ability to see the relationships between patient symptoms and a particular diagnostic label. This is not to say physicians alone can or should do this, but they indeed do this against a different set of contingencies and with a different critical gaze than other providers.

As we look back to the 1950s and 1960s, when the idea of nurses and physicians negotiating the boundaries of clinical care began to solidify into the larger nurse practitioner movement, we see a powerful concept emerge. The idea of a nurse providing increasingly broader arrays of clinical services supported by a foundation of federal support—the interaction of the public and the private—proved extremely powerful for patients. Although the nurse practitioner concept focused the attention of both nurses and physicians on the cultural authority of clinical practice, and the frequently self-absorbed politics of the ownership of particular knowledge and skills, it also, perhaps most importantly, refocused the attention of clinical practice on the patient—as a political entity and as a consumer of clinical practice services. Nurse practitioners were driven by a combination of federal policy, entrepreneurial individuals, and public buy-in. When Wal-Mart began to offer walk-in health clinics in their stores staffed by nurse practitioners with referral agreements with physicians in early 2006 as both an antidote to health care access problems of their customers and as a way to channel business to its own services, one realizes the scale the politics and economics of consumer issues have achieved.[34]

Recent innovative state initiatives also support the political power of patients. They bring together the success of local negotiations of nurses and physicians with the larger goals of improved access to primary-care providers, lower health care costs through health promotion and disease management strategies, and privately financed health insurance options. Part of the Prescription for Pennsylvania, a state health policy initiative announced by Governor Edward Rendell in 2007, relies upon nurse practitioners practicing to their full extent, and in particular providing care to patients who need services on weekends and nights, and who use emergency rooms for common problems such as sore throats and immunizations.[35] Obtaining basic health care in emergency rooms is expensive and time consuming, and patients become powerful policy advocates as they are exposed to the inadequacies of the health care system. Efforts like this state plan may offer more substantial ways of reconceptualizing clinical practice to reach large groups of people who need health services, and provide the opportunity for patients, nurses, and physicians to partner together to meet these goals.

The changes that occurred in the 1960s and 1970s did indeed make room in the clinic for nurse practitioners to provide the care their patients need. This is a virtual space where negotiations with physician colleagues takes place, a physical space to practice, and a political space to form relationships with individual patients and institutions. But the space, perhaps, truly belongs to the patients. It is here where they, no matter how powerless they may feel when they seek services or how small or large their resources, negotiate clinical care and, indeed, find "room in the clinic" for themselves and their families.

A Note on Archival Sources

I used a number of archival sources for this book. Some of them were well processed, such as the ANA collection in the Howard Gotlieb Archival Research Center at Boston University (except for one or two boxes of more recent materials) and the Digital Collection of the Physician Assistant History Center, Duke University Medical Center Archives, although this collection has undergone significant changes since I first encountered it. Others were newly donated, partially processed, or unprocessed. Listed below are the archival sources used, and their status at the time of research. For collections in the process of being archived, the archivists at the particular centers kindly allowed me access to the materials.

Barbara Bates Center for the Study of the History of Nursing, School of Nursing, University of Pennsylvania, Philadelphia, PA

> The Shirley Smoyak Collection, unprocessed
> The Hildegard E. Peplau Papers, processing in progress
> The Carol Hayes Christiansen Collection, unprocessed
> The Dorothy Smith Collection, processed
> The Jessie Scott Collection, processed

Joan Lynaugh Personal Collection, Bryn Mawr, PA. Collection unprocessed

> Barbara Bates Papers

Center for Nursing Historical Inquiry, School of Nursing, University of Virginia, Charlottesville, VA

NAPNAP Collection, processing in progress; not all boxes have file numbers or box numbers.
Jacquette Collection, processing in progress
Brodie Photographic Collection

The Barbara Dunn Personal Collection, Richmond, Virginia. This is a personal collection and I was allowed access to copies of originals.

Pennsylvania State Board of Medical Examiners and Licensure (PSBMEL) (now, State Board of Medicine), and Pennsylvania State Board of Nursing, Office of the Commissioner of Professional and Occupational Affairs, Harrisburg, PA; unnumbered and unprocessed.

The George T. Harrell Medical History Society and Archives, University of Florida Gainesville, FL; processed.

Samuel Proctor Oral History Program (SPOHP), University of Florida. Most of the oral history interviews are transcribed and online.

The Loretta Ford Personal Collection, Wildwood, FL; accessed via copies from owner.

The Howard Gotlieb Archival Research Center, Boston University, Boston, Massachusetts; all materials processed except for more recent materials (1972–73).

The American Nurses' Collection
The Luther Christman Collection

The American Nurses Association Library, Silver Springs, Maryland; processed.

Duke University Medical Center Archives; digitalized and online.

Physician Assistant History Center, Digital Collection

Fellowship of the American Academy of Nurse Practitioners, Group Project, "Stories from the Early Days of Becoming a Nurse Practitioner"; written data submitted to Barbara Resnick and analyzed by Barbara Resnick, Barbara Sheer, Donna McArthur, Judith Lynch, Judith Longworth, Elias Provencio-Vasquez, 2000–2002; a series of written responses by nurse practitioners to questions posed by the researchers.

Notes

Introduction

1. The use of the concept of a social movement is supported by Leila Rupp, *Worlds of Women: The Making of an International Women's Movement* (Princeton, NJ: Princeton University Press, 1997), 6. See also Jeremy Brecher, Tim Costello, and Brandan Smith, *Globalization from Below: The Power of Solidarity* (Cambridge, MA: South End Press, 2000). I also rely on a broad representation of technology from a social construction perspective, as a system of skills, tools, and knowledge to do things, all residing within the social context of the particular time. For example, see Wiebe E. Bijker and Trevor J. Pinch, "SCOT Answers, Other Questions. A Reply to Nick Clayton," *Technology and Culture* 43 (2) (April 2002): 361–369.

2. Rosemary Stevens, *American Medicine and the Public Interest: A History of Specialization*, updated edition with a new introduction (Berkeley: University of California Press, 1998), xvi.

3. Rick Mayes, "The Origins, Development, and Passage of Medicare's Revolutionary Prospective Payment System," 62 (1) (January 2007): 21–55.

4. Physician assistants are trained in intensive programs that last on average about twenty-six months, certified (and recertified every six years) by the National Commission on Certification of Physician Assistants in conjunction with the National Board of Medical Examiners, and licensed by each state. See American Academy of Physician Assistants, "Information about PAs and the PA Profession," http://www.aapa.org/geninf01.html (accessed October 10, 2006).

   Physician assistants also conduct physical exams, diagnose and treat illnesses, order and interpret tests, and counsel patients on preventive health care. They are legally permitted to prescribe in all states. Physician assistants, like nurse practitioners, claim autonomy in clinical decision making, although physician assistants make this claim as part of their medical practice. This is the key difference between physician assistants and nurse practitioners: physician assistants practice medicine while nurse practitioners practice nursing—a very complicated differential that illustrates the complexity of the time period.

5. D. Goodman and the Committee on Pediatric Workforce, "The Pediatrician Workforce: Current Status and Future Prospects," *Pediatrics* 116 (2005): 156–173.

6. American Academy of Nurse Practitioners, "U.S. Nurse Practitioner Workforce 2004," http://www.aanp.org/NR/rdonlyres/exenwjn13eybaktqli266uvk4kw364gapgzjhyy vey2d7fziiv2uhd55atxojxgdjrp3q5vu6e6akp/NPStateWorkforceData1204.pdf (accessed April 29, 2007). According to the National Sample Survey of Registered Nurses conducted by the U.S. Department of Health and Human Services (DHHS), Health Resources and Services Administration (HRSA) in 2004, there are 240,461 nurses prepared (rather than practicing) as nursing practitioners. See *"Preliminary Findings"*, 14, ftp://ftp.hrsa.gov/bhpr/nursing/rnpopulation/theregisterednurse population.pdf (accessed April 29, 2007). The Sample Survey of Registered Nurses is conducted every four years.

7. There is a growing body of historical research that examines nursing and its place in health care. Examples include Barbara Brush, "Exchanges or Employees?

The Exchange Visitor Program and Foreign Nurse Immigration to the U.S., 1945–1990," *Nursing History Review* 1 (1993): 171–181; Karen Buhler-Wilkerson, *No Place Like Home: A History of Nursing and Home Care in the U.S.* (Baltimore: Johns Hopkins University Press, 2001); Patricia D'Antonio, *Founding Friends: Families, Staffs and Patients at the Friends Asylum in 19th-Century Philadelphia* (Bethlehem, PA: Lehigh University Press, 2006); Joan Lynaugh and Barbara Brush, *American Nursing: From Hospital to Health Systems* (Cambridge, MA: Blackwood Press, in conj. with the Milbank Memorial Fund, 1996).

8. Martin Dinges, "Social History of Medicine in Germany and France in the Late Twentieth Century: From the History of Medicine toward a History of Health," in *Locating Medical History: The Stories and Their Meanings*, ed. Frank Huisman and John Harley Warner (Baltimore: Johns Hopkins University Press, 2004), 209–236. See also Arlene Keeling, *Nursing and the Privilege of Prescription* (Columbus: Ohio State University Press, 2007).

9. Joan Lynaugh, personal communication with author, January 13, 2006. Lynaugh's conceptualization of nurse practitioners is both structural and metaphorical and borrows from Virginia Woolf's essays on the historical place of women as writers and as subjects in fictional literature; see *A Room of One's Own* (New York: Harcourt Brace and Co., 1929; New York: Harcourt Brace Modern Classics, 1991).

10. George James, "Medical Advances in the Next Ten Years: The Implications for the Organization and Economics of Medicine," *Bulletin of the New York Academy of Medicine* 41 (1) (January 1965): 14–26; Leonard Stein, D. T. Watts, and T. Stein, "The Doctor-Nurse Game Revisited," *New England Journal of Medicine* 322 (8) (1990): 546–549.

11. Ann C. Greiner and Elisa Knebel, eds., Committee on the Health Professions Education Summit, *Health Professions Education: A Bridge to Quality* (Washington, DC: National Academy of Sciences Press, 2001), 31.

12. Greiner and Knebel, "Executive Summary," in ibid., 1–16.

13. Ibid.

14. Arlyss A. Rothman and Edward H. Wagner, "Chronic Illness Management: What Is the Role of Primary Care?" *Annals of Internal Medicine* 138 (3) (February 4, 2003): 256–261.

15. Feminist scholar Liz Stanley discusses groups emerging within various professional organizations, but this could be equally applicable to the health care professions. See Liz Stanley, "Writing the Borders: Episodic and Theoretic Thoughts on Not/Belonging," in *Knowing Feminisms*, ed. Liz Stanley (London: Sage, 1997), 172–183, quote on 179.

16. U.S. Department of Health and Human Services, Human Resources and Service Administration, "2004 Sample Survey of Registered Nurses: Preliminary Findings," http://bhpr.hrsa.gov/healthworkforce/reports/rnpopulation/preliminaryfindings.htm (accessed August 26, 2006).

17. The materials provided by Dr. Coralease Ruff, Howard University, Washington, DC, are the exception. She provided a copy of Howard's 1992 funding proposal for their Family Nurse Practitioner Program (Ruff is noted on the proposal as the project director). Howard University is a historically black private academic institution. Its first nurse practitioner program, family nurse practitioner, began in 1985, and in the next five years twenty-five students—nineteen African Americans, two Africans, and four Asians—were admitted to the program. See proposal to the U.S. Department of Health and Human Services, Public Health Service, "Family Nurse Practitioner Program at Howard University," April 15, 1991, 21.

No programs in historically black institutions are listed in the 1972 report, *Selected Training Programs for Physician Support Personnel*, DHEW, PHS, BHM, DHEW Pub. #NIH 72–183 (Washington, DC: Government Printing Office, May 1972, revised) as either in operation or planned. Individuals of various races were enrolled in the programs listed (see chapter 4). By the mid-1980s, when Howard began its program, only one other historically black institution had a nursing master's program—Hampton University, Hampton, VA. Other schools may have admitted blacks, American Indians, Hispanics, and Asians, but this was on an individual basis and the numbers would have been small until the 1980s, after the time period covered in this book.

18. In the text I kept the original gender designation found in the documents.

19. These interviews were conducted by Sadie Mitchell, PhD, RN, and Keisha Walker, MSN. None of the women interviewed practiced as nurse practitioners before the 1980s, although all but one were practicing nurses in the earlier decades.

20. On the idea of gender and political culture, see Nancy Cott, Gerda Lerner, Kathryn Kish Sklar, Ellen DuBois, and Nancy Hewitt, "Considering the State of U.S. Women's History," *Journal of Women's History* 15 (1) (2003): 145–163. See also Mari Yoshihara, "Tackling the Contested Categories: Culture, Race and Nation in American Women's History," *Journal of Women's History* 15 (1) (2003): 164–166. Yoshihara examines the idea of cultural representation and the power to engage in negotiations.

21. Alice Kessler Harris, *In Pursuit of Equity: Women, Men and the Quest for Economic Citizenship in 20th-Century America* (New York: Oxford University Press, 2001), quote 5; Sally Gregory Kohlstedt, "Women in the History of Science: An Ambiguous Place," *Osiris* 10 (1995): 39–60; Eileen Boris, "You Wouldn't Want One of Em Dancing with Your Wife": Racialized Bodies on the Job in World War II," *American Quarterly* 50 (1) (March 1998): 77–108. Boris uses the term "racialized gender" to signify the interaction between race, gender identity, and class hierarchy, all contextual components that influence the contemporary health care system.

22. For an example of the complicated gender politics in traditionally women's occupations, see Beth Linker, "Strength and Science: Gender, Physiotherapy, and Medicine in Early-Twentieth-Century America," *Journal of Women's History* 17 (3): 105–132.

Chapter 1   "Oh the Opportunities, the Possibilities . . . !"

1. Portions of this chapter are adapted with permission from the publishers: Julie A. Fairman, "Delegated by Default or Negotiated by Need: Physicians, Nurse Practitioners, and the Process of Clinical Thinking," *Medical Humanities Review* 13 (1) (1999): 38–58; Julie Fairman, "The Roots of Collaborative Practice: Nurse Practitioner Pioneer Stories," *Nursing History Review*, 10 (2002): 159–174; and "Review Essay: Not All Nurses Are Good, Not All Doctors are Bad . . .," *Bulletin of the History of Medicine* 78 (2) (2004): 451–60, 2004. Joan Lynaugh uses the phrase "passageways of care" in "Narrow Passageways: Nurses and Physicians in Conflict and Concert since 1875," in *The Physician as Captain of the Ship: A Critical Reappraisal*, ed. Nancy M. P. King et al. (Boston: D. Reidel, 1988), 23–38.

2. Ellen Baer, "The Feminist Disdain for Nursing," *New York Times*, Op. Ed., February 23, 1991.

3. Andrew Abbott, *The System of Professions: An Essay on the Division of Expert Labor* (Chicago: University of Chicago Press, 1988), 143–157.

4. Anselm Strauss, *Negotiations, Varieties, Context, Processes, and Social Order* (San Francisco: Jossey-Bass, 1979); Roland Svensson, "The Interplay between Doctors

and Nurses—A Negotiated Order Perspective," *Sociology of Health and Illness* 18 (3) (1996): 379–398.

5. Barbara Bates, "Specialty of Patient Care," original manuscript, presented at the University of Kentucky, School of Nursing, Lexington, KY, February 14, 1968, quote on 9, Barbara Bates Collection, Barbara Bates Center for the Study of the History of Nursing, University of Pennsylvania, School of Nursing, Philadelphia (Bates Collection).

6. For a discussion about the tensions between local practices and the politics of national organizations, see Fairman, "Delegated by Default."; Julie A. Fairman and Patricia D'Antonio, "Virtual Power: Gendering the Nurse-Technology Relationship," *Nursing Inquiry* 6 (3) (1999): 178–186.

7. Quote by Sanford A. Marcus, "News," *Modern Medicine,* March 27, 1974, no pagination. Marcus was the president of the Union of American Physicians.

8. See Fairman, "Delegated by Default"; "The Roots of Collaborative Practice"; "Review Essay." The victimization argument is used by Thetis Group and Joan I. Roberts, *Nursing, Physician Control and the Medical Monopoly: Historical Perspectives on Gendered Inequality in Roles, Rights, and Range of Practice* (Bloomington: Indiana University Press, 2001).

9. Alan Rosenstein, "Nurse-Physician Relationships: Impact on Nurse Satisfaction and Retention," *American Journal of Nursing* 102 (6) (2002): 26–34.

10. The word "collaboration" is drawn from Latin—to work—and is defined by the *American Heritage Dictionary* as "to work together, especially in a joint intellectual endeavor," such as patient care (*The American Heritage Dictionary of the English Language,* 4th edition (Boston: Houghton Mifflin, 2000), S.V. "Collaborate.") See also Judith Baggs and Madeline Schmitt, "Collaboration between Nurses and Physicians," *Image* 20 (1988): 145–149; Judith Gedney Baggs and Madeline H. Schmitt, "Nurses' and Resident Physicians' Perceptions of the Process of Collaboration in an MICU," *Research in Nursing and Health* 20 (1997): 71–80. Essentially, collaborative practice incorporates interpersonal interactions based upon socialization and interpersonal factors, and many researchers draw their models from the sociology and labor relations conflict-resolution process models from the 1950s to the late 1970s.

    This word is highly political and its meaning shifts across time and place. As late as 1993, the American Nurses' Association (ANA) and American Medical Association (AMA) negotiated a definition of collaboration to be used as a broad-based dimension of nurse-physician professional relationships. The ANA adopted the definition in 1994 but the AMA refused because it did not make physician supervision a required component; American Nurses' Association, "Collaboration and Independent Practice: Ongoing Issues for Nursing. Executive Summary," *Nursing Trends and Issues* 3 (5) (1998): 1–8.

11. Julie Fairman and Joan Lynaugh, *Critical Care Nursing: A History* (Philadelphia: University of Pennsylvania Press, 1998); Elizabeth Norman, *We Band of Angels: The Untold Story Of American Nurses Trapped on Bataan by the Japanese* (New York: Random House, 1999); Julie Fairman, "Alternate Visions: The Nurse-Technology Relationship in the Context of the History of Technology," *Nursing History Review* 6 (1998): 129–146; Arlene Keeling, "Blurring the Boundaries between Medicine and Nursing: Coronary Care Nursing, circa the 1960s," *Nursing History Review* 12 (2004): 129–164; Arlene Keeling, *Nursing and the Privilege of Prescription, 1893–2000* (Columbus: Ohio State University Press, 2007).

12. Leonard Stein, "The Doctor-Nurse Game," *Archives of General Psychiatry* 16 (June 1967): 699–703.

13. Judith Walzer Leavitt, "Strange Young Women on Errands: Obstetric Nursing between Two Worlds," *Nursing History Review* 6 (1998): 3–24.

14. Sherna B. Gluck, Daphne Patai, ed., *Women's Words: The Feminist Practice of Oral History* (New York: Routledge, 1991). They speak to the power of language to construct hierarchies.

15. Benjamin Baez, "Outsiders Within?" *Academe* 89 (4) (2003): 41–45. Baez is writing about dominant cultures, whiteness, and uses this argument to critique taking on the mantel of "outsider."

16. The idea of a "rhetorical force-multiplier" is used by Cotton Seiler in "Dying Is Easy, Comedy Is Hard," his review of *Pragmatism, Feminism, and Democracy* by James Livingston, *American Quarterly* 55 (March 2003): 121–130, quote 123. The ANA used this technique throughout the last several decades. It issued proclamations and policy statements portraying organized medicine as highly obstructionist in issues ranging from federal funding for education for nurses to economic welfare activities. The AMA also used this tactic in its fight against chiropractors in the early 1960s. See Howard Wolinsky and Tom Brune, *The Serpent on the Staff: The Unhealthy Politics of the American Medical Association* (New York: G. P. Putnam's Sons, 1994), 125–130.

17. Margarete Sandelowski, *Devices and Desires: Gender, Technology, and American Nursing* (Chapel Hill: University of NC Press, 2000).

18. Fairman and Lynaugh, *Critical Care Nursing*.

19. Barbara Bates, "Physician and Nurse Practitioner: A Drama of Conflict, and Reward," original manuscript, 1975, 1–13, Bates Collection. This manuscript was revised and published in *Annals of Internal Medicine* 82 (May 5, 1975): 702–706.

20. The idea of educated allies is derived from an article by Patricia D'Antonio, "Legacy of Domesticity," *Nursing History Review* 199 (1) (1993): 229–246. In this paper she describes how mid-nineteenth-century physicians needed someone competent to carry out prescriptions and treatments, believing their position as healer would be strengthened if competent people could make them look better. I have revised the concept somewhat to capture a more active form, one in "helpful association with another." (Definition from *The American Heritage Dictionary of the English Language*, 4th edition, s.v. "ally.")

21. See C.P., line 147 to 153, fellowship of the American Academy of Nurse Practitioners (AANP), group project, "Stories from the Early Days of Becoming a Nurse Practitioner," written data submitted to Barbara Resnick and analyzed by Barbara Resnick, Barbara Sheer, Donna McArthur, Judith Lynch, Judith Longworth, Elias Provencio-Vasquez, 2000–2002. See also published manuscript of data analysis, Barbara Resnick et al., "The World Is Our Oyster: Celebrating Our Past and Anticipating Our Future," *Journal of the American Academy of Nurse Practitioners* 14 (1) (2002): 484–492.

22. Barbara Bates and Joan Lynaugh, "The Medical Nurse Practitioner," paper presented at the University of Rochester School of Medicine and Dentistry family medical program, "The New Medical Practice," Rochester, NY, April 4, 1971 (dated March 1971), Bates Collection, quote 2.

23. There is very little historiography pertaining to the nurse practitioner movement in general. Exceptions are Barbara Brush and Elizabeth Capezuti, "Revisiting 'A Nurse for All Settings': The NP Movement, 1965–1995," *Journal of the American Academy*

of Nurse Practitioners 8 (1) (January 1996): 5–11; Resnick et al., "The World Is Our Oyster."

24. President's Commission on the Health Needs of the Nation, Building America's Health, vol. 1 (Washington, DC: Government Printing Office, 1952).

25. Surgeon General's Consultant Group, Subcommittee on Paramedical Personnel in Rehabilitation and Care of the Chronically Ill, *Mobilization and Health Manpower,* sect. *II,* (Washington, DC: Government Printing Office, 1956).

26. Surgeon General's Consultant Group on Medical Education, *Physicians for a Growing America,* Public Health Service Pub. #709 (Washington, DC: Government Publishing Office, 1959).

27. President's Commission on Heart Disease, Cancer, and Stroke, *Report to the President: A National Program to Conquer Heart Disease, Cancer, and Stroke, vols. 1 and 2* (Washington, DC: Government Printing Office, 1964–1965); Lowell T. Coggeshall, *Planning for Medical Progress through Education* (Evanston, Ill: Association of American Medical Colleges, 1965).

28. These strategies are described in numerous articles of the 1950s and 1960s. The best overviews are found in Alfred Yankauer, John Connelly, and Jacob Feldman, "Allied Health Worker Utilization in Pediatric Practice in Massachusetts and in the United States," *Pediatrics* 42 (5) (November 1968): 733–742; idem, "Task Performance and Task Delegation in Pediatric Office Practice," *American Journal of Public Health* 59 (7) (July 1969): 1104–1117.

29. Horace Cotton, "The Physician's Business," *Pennsylvania Medicine* 71 (11) (1968): 75–79.

30. Yankauer, Connelly, and Feldman, "Allied Health Worker Utilization."; idem, "Task Performance and Task Delegation." For the use of the term "office girl," see Cotton, "The Physician's Business."

31. Hall's June 23, 1971, inaugural address found in AMA House of Delegates, Proceedings, 120th Annual Convention, Atlantic City, NJ, June 20–24, 1971, 44.

32. See, for example, Earl Siegel and Sylvia C. Bryson, "A Redefinition of the Role of the Public Health Nurse in Child Health Supervision," *American Journal of Public Health* 53 (7) (July 1963): 1015–1024; Nancy Martin, "Freeing the Doctor from Well-baby Care," *Medical Economics* 44 (4) (November 13, 1967): 118–124, 127; John P. Connelly, John D. Stoeckle, Edna S. Lepper, and Ruth M. Farrisey, "The Physician and the Nurse—Their Interprofessional Work in Office and Hospital Ambulatory Settings," *New England Journal of Medicine* 275 (14) (October 6, 1966): 765–769.

33. Faye Davies, telephone interview by M. J. Murphy, March 14, 1997. M. J. Murphy served as a research assistant in 1997.

34. Bonita Roche, telephone interview by M. J. Murphy, October 4, 1997.

35. Loretta Ford, interview by Julie Fairman, Gainesville, FL, January 19, 2006, lines 25–31.

36. Ibid., lines 1532–1535.

37. Ibid., lines 44–51.

38. Ibid., lines 309–316.

39. Ibid., lines 210–214. The nursing health conferences were clinics run by nurses, usually public or community health nurses, with minimal physician supervision. These conferences were typically in very poor rural areas where it was difficult to get physician oversight or supervision. The state of Colorado convened the meeting to strategize about models of care to improve access for patients in these areas.

40. Ibid., lines 251–252.

41. Ibid., lines 253–255.

42. Joan Lynaugh described this response by a student, personal communication, June 12, 2005.

43. Davies, telephone interview.

44. Bates, "Physician and Nurse Practitioner," quote 4.

45. Many terms are used in the literature to describe the process of clinical thinking. Once example is "clinical judgment." See Alvan R. Feinstein, *Clinical Judgment* (Baltimore: Williams and Wilkins, 1967); H. Tristram Engelhardt Jr., Stuart F. Spicker, and Bernard Towers, *Clinical Judgment: A Critical Appraisal* (Boston: D. Reidel, 1977). Another example is "diagnostic reasoning." The terms actually connote very similar concepts. Feinstein's idea of clinical judgment, however, relied more heavily on symptom grouping and categorization (using mathematical principles) for the purpose of rationalizing treatment decisions and developing an accurate prognosis. I prefer to use clinical thinking as suggested by Barbara Bates: *A Guide to Physical Examination and History Taking,* 6th edition (Philadelphia: J. B. Lippincott, 1995), 635–648. Bates's presentation combines rationalization with flexibility to accommodate patient individuality and social circumstances in treatment decisions.

46. Eliot Freidson, *Professional Dominance: The Social Structure of Medical Care* (New York: Atherton Press, 1970), xi.

47. Charles Rosenberg speaks specifically about the power of diagnosis to "rationalize, mediate, and legitimize relationships between individuals and institutions in a democratic society." These words resonate for the entire process of clinical thinking, of which diagnosis is one embedded part. See Charles Rosenberg, "Introduction: Illness, Society, and History," in *Framing Disease: Studies in Cultural History*, ed. Charles Rosenberg and Janet Golden (New Brunswick, NJ: Rutgers University Press, 1992), xiii–xxvi.

48. Bates, "Physician and Nurse Practitioner: Conflict and Reward," *Annals of Internal Medicine* 82 (May 5, 1975): 702–706.

49. For descriptions of nurses involved in informal decision making, see Stein, "The Doctor-Nurse Game"; Rose L. Coser, *Life on the Ward* (E. Lansing: Michigan State University Press, 1962); Rose L. Coser, Howard Becker, B. Greer, Everett C. Hughes, and Anselm Strauss, *Boys in White: Student Cultures in Medical Schools* (Chicago: University of Chicago Press, 1961); Keeling, *Nursing and the Privilege of Prescription*.

50. Nurses staffed the first-aid room until they were found out by local physicians. They then tried using standing orders as a front before giving up their control. See Karen Buhler-Wilkerson, *No Place Like Home: A History of Nursing and Home Care in the United States* (Baltimore: Johns Hopkins University Press, 2001), 109–110.

51. Michael Grey, *New Deal Medicine: The Rural Health Programs of the Farm Security Administration* (Baltimore: Johns Hopkins University Press, 1999), 92–96; Arlene Keeling and Jerry Bigbee, "The History of Advanced Practice Nursing in the United States," in *Advanced Practice Nursing: An Integrative Approach*, 3rd edition, ed. Anne B. Hamric, Judith Spross, and Charlene M. Hanson (St. Louis, MO: Elsevier/Saunders, 2005), 3–45. There are many more examples, such as the nurses of the frontier nursing service in Appalachia, and nurses working on reservations. See Keeling, *Nursing and the Privilege of Prescription*, chapters 3 and 4.

52. See Wilbur H. Watson, *Against the Odds: Blacks in the Profession of Medicine in the United States* (New Brunswick, NJ: Transaction Publishers, 1999). Watson describes back-porch nursing during the late nineteenth century in Tuskegee, Alabama, as

a deliberate practice associated with the John A. Andrew Memorial Hospital, which did not have an outpatient medical clinic when it opened in 1908 (69–70).

53. For a discussion on decision-making authority in intensive care units, see Fairman and Lynaugh, *American Critical Care*, chapter 4.

54. Walsh McDermott, "Absence of Indicators of the Influence of Its Physicians on a Society's Health," *American Journal of Medicine* 70 (April 1981): 833–843, quote on 837.

55. Ibid., 838.

56. These parameters were and remain important, as recent contemporary epidemics make clear, but their value is limited when applied to health and chronic illness therapeutics that require supportive and behavioral interventions.

57. Edward Shorter, "The History of the Doctor-Patient Relationship," in *Companion Encyclopedia of the History of Medicine*, vol. 2, ed. William F. Bynum and Roy Porter (London: Routledge, 1993), 783–800, quote on 794.

58. See William Morgan and Barbara Bates, "Should Nurses Do Physical Examinations?" *Annals of Internal Medicine* 75 (2) (1971): 314.

59. McDermott, "Absence of Indicators," 839.

60. Alan H. Rosenstein, "Consumerism and Health Care: Will the Traditional Patient-Physician Relationship Survive?" *Postgraduate Medicine* 79 (1986): 13–28; study cited on 16.

61. Richard Edlick, telephone interview by Julie Fairman, August 28, 2000. Edlick is a physician who developed the emergency medical system for the state of Virginia in the 1970s.

62. Corene Johnson, telephone interview by M. J. Murphy, September 20, 1997.

63. Many scholars acknowledge negotiations can occur when parties do not share the same status or power. See Anselm Strauss, Shizuko Fagerhaugh, Barbara Suczek, and Carolyn Wiener, *Social Organization of Medical Work* (Chicago: University of Chicago Press, 1985); Eliot Friedson, *Professionalism Reborn* (Chicago: University of Chicago Press, 1994). For negotiations in particular settings where power between negotiators is also uneven, see Rue Bucher and Leonard Schatzman, "Negotiating a Division of Labor among Professionals in the State Mental Hospitals," *Psychiatry* 27 (1964): 266–77; Julie Fairman, "Watchful Vigilance: Nursing Care, Technology, and the Development of Intensive Care Units," *Nursing Research* 41 (January/February 1992): 56–60.

64. Davies, telephone interview.

65. Most of the nurse practitioner programs relied upon physicians as instructors and mentors during the early years because there were not enough nurses to teach these courses. See American Academy of Nurse Practitioners, Group Project, lines 325–326.

66. Ibid., lines 340–343.

67. Ibid., lines 271–281.

68. Johnson, telephone interview.

69. Denise Geolot, telephone interview by Julie Fairman, January 5, 2000. Denise Geolot went on to become the director, Division of Nursing, Health Resources and Services Administration. Linda Davies, another early Virginia nurse practitioner, also speaks of the support she had from physicians. Linda Davies, interview by Julie Fairman, Charlottesville, VA, July 22, 2000.

70. Roche, telephone interview.

71. American Academy of Nurse Practitioners, Group Project, lines 550–553.

72. Geolot, telephone interview.

73. Roche, telephone interview.

74. Ibid.

75. Ibid.

76. L. Davies, interview.

77. Keeling, *Nursing and the Privilege of Prescription*.

78. See various entries in the minutes of the State Board of Medical Education and Licensure, State of Pennsylvania, Office of Occupational and Health Affairs, Harrisburg, PA. See, for example, entries of October 10, 1971; October 22, 1971; January 6, 1972; December 4, 1973; March 15, 1974; and April 24, 1974.

79. Diane Purcell, telephone interview by M. J. Murphy, October 12, 1997.

80. Ibid.

81. Barbara Bates, "Twelve Paradoxes: A Message for Nurse Practitioners," *Nursing Outlook*, 22 (1974): 686–688.

82. Purcell, telephone interview.

83. Barbara Medoff Cooper, interview by M. J. Murphy, October 23, 1997, Philadelphia.

84. Ibid.

85. See Deidre Wicks, *Nurses and Doctors at Work: Rethinking Professional Boundaries* (Buckingham, UK: Open University Press, 1998), 1–5. The power in the ability to make choices is presented by Ruth Schwartz Cowan, *More Work for Mother: The Ironies of Household Technology from the Open Hearth to the Microwave* (New York: Basic Books, 1983); Fairman, "Alternate Visions."

86. George E. Ferrar Jr., "Keynote Address," 1969 Officers' Conference, Pennsylvania Medical Society, *Pennsylvania Medicine*, June 1969, 9–10. Italics in original.

87. Geolot, telephone interview.

Chapter 2 Following the Money

1. Andrew Abbott, *The System of Professions: An Essay on the Division of Expert Labor* (Chicago: University of Chicago Press, 1988).

2. Susan Reverby, "From Papers to Person," in *Virginia Henderson: Signature for Nursing*, ed. Eleanor Krohn Herrmann (Indianapolis, IN: Sigma Theta Tau International, 1998), 85–87.

3. Barbara Bates, "Can a Screening Unit Do It?" Rough draft, paper presented at the 165th annual convention, Medical Society of the State of New York, New York, NY, February 16, 1971, 7, Barbara Bates Collection, Barbara Bates Center for the Study of the History of Nursing, University of Pennsylvania, School of Nursing, Philadelphia (Bates Collection). Rosemary Stevens also addresses the need for strategic planning in *American Medicine and the Public Interest*, Updated Edition with a New Introduction (Berkeley: University of California Press, 1998).

4. William G. Rothstein, *American Medical Schools and the Practice of Medicine: A History* (New York: Oxford University Press, 1987), quote 187. There are several well-documented histories of medical education, and the purpose of this chapter is not to repeat these arguments but to place the nurse practitioner movement within these contextual changes. See, for example, Stevens, *American Medicine and the Public Interest*; and Kenneth M. Ludmerer, *Time to Heal: American Medical Education from the Turn of the Century to the Era of Managed Care* (New York: Oxford University Press, 1999).

5. Stevens, *American Medicine and the Public Interest*. See particularly chapter 16.

6. Ibid.; Stevens, *In Sickness and in Wealth: American Hospitals in the Twentieth Century* (New York: Basic Books, 1989).

7. This trend changed in the early 1970s. The Health Professions Educational Assistance Program made training funds available to specialties other than psychiatrists and physiatrists, including family practice specialists. See Louis M. Rousselot, "Federal Efforts to Influence Physician Education: Specialization Distribution Projections and Options," *Journal of the American Medical Association* 55 (August 1973): 123–130.

8. Richard Edlick, telephone interview by Julie Fairman, August 28, 2000.

9. U.S. Department of Health, Education and Welfare (DHEW), *Health Resources Statistics*, 1969, PHS Pub. #1509 (Washington, DC: Government Printing Office, 1969), cited in Staff Report, Committee on Ways and Means, *Basic Facts on the Health Industry. Prepared for the Use of the Committee on Ways and Means*, 92nd Cong., 1st sess. (Washington, DC: Government Printing Office, June 28, 1971), 7. These figures include both osteopaths and chiropractors. The physician ratio (allopathic) fell from 134 to 133 per 100,000 population from 1950 to 1959.

10. Office of Defense Mobilization, *Mobilization and Health Manpower*, Report of the Health Resources Advisory Committee (Washington, DC: Government Printing Office, January 1955); Frank Bane, *Physicians for a Growing America*, Surgeon General's Consultant Group on Medical Education, PHS Pub. #709 (Washington, DC: Government Printing Office, 1959); U.S. Department of Health, Education, and Welfare, Final Report of the Secretary's Consultants on Medical Research and Education, *The Advancement of Medical Research and Education through the Department of Health, Education, and Welfare* (Washington DC: Government Printing Office, 1958) (known as the Bayne-Jones Report).

11. See, for examples in the popular press, "The Plight of the U.S. Patient," *Time*, February 21, 1969, 53; "The Crisis in American Health Medicine," *Harper's Magazine*, October 1960, 123; "It's Time to Operate," *Fortune*, January 1970, 79.

12. Stevens, *American Medicine and the Public Interest*, quote 357. Stevens argues against the "Machiavellianism" of economic restrictionism as the reason for the AMA's resistance to federal funding for medical education. This, she notes, may have been a part of the AMA's reason for resistance, but only as a set of symptoms surrounding professionalism that emerged after the Flexner decades. The AMA eventually lost its battle over federal funding and offered its support.

13. There was earlier federal support for medical schools, but it was primarily to produce medical scientists rather than clinical practitioners. Examples included monies as part of the development of the National Science Foundation in 1950 (P.L. 81–507) and the National Defense Education Act of 1958 (P.L. 85–864).

President Kennedy first proposed a four-year scholarship program and a ten-year federal matching-grants construction program to build and rehabilitate medical and dental schools. Supporters struggled to bring this proposal to the hearing stage after tepid response from Republicans and the AMA. In 1962 it was resubmitted when the house substituted a five-year student loan program for the scholarship aid, and broadened the coverage to include teaching facilities for pharmacists, optometrists, podiatrists, and nurses. The 1962 version of the act never reached the House floor, although there was some last-minute political maneuvering to do so if another one of the administrations bills (the College Aid Bill, HR 8900) died. Nevertheless, the Senate version, although discussed in hearings in 1961, never received action in 1962. During the same year, the AMA developed its own loan program for needy students, providing $10,000 over a seven-year period, to be paid back when recipients started their practice. The federal bill was finally signed into law in September 1963 and expanded in 1964 to include optometry students

(P.L. 88–654). Scholarships were eventually added in 1965 (P.L. 89–290). A forgiveness principle was added in 1966 for practitioners in special areas designated by the Secretary of Health, Education and Welfare (P.L. 89–7550). In 1968, the various provisions included in earlier NTAs were added to the Health Manpower Act (P.L. 90–490). See U.S. Congress, *Congressional Quarterly Almanac*, 89th Cong., 1st sess., 1965, vol. 21 (Washington, DC: Congressional Quarterly Service), 272, 334; U.S. Congress, *Congressional Quarterly Almanac*, 87th Cong., 2nd sess., 1962, vol. 18 (Washington, DC: Congressional Quarterly Service), 229; U.S. Congress, *Congressional Quarterly Almanac*, 87th Cong., 1st sess., 1961, vol. 17 (Washington, DC: Congressional Quarterly Service), 266. See also Stevens, *American Medicine and the Public Interest*, 367.

14. The AMA successfully fought increased medical school admissions until the passage of the 1963 act, henceforth the number of graduates did not increase greatly until about 1965, two years later. This span is significant because many two-year medical schools converted to four-year programs with support of federal money. Most of these were in rural areas. Between 1960 and 1964, the number of graduates typically increased from between one hundred to five hundred students per year. Figures derived from Ludmerer, *Time to Heal*, table 7, 212.

15. AMA, *Distribution of Physicians in the United States, 1971. Regional, State, County, and Metropolitan Area* (Chicago: American Medical Association, 1972), 10–18.

16. Specialization, as Rosemary Stevens has noted, "with its strong professional, organizational, and political connotations . . . is the fundamental theme for the organization of medicine in the twentieth century"; Stevens, *American Medicine and the Public Interest*, 9.

17. Ibid., table 1, 162; James Cooper and Karen Heald, "Is There a Doctor Shortage?" *Journal of the American Medical Association* 227 (12) (March 25, 1974): 1410–1411.

18. Patricia Kendall, "Medical Specialization: Trends and Contributing Factors," in *Psychosocial Aspects of Medical Training*, ed. R. H. Coombs and C. E. Vincent (Springfield, IL: C. Thomas, 1971), 461.

19. The armed forces also endorsed the shift toward physician specialization through its funding of specialist training, as did hospitals, health insurers, and government agencies, which required specialty certification as evidence of competence. See the American Board of Medical Specialties, *Annual Report and Reference Handbook—1984* (Evanston, IL: American Board of Medical Specialties, 1984), 7–22, 53–54.

20. William Stewart and Maryland Pennell, "Pediatric Manpower in the United States and Its Implications," *Pediatrics* 31 (February 1963): 316–317.

21. For an overview, see Rashi Fein, *The Doctor Shortage: An Economic Diagnosis* (Washington, DC: Brookings Institution, 1967).

22. Illustrative advertisements found in the "Practice Opportunities" section, *Pennsylvania Medicine*, February 1966, 68. The calculation of 50 percent is drawn from the advertisements in each month's issues. It is probably a low estimate as many of the requests were unspecific.

23. George E. Ferrar Jr., "Keynote Address," Pennsylvania Medical Society, 1969 Officers' Conference, *Pennsylvania Medicine*, June 1969, 10.

24. National Academy of Sciences, Institute of Medicine, "Study Proposal: An Analysis of the Functions and Roles of Primary Health Care Manpower," final draft with cover letter to Alan Fisher from Karen Grimm (staff office), February 4, 1974, 1, Shirley Smoyak Collection, Barbara Bates Center for the Study of the History of Nursing, School of Nursing, University of Pennsylvania, Philadelphia, (Smoyak

Collection). Stevens also discusses the piecemeal development of these programs and the resulting fragmentation of health services in *American Medicine and the Public Interest*, 517–522.

25. Edward Shorter, "The History of the Doctor-Patient Relationship," in *Companion Encyclopedia of the History of Medicine*, vol. 2, ed. William F. Bynum and Roy Porter (London: Routledge, 1993), 783–800, quote on 793.

26. Terrance Keenan, Linda Aiken and Leighton E. Cluff, *Nurses and Doctors: Their Education and Practice* (Cambridge, MA: Oelgeschlager, Gunn and Hain, 1981).

27. The Health Disease, Cancer and Stroke Amendments of 1965 (P.L. 89–239) created the regional medical programs. The guidelines were published in 1966, and six months later, fifty-four regions organized themselves into academic and community service centers. Fifty of them received planning grants given by the surgeon general as authorized by the National Advisory Council of the NIH, under which the program was housed (and eventually, the Public Health Service). The provisions were extended in 1968, and again in 1970. Kidney disease was added to the focus in 1970. See Stephen P. Strickland, *The History of Regional Medical Programs: The Life and Death of a Small Initiative of the Great Society* (Lanham, MD: University Press of America, 2000), 41, 107.

28. The comprehensive care movement began in the early 1950s as a social advocacy response by medical educators and certain academic centers to the growing sense of inadequate ambulatory care in hospitals and community clinics. At least ten schools, (Cornell, University of Colorado, Western Reserve (later Case Western Reserve) University, University of North Carolina, Temple University, University of Albany, University of Louisville, University of Oklahoma, Washington University, Saint Louis University, and Vanderbilt University) established programs in 1952. These programs included both theory components and clerkships that focused on primary and preventive care, with an emphasis on family and developmental theory, establishing long-term relationships with families, and utilizing a team approach to services. Most of these programs, although popular at first, were eventually phased out by the mid-1970s, as both students and faculty found them less appealing in contrast to the typical tertiary care–based curriculum. Several facets of the programs, such as family-based practice, eventually migrated into traditional medical programs. See George G. Reader and Rosemary Soave, "Comprehensive Care Revisited," *Milbank Memorial Fund Quarterly* 54 (1976): 412–415; Parnie S. Snoke and Richard Weinerman, "Comprehensive Care Programs in University Medical Centers," *Journal of Medical Education* 40 (7) (July 1965): 625–657.

29. Staff, "Prescription for the Medical Manpower Shortage," *Pennsylvania Medicine*, April 1969, 71–82, quote on 72.

30. For a fuller description of community-based medical schools, see Irving J. Lewis and Cecil G. Sheps, *The Sick Citadel: The American Academic Medical Center and the Public Interest* (Cambridge, MA: Oelgeschlager, Gunn and Hain, 1983), 149–153; Rothstein, *American Medical Schools*, 228–230; Ludmerer, *Time to Heal*, 212–213.

31. Barbara Bates, "Medical and Nursing Education to Meet Community Health Needs," paper presented at the New York State Nurses' Association Convention, Syracuse, New York, October 31, 1967, Bates Collection, quote on 7.

32. Quotes are from a study conducted by Robert Aldrich and the Education Committee of the American Pediatric Society, *Survey of Pediatricians in the U.S. 1958*, cited

by S. Z. Levine in the 1960 presidential address of the society: "Pediatric Education at the Crossroads," *American Journal of Diseases of Children* 100 (5) (1960): 651–655, quote on 653.

33. Association of American Medical Colleges, *Physicians for the Twenty-First Century* (Washington, DC: Association of American Medical Colleges, 1984), 6–12, 27–30.

34. Kerr L. White, Franklin Williams, and Bernard G. Greenberg, "The Ecology of Medical Care," *New England Journal of Medicine* 265 (18) (1961): 885–881.

35. Allen C. Johnson, Hilda H. Kroeger, Isidore Altman, Dean A. Clark, and Cecil G. Sheps, "The Office Practice of Internists III, Characteristics of Patients," *Journal of the American Medical Association* 193 (11) (1965): 916–922.

36. DHEW, Public Health Service (PHS), *Nursing Resources: A Progress Report of the Program of the Division of Nursing Resources*, PHS Pub. 551 (Washington, DC: Government Printing Office, 1958), chart 3. For the concept of jurisdictional dominance and the importance of the workplace in establishing professional exclusivity, see Abbott, *The System of Professions*, 117–142; Arlene Keeling, *Nursing and the Privilege of Prescription, 1893–2000* (Columbus: Ohio State University Press, 2007), 97–99.

37. Isabel Stewart was also the chair of the Committee on Curriculum of the National League for Nursing Education (NLN), which published *A Curriculum Guide for Schools for Nursing* in 1937. The curriculum was the culmination of a gradual change in nursing education originating at the turn of the century, from a training system based on rudimentary case methods to a functional, rule-based efficiency method. For a more detailed analysis of Stewart's method and influence on hospital nursing, see Julie Fairman, "Thinking about Patients: Nursing Science in the 1950s," *Reflections* 23 (3) (3rd/4th Quarter, 1997): 30–32. Also see Susan Reverby, "A Legitimate Relationship: Nursing, Hospitals, and Science in the Twentieth Century," in *The American General Hospital: Communities and Social Contexts*, ed. Diana Long and Janet Golden (Ithaca, NY: Cornell University Press, 1989), 135–156. Although there are many definitions of functional method, I have used the perspective drawn from Frances Reiter, "The Nurse-Clinician," *International Nursing Review* 13 (4) (1996): 62–73.

38. National League for Nursing, *Report on Hospital Schools of Nursing, 1957* (New York: NLN, 1959), 18.

39. M. Lucille Kinlein, "Independent Nurse Practitioner," *Nursing Outlook* 20 (1) (1972): 22–24, quote on 22. Kinlein practiced independently as a generalist nurse beginning in 1971.

40. Esther Lucile Brown, *Nursing for the Future: A Report Prepared for the National Nursing Council* (New York: Russell Sage Foundation, 1948); idem, *Newer Dimensions of Patient Care*, Parts 1–4 (New York: Russell Sage Foundation, 1965); Hildegard Peplau, *Interpersonal Relations in Nursing: A Conceptual Frame of Reference for Psychodynamic Nursing* (New York: G. P. Putnam's Sons, 1952); and later, Virginia Henderson, "The Nature of Nursing," *American Journal of Nursing* 64 (1964): 62–68. Henderson began to think about clinically based nursing practice in the 1940s but did not publish many of her thoughts until after she left Teachers College in the 1950s.

41. Henderson, "The Nature of Nursing." Henderson published many other important articles and texts, but this essay is the most often quoted and best representative of the changes occurring in nursing during this time period.

42. Brown, *Nursing for the Future;* idem, *Newer Dimensions;* Peplau, *Interpersonal Relations;* Henderson, "The Nature of Nursing."

43. Mildred Montag, *Community College Education for Nursing: An Experiment in Technical Education in Nursing* (New York: McGraw-Hill, 1959).

44. Edith Lewis, "The Associate Degree Program," *American Journal of Nursing* 64 (5) (1964): 78–81. See also Susan Rimby Leighow, *Nurses' Questions, Women's Questions* (New York: Peter Lang, 1996), 59, figure 7.

45. Patricia D'Antonio, "Women, Nursing, and Baccalaureate Education in 20th Century America," *Journal of Nursing Scholarship* 36 (4) (2004): 379–384.

46. Lewis, "The Associate Degree Nurse," table, 80.

47. Hildegard Peplau, "Present Day Trends in Psychiatric Nursing," *Neuropsychiatry* 3 (1956): 190–204. Peplau began the first graduate program in psychiatric-mental health nursing at Rutgers University, New Brunswick, NJ, in 1957.

48. Hildegard Peplau, "Interpretation of Clinical Observations," original manuscript with marginalia, presented to the class on interdisciplinary communication in psychiatry of the Nebraska Psychiatric Institute, University of Nebraska, College of Medicine, Omaha, January 2–3, 1958, 11–12, Hildegard E. Peplau Papers, Barbara Bates Center for the Study of the History of Nursing, University of Pennsylvania, School of Nursing, Philadelphia (Peplau Collection).

49. For a comprehensive overview of nursing education delivered by nurse training schools, see Joan Lynaugh and Barbara Brush, *American Nursing: From Hospital to Health Systems* (Malden, MA: Blackwell Publishing in conj. with the Milbank Memorial Fund, 1996), chapter 1.

50. Frances Reiter, "The Improvement of Nursing Practice," speeches presented at the American Nurses' Association Section, Regional Conferences for Professional Nurses (Kansas City, MO: ANA, 1961), 3–11; Reiter, "The Nurse-Clinician," 62–71.

51. For a general view of Dorothy Smith's philosophy and practice, see *The Collected Works of Dorothy M. Smith, 1948–1967* (Gainesville: College of Nursing Section, University of Florida Alumni Association, 1968).

52. Loretta Ford, Marguerite Cobb, and Margaret Taylor, *Defining Clinical Content of Graduate Nursing Programs: Community Health Nursing* (Boulder, CO: Western Interstate Commission for Higher Education, 1967); Loretta Ford and Henry Silver, "The Expanded Role of the Nurse in Child Care," *Nursing Outlook* 15 (1967): 43–45.

53. Laura L. Simms, "The Clinical Nursing Specialists," *Journal of the American Medical Association* 198 (1966): 675–678.

54. For statistics, see D'Antonio, "Women, Nursing, and Baccalaureate Education," 379–384.

55. Virginia Henderson coauthored *Textbook of the Principles and Practice of Nursing* with Bertha Harmer (who began the series and completed solo revised editions in 1922, 1928, and 1934) in 1939 (New York: Macmillan). Henderson revised the text in 1955, and again in 1978, this time with Gladys Nite and others, also issued by Macmillan.

56. For description of theories see, Jacqueline Fawcett, *Analysis and Evaluation of Conceptual Models of Nursing* (Philadelphia: F. A. Davis, 1984).

57. Bonnie Bullough, "Is the Nurse Practitioner Role a Source of Increased Work Satisfaction?" *Nursing Research* 23 (January February 1974): 14–19; Charles Lewis and Barbara Resnik, "Nurse Clinics and Progressive Ambulatory Patient Care," *New England Journal of Medicine* 277 (23) (December 7, 1967): 1236–1241.

58. In the mental illness field, social workers and psychologists also opposed nursing specialization because they feared competition. In contrast, many physicians

welcomed specialization in the field of psychiatry as long as these nurses practiced in psychiatric institutions (and not private practices), a place many physicians found uninteresting. See Barbara J. Callaway, *Hildegard Peplau: Psychiatric Nurse of the Century* (New York: Springer, 2002). Dorothy Mereness taught at New York University and was the dean of the School of Nursing at the University of Pennsylvania from 1965 to 1977. For Rogers's opinions, see Martha Rogers, "Nursing: to Be or Not to Be?" *Nursing Outlook* 20 (1972): 42–46.

59. See Dorothy Mereness, "Recent Trends in Expanding Roles of the Nurse," *Nursing Outlook* 18 (May 1970): 30–33.

60. Jerome Lysaught, telephone interview by Julie Fairman, October 29, 1999. Jerome Lysaught was a professor of education at the University of Rochester, Rochester, NY, when he was chosen to direct the national commission.

61. For exemplars of economic implications of practice initiatives on training schools and academic programs, see Rita A. Seeger Jablonski, "Sparks to Wildfires: The Emergence and Impact of Nurse Practitioner Education at Virginia Commonwealth University, 1974–1991," *Nursing History Review* 11 (2003): 167–187.

62. Exceptions to the education and administration focus of graduate education included the aforementioned programs at New York Medical College, University of Colorado, and Rutgers University. Yale University had one of the earliest graduate programs focused on clinical practice. Yale offered graduate programs for nursing since 1926 in areas such as education and administration, in addition to a clinically focused graduate program in public health. In 1949 Yale began an advanced program in psychiatric nursing, one of the first clinically oriented graduate programs besides public health in the country. See http://www.med.yale.edu/library/nursing/historical/chronology/1942.html (accessed September 20, 2007).

63. Lysaught, interview.

64. For an in-depth and insightful discussion of academic nursing programs and their focus on clinical practice, see Joan E. Lynaugh, "Academic Nursing Practice: Looking Back," in *Academic Nursing Practice: Helping to Shape the Future of Health Care*, ed. Lois K. Evans and Norma M. Lang (New York: Springer, 2004), 20–37.

65. U.S. Department of Health, Education, and Welfare, Report of the Surgeon General's Consultant Group on Nursing, *Toward Quality in Nursing: Needs and Goals*, Public Health Service Pub. #992 (Washington, DC: Government Printing Office, 1963), 46–72. This report became the cornerstone for President Lyndon Johnson's 1963 health message in which he requested legislation to expand the 1956 Health Amendments Act (P.L. 84–911) that established nurse traineeship programs. The 1963 report weighed in on the nursing education debate by recommending massive federal funding for nursing education and, with an innovative brushstroke, recommended the baccalaureate program as the foundational level for nursing education. Based partially on this report, President Johnson submitted his first bill to Congress in 1963 authorizing appropriation of federal funds for nurse training. This bill, Nurse Training Act (NTA), after much discussion in the House, was tabled but resubmitted and passed in 1964. For the 1964 NTA, see U.S. Congress, *Congressional Quarterly Almanac*, 88th Cong., 2nd sess., 1964, vol. 20 (Washington, DC: Congressional Quarterly Service, 1964), 244–245. See also Lynaugh, "Academic Nursing Practice," 20–37.

66. The NTA of 1964 (P.L. 88–581) added Title VIII to the Public Service Act of 1956, and included almost $283 million over five years for construction grants for teaching

facilities, student loans, and traineeships for students across all levels of programs. As perhaps an exemplar of the organization's difficulty reconciling its focus on workforce issues or professionalization, the ANA lobbied hard for the bill in general, but prioritized support for baccalaureate programs in particular, and decreased funding for diploma programs, although most of its constituents were diploma graduates. Their proposed amendments were defeated, due in part to major lobbying efforts of the American Hospital Association (AHA) and the AMA, who supported hospital diploma programs and invoked the nursing shortage as a national health crisis. See U.S. Congress, *Congressional Quarterly Almanac*, 88th Cong., 2nd sess, 244–245.

67. Many speculate that the anonymous donor was Mary Rockefeller, who was very interested in health care and nursing. The funding groups, through contacts with the Kellogg Foundation, invited W. Allen Wallis, president of the University of Rochester, to head the study. The Flexner report was one of the major historical reform mechanisms in medical education. Over eighteen months, educator Abraham Flexner visited 155 medical schools around the country and issued a report based on his assessments of admission criteria, curricula, and facilities. Although many lower-rated schools were already closing before Flexner issued his report, it further supported more rigorous medical-education standards based on scientific standards and clinical experience. See Abraham Flexner, *Medical Education in the United States and Canada: A Report to the Carnegie Foundation for the Advancement of Teaching*, Bulletin No. 4 (New York: Carnegie Foundation for the Advancement of Teaching, 1910).

68 See National Commission for the Study of Nursing Education, *Abstract for Action: Appendices* (New York: McGraw-Hill, 1971).

69. National Commission For the Study of Nursing Education, *Abstract for Action* (New York: McGraw-Hill, 1970).

70. Episodic nursing care was essentially curative and restorative and most often practiced in hospitals or impatient settings. Distributive care was practiced in communities or clinics and focused on health maintenance and promotion.Ibid., 91–92.

71. Lowell T. Coggeshall, Executive Council of the Association of American Medical Colleges, *Planning for Medical Progress through Education* (Evanston, IL: Association of American Medical Colleges, 1965).

72. At the time of the report, the relationship between the NLN and the ANA was quite tense, and each organization was experiencing its own financial and organizational conflicts. The Lysaught Commission was probably not high on their priority list at the time even though both organizations worked to gather the money to undertake the study. For example, there is scant mention of the report in ANA executive board minutes during the time period before and after it was released.

73. *Abstract for Action: Appendices*.

74. Lysaught, telephone interview. The Daughters of Charity were affiliated with almost three hundred hospitals during this time period, and they already began to close their training schools before the report in 1965. In contrast, the earlier report of the Council of the Conference of the Catholic Schools of Nursing in 1963 supported continuation of the training schools and improving the quality of the baccalaureate education programs in academic institutions. See *Abstract for Action*, 125.

75. Edith P. Lewis, editorial, "In Perspective," *Nursing Outlook* 20 (3) (March 1972): 1.

76. Edith P. Lewis to Karen Buhler-Wilkerson, November 12, 1998, Joan Lynaugh Personal Collection, Bryn Mawr, PA (Lynaugh Collection).

77. Josephine Goldmark, *Nursing and Nursing Education in the United States: Report of the Committee for the Study of Nursing Education* (New York: Macmillan, 1923).

78. Joan E. Lynaugh, "Academic Nursing Practice," 20–37. For an overview of the various reports, see *Abstract for Action: Appendices*, 130–133.

79. For example, see Mary Sarnecky, *A History of the U.S. Army Nurse Corps* (Philadelphia: University of Pennsylvania Press, 1999), 290–319. The Army Nurse Corps was a leader in nursing education and sent enlisted nurses to civilian baccalaureate and graduate programs before the professional nursing organizations began to rally for collegiate education.

80. Rimby Leighow, *Nurses Questions*, figure 6, 54. By 1960 about 20 percent of nursing students were enrolled in baccalaureate programs, and by 1970 about 30 percent. In 1980, 40 percent of students were enrolled in baccalaureate programs.

81. P.L. 88–129 was intended primarily for medical education, but the act also initially authorized funds for schools of nursing, dentistry, osteopathy, pharmacy, podiatry, and public health. Optometry schools were added in 1964. When the NTA was passed in 1964, nurses were removed from the 1963 act. DHEW, PHS, Division of Nursing, *First Report to the Congress, 1 February 1977, The Nurse Training Act of 1975* (Washington, DC: DHEW, Human Resources Administration 78–38, 1978), 146.

82. Kimi Taguchi Hara, "Memo #2," June 1964, 6, box 128, folder 2. From the ANA Collection in the Howard Gotlieb Archival Research Center at Boston University, Boston, (ANA Collection). Taguchi Hara was chair of the Maternal and Child Nurse Conference Group. The act provided money for special projects to improve and expand training programs preparing nurses to practice in settings other than hospitals.

83. Taguchi Hara, June 1964, 5. The institute operated from 1949 to 1979 and trained both doctors and nurses to care for premature infants. See Joellen W. Hawkins and Linda L. Bellig, "Evolution of Advanced Practice Nursing in the United States: Caring for Women and Newborns," *Journal of Obstetric, Gynecologic, and Neonatal Nursing* 29 (1) (January/February 2000): 83–89.

84. Denise Geolot, "Federal Funding of Nurse Practitioner Education: Past, Present and Future," *Nurse Practitioner Forum* 1 (3) (December 1990): 159–162. According to Geolot, these early demonstration projects were funded by the Commonwealth Fund, but the evaluation portion of the project was funded by the Division of Nursing. For examples of other programs, see Keeling, *Nursing and the Privilege of Prescription*, 132–135.

85. See Strickland, *The History of Regional Medical Programs*, 41, 107. For a discussion of federal funding of nursing education, see Lynaugh and Brush, *American Nursing*, chapter 1.

86. Madeline Leininger, D. E. Little, and Doris Carnevali, "PRIMEX," *American Journal of Nursing* 72 (July 1972): 1274–1277; Elizabeth A. Walker, "PRIMEX—The Family Nurse Practitioner Program," *Nursing Outlook* 20 (1) (1972): 28–31.

87. The 1975 act was designated P.L. 94–63, new subpart Y, Section 822, of the Public Health Service Act, Title IX. Geolot, "Federal Funding of Nurse Practitioner Education," 159–162.

88. See Abbott, *The System of Professions*, 125–135, for a discussion of the influence of the workplace in professional jurisdictional differentiation.

89. Elizabeth Cameron, interview by Julie Fairman, Philadelphia, May 16, 1996.

90. Barbara Rollins, telephone interview by Joan Lynaugh, March 23, 1990.

Chapter 3   Psychology Girls and Clandestine Groups

1. See Thomas P. Hughes, *Networks of Power: Electrification in Western Society, 1880–1930* (Baltimore, MD: Johns Hopkins University Press, 1983). His work analyzes large technological systems and in previous writing has considered health care as one such system.
2. Terrance Keenan, Linda Aiken, and Leighton E. Cluff, *Nurses and Doctors: Their Education and Practice* (Cambridge, MA: Oelgeschlager, Gunn and Hain, 1981). Linda Aiken was a student at the College of Nursing, University of Florida, while Dorothy Smith was dean.
3. Joan Lynaugh, personal communication, January 22, 2006.
4. Report of the Committee on Nursing, University of Rochester Medical Center, January 31, 1969, 8; Joan Lynaugh Personal Collection, Bryn Mawr, Pennsylvania (Lynaugh Collection).
5. U.S. Department of Health, Education and Welfare (DHEW), *Extending the Scope of Nursing: A Report of the Secretary's Committee to Study Extended Roles for Nurses* (Washington, DC: Government Printing Office, 1971).
6. The armed forces were early supporters of the expanded role for nurses, realizing their value as manpower resources in well-child care and family practice. The first program, adult ambulatory care, opened at Fort Benning, Georgia, in January 1972 and graduated its first class six months later in June 1972. The air force program was already in place by 1971, as was a navy nurse baccalaureate program. See Cynthia A. Gurney, *Thirty-three Years of Army Nursing: An Interview with Brigadier General Lillian Dunlap* (Washington, DC: U.S. Army Nurse Corps, 2001), 206–211.
7. Esther Lucile Brown, *Nursing Reconsidered: A Study of Change*, part 1 (Philadelphia: J. B. Lippincott, 1970), 52.
8. See John M. Maclachlan, *Planning Florida's Health Leadership*, vols. 1–5 (Gainesville: University of Florida Press, 1954).
   The label "health center" was purposefully chosen by the medical center study group to reflect interdisciplinary practice and patient care and the required integration of teams needed to provide disease prevention and health promotion. See *Planning*, vol. 1, 26.
9. Thomas J. Peters and Robert H. Waterman Jr., *In Search of Excellence: Lessons from America's Best Run Companies* (New York: Harper Row, 1982). Peters, a business entrepreneur, used the term in his book, but it has earlier origins in the engineering and technical fields, particularly aeronautics. See http://www.lockheedmartin.com/wms/findPage.do?dsp=fec&ci=16504&rsbci=15047&fti=0&ti=0&sc=400 (accessed June 20, 2007).
10. *Planning*, vol. 1, 14. The medical school in particular was designed to produce physicians for primary care and, later, family practice in response to the state's changing demographics. See the proposal developed for the Commonwealth Fund, "The University in Medicine: An Experiment in Interdisciplinary Cooperation. A Proposal," manuscript, 23–24, George T. Harrell Medical History Society and Archives, University of Florida, Gainesville (Harrell Archives).
11. See George T. Harrell interview with Samuel Proctor, July 26, 1982, UFHC #7, 115, Samuel Proctor Oral History Program (SPOHP), University of Florida, Gainesville. George Harrell was hired as dean of the medical school in 1954.
12. Dorothy Smith to Carol Hayes, April 21, 1956, box 1, file 8, Dorothy Smith Collection, Barbara Bates Center for the Study of the History of Nursing, School of Nursing, University of Pennsylvania, Philadelphia (Smith Collection). Italics in original.

13. Linda Aiken, "Dorothy M. Smith—Pioneer," handwritten memorial tribute, undated, box 2, file 22, Smith Collection.

14. The original model for medical education recommended by the medical center study was a 2–4–2 program—the first two years of general education (the junior and senior year of general university education), followed by a four-year combination of liberal arts, medical subjects, and some clinical experience, followed by two years of clinical education, and ending with a senior clerkship with local practitioners. This program was meant to train primary care physicians for rural and small communities in Florida.

15. Dorothy Smith to the Faculty, "Memo: Education and Nursing," December 17, 1962, box 6, file 19, Smith Collection.

16. Dorothy Smith to Linda Aiken, August 30, 1990, box 1, file 5, Smith Collection.

17. Francis Reiter became the first dean of the Graduate School of Nursing, New York Medical College, in 1960. She used the term "nurse clinician" initially in 1943, and later in 1966 to describe nurses who developed an intellectual and clinical competence to care for patients across all levels of patient needs. See Frances Reiter, "The Nurse-Clinician," *International Nursing Review* 13 (4) (1966): 62–71.

18. Other notable later efforts to integrate practice and education included Luther Christman's work at Vanderbilt University School of Nursing in Tennessee; Cynthia Kensella at Mt. Sinai Medical Center in New York City; Loretta Ford at the University of Rochester, NY; and Rozella M. Schlotfeldt and Janetta MacPhail at Case Western Reserve University in Cleveland, OH. Most of these programs opened in the later 1960s and 1970s and many of the developers came to visit Smith and her faculty at the University of Florida. See Brown, *Nursing Reconsidered*, 114–117.

19. Betty Hilliard, interview by Ann Smith, February 2, 2001, SPOHP, University of Florida College of Nursing, UFCN-2, 29. Dorothy Smith hired Hilliard as a nursing instructor in 1961. Ann Smith conducted the oral histories for the College of Nursing as part of the Samuel Proctor Oral History Program (SPOHP). She was a former nursing faculty member.

20. Cynthia Parks, "New Look at Nursing: Brains Not Bedpans," *Florida-Times Union*, Jacksonville, Florida, July 4, 1965, 50. The reporter's use of the term "psychology girls" in this piece holds positive connotations because it praises them for their intellect. Although the news reports were favorable, there still remained a level of ridicule in the language the reporters used and disbelief in the usefulness of the program.

21. Harrell had a somewhat different perspective. He claimed he insisted on the joint position of dean and chief of nursing to prevent a two-tiered care system—students learning one way of practice in the school and another way in the hospital. See Harrell, SPOHP, 110. Smith's views were presented in a letter to Carol Hayes, circa 1970, Smith Collection. Carol Hayes was hired in 1956 as one of the first nursing faculty.

22. Smith to Hayes, circa 1970, Smith Collection.

23. Dorothy M. Smith, "Practice—A Part of Teaching," *Nursing Outlook* 7 (3) (March 1959): 134–135.

24. The hospital became the W. A. Shands Teaching Hospital in 1965, named after Senator William A. Shands, Gainesville, Florida.

25. Smith to Hayes, circa 1970, Smith Collection.

26. Hilliard, SPOHP, 28. See also Dorothy Smith, "Position Paper on Nursing and Practice and Nursing Education at the University of Florida," March 22, 1968, Smith Collection.

27. Smith to Hayes, circa1970, Smith Collection. Loretta Ford, the dean of the School of Nursing, University of Rochester, implemented a similar model when she began her tenure there. See Loretta Ford, "The University of Rochester Model," in *Nurses and Doctors: Their Education and Practice*, 69–84.

28. By 1953, only 3 percent of Florida nurses held a bachelor of science degree. Ninety-five percent of nurses working in Florida completed a three-year nursing diploma program. See *Planning*, vol. 4, 92–96.

29. Smith to Aiken, August 19, 1990, box 1, series 1, file 5, Smith Collection.

30. Smith to Hayes, August 6, 1959, box 1, series 1, file 12, Smith Collection.

31. Dorothy Smith to Edmund F. Ackell, March 11, 1970, Smith Collection. Ackell was health center provost and vice president for health affairs at the University of Florida from 1969 to 1974.

32. Jennet Wilson, telephone interview by Julie Fairman, September 20, 2000, 4. Wilson was an early College of Nursing faculty member hired by Dorothy Smith.

33. Dorothy Smith, "Living Legend Acknowledgement Speech," October 14, 1996, American Academy of Nursing, Orlando, Florida, series 1, file 2, Smith Collection.

34. Quote from a speech Smith gave at Emory University School of Nursing, Atlanta, Georgia, September 18, 1992, manuscript, box 1, series 1, file 5, Smith Collection. An earlier exemplar is her "Speech to the General Duty and Private Duty Nurse Section," annual convention of the Florida State Nurses' Association, Clearwater, Florida, October 18, 1957, box 2, series 2, file 3, Smith Collection.

35. Smith, Florida State Nurses' Association, Smith Collection.

36. Smith to Aiken, April 6, 1987, Smith Collection.

37. Ibid.

38. Smith to Hayes, January 16, 1956, box 1, file 8, Smith Collection.

39. Smith to Hayes, dated January, 1956, box 1, file 8, Smith Collection.

40. Lucille Mercadante, interview by Ann Smith, March 28, 2001, SPOHP, UFCN-2, 26. Mercadante was associate dean of nursing practice, 1959–1967.

41. Ibid., 16.

42. The Cardex was a collection of patient data cards held together in a metal frame. Nurses wrote on them, usually in pencil, and changed them as the plan of care evolved. Cardex had been in use since the late 1950s, but gained popularity as Lawrence Weed's problem-oriented record integrated some of the structural components. Smith was an admirer of Weed's system long before many of his own colleagues. See Lawrence Weed, "Medical Records That Guide and Teach, Part I, Part II," *New England Journal of Medicine* 278 (11, 12) (March 14, 21, 1968): 593–600, 652–657.

43. Mercadante, SPOHP, 23.

44. Dorothy Smith to the Faculty, "Graduate Programs in the College of Nursing," November 20, 1962, 5, box 6, file 19, Harrell Archives.

45. Smith to Aiken, July 22, 1993, box 1, file 6, Smith Collection.

46. Harrell discusses the political battles he faced from the larger university over faculty positions, funding for various innovations such as the ambulatory care unit (which opened after Harrell left the university), and from local and state medical associations. See Harrell, SPOHP, 117, 136.

47. J. Wayne Reitz left the presidency in 1967; George Harrell left in 1964 and went on to develop the medical school at Hershey Medical Center, Hershey, PA. Sam Martin left in 1968.

48. See selected minutes of the Health Center Council, July 22, 1964; October 19, 1969, series 6, Harrell Archives.

49. Smith to Ackell, March 11, 1970, 8, Smith Collection.
50. Anonymous to Edmund F. Ackell, hand dated 1969, file Nursing-Dean, 69–70, Harrell Archives. Smith responded with a memo predicting the "possible crisis" in nursing care when the new pediatric intensive care unit opened. It was to be staffed by the current pediatric nursing staff, which was already short. Smith to Ackell, memo, December 17, 1969, file Nursing-Dean, 69–70, Harrell Archives.
51. Smith to Ackell, March 11, 1970, 1, Smith Collection. Smith did not have quite the same close relationship with Ackell as she did with Martin. For example, chair of physiology Arthur B. Otis wrote that the department agreed to admit nursing students to a course in human physiology in 1971 only after Provost Ackell promised a postdoctoral position for a year and then a permanent position to teach the course. Ackell provided the manpower to "get the dean of nursing off his back." See Arthur B. Otis, "History of Physiology Department at University of Florida, 1956–1981," *The Physiologist* 29 (5) Supplement (October 1986): 27–33, quote 30.
52. Smith had been complaining about the budget since 1962. Smith to Ackell, March 11, 1970, 5, Smith Collection.
53. Ibid., 2. See also the report, National Commission for the Study of Nursing and Nursing Education, *Abstract for Action* (New York: McGraw-Hill, 1970).
54. Dorothy Smith to the Faculty, memo, "Faculty Resolution," December 22, 1969, Smith Collection.
55. M. W. to Lamar E. Crevasse Jr., memo, March 25, 1969, 1–2, file EA, College of Nursing, Harrell Archives. Crevasse was the area coordinator for the North Florida regional medical program.
56. Smith to Ackell, memo, April 2, 1969, file EA, College of Nursing, Harrell Archives. Smith's main complaints were that the director believed the nursing students provided little care at the health center, and that he was personally attacking her and individual members of her faculty.
57. Smith to Ackell, memo, July 13, 1970, 1, file EA, College of Nursing, Harrell Archives. In the memo she "relinquish[es] that part of my title which states chief of nursing practice."
58. Smith to Hayes, July 20, 1970, Smith Collection. Smith to Ackell, July 13, 1970, 1, Harrell Archives.
59. William A. Wallis and Emory Morris, who was head of the W. K. Kellogg Foundation at the time, were acquaintances, and the foundation had a long interest in baccalaureate nursing in general. See Joan Lynaugh, "A Special Relationship: Nursing and the W. K. Kellogg Foundation," *Nursing and Health Care* 43 (4) (July 1995): 183–202. Wallis served as president of the National Commission for the Study of Nursing and Nursing Education, which was directed by Jerome Lysaught, a professor in the Graduate School of Education at Rochester. See chapter 2.
60. There is a crossover here between the University of Florida and the University of Rochester. Lucille Mercadante, who was a colleague of Dorothy Smith when she was at Florida, had by this time moved to New York where she worked with Joan O'Brien, dean of the College of Nursing at SUNY Downstate, as a consultant. Mercadante subsequently served as a consultant to the Committee on Nursing, University of Rochester. "Report of the Committee on Nursing," January 31, 1969, 1, Lynaugh Collection.
61. Ibid.
62. Ibid, 16.
63. Ibid., 16–17.

64. Marcia A. Dake, Barbara Bates, Grace White, and M. Sue Kern, "The University of Kentucky Medical Center: One Approach to Health Care," in *Exploring Progress in Nursing Practice*, ed. ANA Staff (New York: ANA, 1966), 21–34. The Frontier Nursing Service had also been operating in Kentucky since the first decades of the twentieth century, and nurses in expanded practices provided most of the services. See Arlene Keeling, *Nursing and the Privilege of Prescription, 1893–2000* (Columbus: Ohio State University Press, 2007), 49–71.

65. Joan Lynaugh, handwritten note circa 1968–1970, Lynaugh Collection.

66. Joan Lynaugh, interview with Julie Fairman, Bryn Mawr, PA, February 20, 2003, lines 73–83.

67. Quotes from handwritten text, yellow notebook pages, "written in 1980, notes for Sr. Mary Johns," Lynaugh Collection.

68 Barbara Bates and Joan Lynaugh, grant proposal to the division of nursing, U.S. Public Health Service, "The Medical Nurse Practitioner: A Planning Proposal for Developing a Curriculum and a Collaborative Nurse-Physician Team," 1971, 15, Lynaugh Collection.

69. Joan Lynaugh, handwritten notes on clinic patients, 1970–1971, Lynaugh Collection. The initials are fictitious to remove patient identifiers.

70. By 1971 there were seven teams, including clinic nurses and the nursing faculty, with support from the Rochester regional medical program, of which Bates was a board member. Bates and Lynaugh, grant proposal, 16, Lynaugh Collection.

71. Letter from V.M. to Nate Lassman and Joan Lynaugh, September 4, 1970, Lynaugh Collection.

72. The program was under the direction of nurse Eleanor Lambertson and physician George Reader, program directors nurse Doris Schwartz, and physician Frederic Kirkham. Lambertson was dean of the School of Nursing, Reader was director of ambulatory care and professor of medicine and public health at Cornell, Kirkham was the medical director of the project, and Schwartz was part of the nursing faculty at City University of New York.

73. Doris Schwartz, "Steps Leading to a PRIMEX Program," speech given at the ANA, May 2, 1972, Detroit, Kathryn Jacquette Collection, Center for Nursing Historical Inquiry, University of Virginia, School of Nursing (Jacquette Collection). Doris Schwartz, interview by Susan Reverby, June 5, 1968, 12–16, Lynaugh Collection.

74. Harriet Kitzman, telephone interview by Julie Fairman, May 26, 2005, lines 69–74. This same kind of informal authority occurred in the early intensive care units in the 1950s and 1960s. See Julie Fairman and Joan Lynaugh, *Critical Care Nursing: A History* (Philadelphia: University of Pennsylvania Press, 1998).

75. Kitzman interview, lines 91–94.

76. Ibid., lines 99–106.

77. Evan Charney and Harriet Kitzman, "The Child-Health Nurse (Pediatric Nurse Practitioner) in Private Practice," *New England Journal of Medicine* 285 (24) (1971): 1352–1357.

78. Kitzman Interview, lines 267–274.

79. Ibid., lines 210–227.

80. Lynaugh interview, lines 83–93.

81. William L. Morgan and Barbara Bates, "Should Nurses Do Physical Examinations?" *Annals of Internal Medicine* 75 (2) (1971): 314.

82. George Engel to Barbara Bates and Joan Lynaugh, April 6, 1973, correspondence, University of Rochester, 1972–75, 76, Lynaugh Collection. Engel is responding to

the article written by Joan Lynaugh and Barbara Bates, "The Two Languages of Nursing and Medicine," *American Journal of Nursing* 73 (1) (1973): 66–69.

83. Dorothy Taylor and Joan Lynaugh to Mrs. Deffenbaugh and Miss Hall, January 14, 1971, Lynaugh Collection. Dorothy Taylor was the assistant director of nursing services for ambulatory care, Betty Deffenbaugh was director of nursing service, and Eleanor Hall was chair of the Department of Nursing of the School of Medicine and Dentistry.

84. Lynaugh interview, line 108.

85. Ibid., lines 117–123.

86. Ibid., lines 126–128.

87. Ibid., lines 136–143.

88. Barbara Bates, interview with Julie Fairman, Bryn Mawr, PA, circa 1999. See also typed sheet "Behavioral Objectives for Practitioners in Physical Examination," rough draft #1, Spring 1971, Lynaugh Collection.

89. Lynaugh interview, lines 148–150.

90. Barbara Bates, handwritten notes, Lynaugh Collection.

91. Lynaugh interview, lines 67–69. They agreed upon a systematic approach to physical examination, working from head to toe, beginning with an examination of the head and neck, and ending with the musculo-skeletal system. For a description, see Joan Lynaugh and Dorothy Taylor to "distribution," "Physical Diagnosis for Nurses," February 25, 1971, 1, Lynaugh Collection.

92. The guidebooks were developed and illustrated by naturalist Roger Tony Peterson almost seventy years ago and published by Houghton Mifflin. See http://www.houghtonmifflinbooks.com/peterson/petersonhome.cfm (accessed June 6, 2006). Bates eventually engaged a professional artist and photographer for the illustrations.

93. The mimeographed texts eventually gave way to over nine editions of *Bates Guide to Physical Examination and History Taking*, starting in 1974, and published by Lippincott. There are currently eleven translations, including Chinese and Russian, pocket guides, video and DVD versions of the text, study guides, and instructor manuals. Bates sent the manuscript to Lippincott's medical division, probably because it was well known to her. David Miller, who was head of nursing publications, was quite enthusiastic because he believed he could sell the text to both medicine and nursing programs (personal email communication, Joan Lynaugh, April 5, 2005). Medical student use noted in a letter from Lawrence E. Young, chairman, Department of Medicine, to Joan Lynaugh and Barbara Bates, January 10, 1972, Lynaugh Collection.

94. U.S. Congress, *Congressional Quarterly Almanac*, 92nd Cong., 1st sess., 1971, vol. 27 (Washington, DC: Congressional Quarterly Service, 1971), 534–537. Also see Denise Geolot, "Federal Funding of Nurse Practitioner Education: Past, Present and Future," *Nurse Practitioner Forum* 1 (3) (December 1990): 159–162.

95. They first submitted a joint proposal in 1969 but were advised by the division officers to resubmit separately.

96. Bates and Lynaugh began to use the terms "physical diagnosis" and "collaboration" in the 1971 Division of Nursing planning grant proposal. The first version of the module text was entitled "Physical Examination."

97. The goals are outlined in an information sheet, dated Summer 1971, "The Medical Nurse Practitioner Program: General Information," Lynaugh Collection. See also Bates and Lynaugh, grant proposal, Lynaugh Collection.

98. Lynaugh, typed notes, July 28, 1971, Lynaugh Collection.
99. Ibid., July 20, 1971.
100. According to Joan Lynaugh (personal communication, June 7, 2006), she and Barbara Bates taught most of the classes, but physicians Milton Luria, Phillip Bonnani, Abe Levy, and others helped in the physical exam part of the course for the first round.
101. Bates and Lynaugh, grant proposal, 26, Lynaugh Collection. For the University of Colorado program, see Loretta Ford and Henry Silver, "The Expanded Role of the Nurse in Child Care," *Nursing Outlook* 15 (1967): 43–45. For the Kansas City program, see Charles Lewis and Barbara Resnik, "Nurse Clinics and Progressive Ambulatory Patient Care," *New England Journal of Medicine* 277 (23) (December 7, 1967): 1236–1241.
102. See Joan Lynaugh and Barbara Bates, annual comprehensive report, 1972–1973, Contract NIH 72–4214, 15, Lynaugh Collection.
103. Lynaugh interview, lines 440–443.
104. Ibid., lines 348–360.
105. For further discussion on this issue, see Frances Hughes et al., "Nurse Practitioner Research: An Historical Analysis," in *Nurses, Nurse Practitioners*, ed. Mathy D. Mezey and Diane O. McGivern (New York: Springer, 2003), 84–108.
106. Lynaugh interview, lines 540–542.
107. In 1973, over 60 percent of certificate nurse practitioner programs required a guarantee of employment from applicants. Only one of the master's programs surveyed demanded employment certification. The requirement declined steadily over the decade, and by 1980 only 22 percent of the certificate programs and none of the master's programs mandated this. See Henry A. Sultz, Maria Zielezny, Jane Mathews Gentry, and Louis Kinyon, *Longitudinal Study of Nurse Practitioners: Phase II*, DHEW Publication No. 78–92 (Hyattsville, MD.: U.S. Department of Health, Education and Welfare, 1978), 12, 36.
108. Joan Lynaugh and Barbara Bates, "Medical Nurse Practitioner: Nursing Education in the Care of Adult Ambulatory Patients and Implementation of the Role in Practice," grant proposal, 1972, 14–20, Lynaugh Collection. Lynaugh and Bates were codirectors, and the grant was submitted to the NIH.
109. M. Lucille Kinlein, "Independent Nurse Practitioner," *Nursing Outlook* 20 (1) (1972): 22–24; idem, *Independent Nursing Practice with Clients* (Philadelphia: J. B. Lippincott, 1977). Kinlein practiced independently as a nurse beginning in 1971. Gertrude Isaacs, "The Family Nurse and Primary Health Care in Rural Areas," *Frontier Nursing Service Quarterly Bulletin* 47 (1972): 3–9. For earlier examples, see Arlene Keeling, " 'Carrying Ointments and Even Pills!' Medicines in the Work of Henry Street Settlement Visiting Nurses, 1893–1944," *Nursing History Review* 14 (2006): 7–30.
110. Lynaugh interview, lines 573–579.
111. N.Y. State Senate Bill No. 1918 was introduced in January 1971 and was supported by the New York State Nurses Association (NYSNA). Many other state nursing organizations during this time, and even earlier, were supporting changes in the practice acts to better reflect the clinical practice of generalist nurses (Karen Ballard of the NYSNA, telephone interview with Rebecca Nanansi, October 20, 2004). Governor Nelson Rockefeller vetoed the 1971 bill on July 7 after appeals by the New York State Medical Association and the Hospital Association of New York who argued that the bill would permit nurses to practice medicine. A new bill, Senate Bill No. 8274, was submitted in 1972 and signed into law by Governor Rockefeller

that year. This bill clarified the difference between nursing diagnosis and medical diagnosis, and specifically noted that nurses did not have the authority to practice medicine. For further discussion, see NYSNA, *Legislative Bulletin*, no. 4 (February 16, 1971), 1.

112. See, for example, Pam King, "Nurse-Practitioners Trained in Rochester," *Rochester Democrat and Chronicle*, Monday, April 19, 1977, 6B.

113. Martha Rogers, "Nursing: To Be or Not to Be?" *Nursing Outlook* 20 (1972): 42–46.

114. Mary Kohnke, "What's in a name. . . . Plenty!" Letters, *Nursing Outlook* 23 (10) (1975): 602–603. Kohnke was responding to an article by Lynaugh and Bates ("Clinical Practicum in Ambulatory Care," *Nursing Outlook* 23 [7] [1975]: 444–448).

115. In the report of the Secretary of Health, Education and Welfare on the supply and distribution of and requirements for nurses, *First Report to the Congress, February 1, 1977, Nurse Training Act of 1975* (Hyattsville, MD: DHEW, 1977), 44, nurse practitioners reported increased salary and status, and the opportunity for collaboration with physicians as the three least important influences on their decision to enter nurse practitioner programs. The three most important factors were the opportunity to have a greater influence on patient care, interest in learning additional skills, and the challenge of the work.

116. Carnegie Commission on Higher Education, *Higher Education and the Nation's Health—Policies of Medical and Dental Education* (New York: McGraw-Hill, 1970).

117. Annual Comprehensive Report, 1972–1973, Lynaugh Collection.

118. See Lynaugh and Bates, grant proposal, 1972, 72–4214, Lynaugh Collection.

119. The total authorization numbers for special projects, under which most nurse practitioner programs were funded under the 1971 NTA, were $20 million, $25 million, and $30 million from fiscal years 1972–75, respectively, and are probably estimates, as other sources list other amounts. These figures do not include traineeship funds, which were between $10 million and $15 million per year over the same time period. See insert, U.S. Department of Health and Human Services (DHHS), Public Health Service, "Chronology of Federal Support for Programs of Nursing Education and Research Administered by the Division of Nursing," *Chronology of Health Professions Legislation, 1956–1979*, Appendix C, DHHS Pub. #80–69 (Washington, DC: Government Printing Office, August 1980) 11. In this insert, special projects are defined as grants or contracts to train nurse practitioners, and to merge training school and collegiate programs, among other things (11).
      The 1971 Comprehensive Health Manpower Training Act of 1971, Section 774(a) (1), also provided money specifically for pediatric nurse practitioners.

120. Henry A. Sultz, Maria Zielezny, Jane Mathews Gentry, and Louis Kinyon, *Longitudinal Study of Nurse Practitioners Phase III*. DHEW Publication No. 80-2 (Bethesda, MD: U.S. Department of Health, Education and Welfare, 1980), 22. In 1977, the American Academy of Nursing advocated baccalaureate education for primary care nurse practitioners, and the discontinuation of all short-term programs by 1980. See American Academy of Nursing, *Primary Care by Nurses: Sphere of Responsibility and Accountability* (Kansas City, MO: ANA, 1977), 3. By 1978 professional nursing organizations such as the National League for Nursing (NLN) believed the nurse practitioner should hold a master's degree and be educated within nursing's formal education structure at the college/university level. The NTAs up to 1975 did not require master's-level training and set up the following criteria for programs: students must be registered nurses who completed a formal program of study designed to prepare them to deliver primary health care; the program must

be at least nine months long, including four months of course work and five months of physician-directed preceptorship. See NLN, "Position Statement on the Education of Nurse Practitioners," approved by the Board of Directors, October 1, 1979, 2.

121. U.S. DHEW, *Nurse Practitioner and Physician Assistant Training and Deployment*, National Center for Health Service Research, Research Digest Series, Hyattsville, MD: May 1977, 1–3. This pamphlet is the report of a descriptive and comparative study of 145 DHEW-sponsored nurse practitioner and physician assistant training programs to determine if the objectives and congressional expectations were achieved.

122. Harriet J. Kitzman, Bethel A. Powers, and Madeline H. Schmitt, "The School of Nursing: Integrating Practice, Research and Education," in *75 Years of Achievement, 1925–2000, The University of Rochester Medical Center: Teaching, Discovering, Caring*, ed. Jules Cohen and Robert J. Joynt (Rochester, NY: University of Rochester Press, 2000), 233–298.

123. By 1971 alone, New York City had programs at the Loeb Center for Nursing and Rehabilitation, Montefiore Hospital and Medical Center, Brooklyn Hospital, New York–Cornell Medical Center, State University of New York, Downstate Medical Center, among others.

124. Staff, Health Resources Administration, *Nurse Practitioners*, report prepared for Dr. Henry A. Foley, September 27, 1979, 13, Helen Osgood Collection, Center for Nursing Historical Inquiry, University of Virginia, School of Nursing, Charlottesville. Foley was an administrator in the Health Resources Administration in 1979, and became a special assistant to the surgeon general in 1982. For state distribution, see Sultz et al., *Longitudinal Study of Nurse Practitioners—Phase III*, 52.

125. Although funding for nursing education in general began to decrease with the 1975 NTA, this act and the 1979 NTA amendments included discrete authorities and authorizations for appropriations for this purpose. See Sultz et al. *Longitudinal Study of Nurse Practitioners—Phase III*, 48. The 1975 NTA was the first legislation with a specific authority to support nurse practitioner and nurse midwifery education via a separate program (Sec. 822 of the PHS Act) of grants and contracts to meet the cost of projects to plan, develop, operate, significantly expand, or maintain programs. Both master's and certificate programs were eligible for support as long as they met the secretary's guidelines. See Geolot, "Federal Funding of Nurse Practitioner Education," 159–162. From 1975, with the passage of the NTA to fiscal year 1980, $50 million was invested in nurse practitioner training.

Chapter 4   Stealing the Spell Book

1. *Fantasia* was released in 1940 by the Walt Disney Corporation, and used the symphonic poem composed in 1897 by Paul Dukas. His music was inspired by Goethe's 1797 ballad, "Der Zauberlehrling." http://www.answers.com/topic/the-sorcerer-s-apprentice (accessed May 22, 2007).

2. Susan Reverby also uses the tale of the sorcerer's apprentice to discuss physician assistants, albeit in a different context in "The Sorcerer's Apprentice," in *Prognosis Negative: Crisis in the Health Care System*, ed. David Kotelchuck (New York: Vintage Books, 1976), 215–228.

3. In this chapter I will use the current term "physician assistant" unless in the context of a direct quote or reference title. The term "physician's assistant" was also in use in the 1970s.

4. In this chapter, family practice and general practice will be used interchangeably, as it was in most of the literature of the time. The terms generally became more

differentiated in the mid-1960s as various groups maneuvered for a family practice specialty board. By 1966, the terms were differentiated by function and content— family practice referred to the function of the practitioner, while general practice referred to the content of the practice. The family practitioner drew skills from one or more medical specialties while the general practitioner drew from two or more. In a group practice, the general practitioner could serve as a family practitioner. For the differentiation, see AMA, *Meeting the Challenge of Family Practice. The Report of the ad hoc Committee on Education for Family Practice of the Council on Medical Education American Medical Association* (Chicago: AMA, 1966), 7–10.

5. Family practice is included in this chapter because the physician assistant developed into a more viable occupation somewhat in tandem to the reorganization of general practice.

6. From the early twentieth century, general practitioners constantly reconfigured themselves to survive economically and professionally in an increasingly specialized health system. Examples include reshaping work and work space into "cancer offices," and integrating early-detection screening and counseling services into practice. Family practice could be seen as part of this continuum to remain viable. See Robert Aronowitz, "Do Not Delay: Breast Cancer and Time, 1900–1970," *Milbank Memorial Quarterly* 79 (3) (September 2001): 335–386.

7. Janice Radway, "What's in a Name?" *American Quarterly* 51 (1) (March 1999): 1–32.

8. Richard A. Smith, "MEDEX," *Journal of the American Medical Association* 211 (March 1970): 1843–1845.

9. Henry Silver, "Use of New Types of Allied Health Professionals in Providing Care for Children," *American Journal of Diseases of Children* 116 (November 1968): 486–490.

10. Laura L. Simms, "The Clinical Nursing Specialist," *Journal of the American Medical Association* 198 (1966): 675–678. The clinical specialist during this time was a cross between a nurse practitioner, nurse educator, and nurse generalist. Differentiating this provider from nurse practitioners is still a topic actively debated in contemporary nursing literature. See Ann B. Hamric, Judith A. Spross, and Charlene M. Hanson, *Advanced Practice Nursing: An Integrative Approach* (Philadelphia, W. B. Saunders, 2004), for the most comprehensive treatment of clinical specialists.

11. See, for example, Gary L. Appel and Aaron Loivin, *Physician Extenders: An Evaluation of Policy-Related Research* (Washington, DC: National Science Foundation, 1975); Len Hughes Andrus and Mary Fenley, "Assistants to Primary Physicians in California," *Western Journal of Medicine* 122 (1) (1975): 80–86. Because of the confusion of names, statistics differentiating the different types of practitioners in the early 1970s are quite unreliable, as there is great overlap and repetition across groups.

12. See for example, Department of Health, Education and Welfare, Comptroller General of the U.S., Report to Congress, *Progress and Problems in Training and Use of Assistants to Primary Care Physicians*, B-164031(5) (Washington, DC: Government Printing Office, 1976); National Academy of Sciences, (NAS), Board of Medicine, ad hoc panel, *New Members of the Physician's Health Team: Physician's Assistants* (Washington, DC: NAS, 1970).

13. National Health Service Corp, U.S. Public Health Service, "Federal Description and Manual for Nurse Practitioners," mimeographed copy, revised August 3, 1974, Kathryn Jacquette Collection, Center for Nursing Historical Inquiry, University of Virginia, School of Nursing, Charlottesville, (Jacquette Collection).

14. For one perspective, see Robert Oseasohn, Edward A. Mortimer Jr., Carol C. Geil, Betty J. Eberle, Ann E. Pressman, and Naomi L. Quenk, "Rural Medical Care: Physician's Assistant Linked to an Urban Medical Center," *Journal of the American Medical Association* 218 (9) (29 November 1971): 1417–1419. See also Vernon W. Lippard and Elizabeth F. Purcell, eds., *Intermediate-Level Health Practitioners* (New York: Josiah Macy Jr. Foundation, 1973).

15. See, for example, "The Physician's Assistant Programs," *RN* 33 (10) (October 1970): 43–46. Expanded nursing role programs also used various labels. In 1973, about 60 percent of the certificate programs and only 13 percent of the master's programs called their graduates nurse practitioners. Most of the master's programs used the label "clinical specialist." Twenty-two percent of programs used the label "nurse associate." By 1980 the programs used more consistent labels, with 84 percent of certificate programs and 50 percent of master's programs using the label "nurse practitioner" to describe their graduates. Only 5 percent of programs used "nurse associate," and these programs were usually pediatric programs. See Harry A. Sultz, O. Marie Henry, Louis J. Kinyon, Germaine M. Buck, and Bonnie Bullough, "Nurse Practitioners: A Decade of Change, Part II," *Nursing Outlook* 31 (4) (July/August 1983): 216–219.

16. Loretta "Lee" Ford discusses receiving recognition for what she and her nurse colleagues were already doing (Loretta Ford, interview with Julie Fairman, January 19, 2006); Joan Lynaugh talks about "not asking for permission" to learn new skills in "The Freedom to Practice Nursing," paper presented at the National Organization of Nurse Practitioner Faculty, Thirtieth Annual Meeting, San Diego, CA, April 22, 2004. Joan Lynaugh Personal Collection, Bryn Mawr, PA (Lynaugh Collection).

17. Bonita Roche, telephone interview by M. J. Murphy, October 4, 1997; Faye Davies, telephone interview by M. J. Murphy, September 24, 1997.

18. See, for example, Robert D. Coye and Marc R. Hansen, "The "Doctor's Assistant," *Journal of the American Medical Association* 209 (4) (28 July 1969): 529–533; Abraham B. Bergman, Jeffrey L. Probstfield, and Ralph J. Wedgwood, "Task Identification in Pediatric Practice," *American Journal of the Diseases of Children* 118 (September 1969): 459–468.

19. *The Oxford English Dictionary*, 2nd ed., s.v. "delegate."

20. Loretta Ford, "Nurse Practitioners: History of a New Idea and Predictions for the Future." in *Nursing in the 1980s: Crises-Opportunities-Challenges*, ed. Linda Aiken (Philadelphia: J. B. Lippincott, 1982), 231–248.

21. Silver, "New Types of Allied Health Professionals"; Henry Silver, Loretta Ford, and Lewis Day, "The Pediatric Nurse-Practitioner Program," *Journal of the American Medical Association* 204 (4) (April 22, 1968): 88–92.

22. Julie Fairman, "The Roots of Collaborative Practice: Nurse Practitioner Pioneer Stories," *Nursing History Review* 10 (2002): 159–174.

23. *Marcus Welby, M.D.* was an evening ABC television series about a general practitioner, showing from 1969 to 1976. Many physicians found his positive image harmful, because patients—one out of four Americans watched the show during the height of its popularity—were disappointed with the discontinuity between image and reality. See http://www.museum.tv/archives/etv/M/htmlM/marcuswelby/marcuswelby.htm (accessed March 4, 2007).

24. Oliver Garceau, *The Political Life of the American Medical Association* (Cambridge, MA: Harvard University Press, 1941), 53–56; Corinne Lathrop Gilb, *Hidden Hierarchies: The Professions and Government* (New York: Harper and Row, 1966), 129–130.

25. See Rosemary Stevens, *American Medicine and the Public Interest*, Updated Edition with a New Introduction (Berkeley: University of California Press, 1998), for an overview of medical specialization.

The AMA was organized somewhat similarly to the ANA, with a house of delegates derived from the state organizations. Until the early 1970s, the delegates were typically general practitioners and the board members were academic physicians, resulting in great tensions within the organization as a whole. The delegates held enormous power to approve or deny resolutions that came from the board of directors and any of the appointed committees. For earlier analysis of membership, see Garceau, *The Political Life of the American Medical Association*, 53–56.

26. See Robert D. Gilette, "Letter to the Editor," *American Medical News*, November 16, 1970, 5. Gilette extols the positive social aspects of the general practitioner.

27. Stevens, *American Medicine and the Public Interest*, 301.

28. American Academy of Family Physicians (AAFP), *Family Practice: Creation of a Specialty* (Kansas City, MO: AAFP, 1980), 25–29.

29. The American Board of Family Practice was approved by the Advisory Board of Medical Specialties (which became the American Board of Medical Specialties in 1971) in February 1969. This board, given authority to offer a certification exam in family practice, was partially an outgrowth of the American Academy of General Practice, founded in 1947.

30. The rotating internship was an imperative for general practice; the straight internship, for specialization. There was also a move by the AMA Council on Medical Education to eliminate rotating internships and move to all straight internships.

31. AMA, *Final Report on Preparation for Family Practice: Report of the Committee on Preparation for General Practice* (Chicago: AMA, June 1959).

32. Stevens, *American Medicine and the Public Interest*, 310–311.

33. Staff, Executive Directors Page, *Bulletin of the American College of Physicians* 6 (July/August 1965): 218.

34. Ibid. See also AMA, *Meeting the Challenge of Family Practice*, 7–10.

35. Charles L. Hudson, "Expansion of Medical Professional Services with Nonprofessional Personnel," *Journal of the American Medical Association* 176 (1961): 839–841. Hudson served as president of the AMA from 1965 to 1967.

36. Ibid.

37. Stead was an energetic and motivated advocate of the program, and his letters and other documents are accessible online from the Physician Assistant History Center, Duke University Medical Center Archives (PAHC).

38. Eugene A. Stead to Charles Frenzel, 21 April, 1964, 1, item 142, PAHC. Online image. Digital archive collection, http://www.pahx.org/pdf/Item142.pdf (originally accessed July 16, 2004). Original materials from the Eugene A. Stead Papers, Duke University Medical Center Archives. Frenzel was the chief administrator of the medical center at the time. Further materials from the Physician Assistant History Center Online Digital Collection will be referenced as PAHC, with collection information. All are from the Eugene A. Stead Papers unless otherwise noted. Access dates and Web site remain the same for all cited material (www.pahx.org/ followed by item number).

39. Stead to Frenzel, April 21, 1964, PAHC.

40. James C. Mau and Eugene Stead to Robert L. Ballentine, September 24, 1964, 1, item 143, PAHC. Mau was the director of health careers in the Department of Medicine at Duke. Ballentine worked for the U.S. Department of Labor. The program eventually received funding from the National Institutes of Health, and Stead

also sought additional funding from the W. K. Kellogg Foundation in 1966 to extend the program to additional rural communities.

41. Ibid.

42. Thelma Ingles, "A New Health Worker," *American Journal of Nursing* 68 (5) (May 1968): 1059–1061. Ingels describes the Duke physician assistant program after a seven-week observation experience. See also Eugene E. Stead, "PA Profession in Review: A Founder's Perspective," *Physician Assistant* 10 (1) (1986): 12, 19, 22. For another vantage point on Stead's difficulty with nursing organizations, see Natalie Holt, "Confusion's Masterpiece: The Development of the Physician Assistant Profession," *Bulletin of the History of Medicine* 72 (2) (Summer 1998): 246–278. Ingles was a professor and chair of the Department of Medical-Surgical Nursing at Duke University from 1949 to 1952, and is credited with starting one of the earlier clinically focused master's programs in nursing in 1958. See http://www.pahx.org/inglesBio.htm (originally accessed July 16, 2004).

43. An interesting picture of Stead may be gained from his letters to the AMA, which are sometimes quite direct and challenging. See, for example, Eugene E. Stead to Walter Bornemeier and William Ruhe, January 7, 1971, item 155, PAHC, Bornemeier was the president of the AMA, and Ruhe was the secretary of the Council on Medical Education.

44. Ingles, "A New Health Worker," quote 1061.

45. Kathleen G. Andreoli, RN, MSN, was an instructor in the Duke physician assistant program. See Kathleen Andreoli and Eugene A. Stead, "Training Physician Assistants at Duke," *American Journal of Nursing* 67 (7) (July 1967): 1442–1443; Roland H. Berg, "More than a Nurse, Less than a Doctor," *Look*, (September 6, 1966), 59–61. Andreoli eventually went on to become dean of the College of Nursing, Rush University, retiring after eighteen years in June 2005.

    Other physician assistant programs, such as Bowman Gray School of Medicine and Wake Forest University, also used nurses as instructors, usually in areas such as child development and community health. See Staff, "A Visit to Bowman Gray," *RN* 33 (10) (October 1970): 47–49.

46. Eugene Stead to James E. Zucker, December 20, 1967, 1, item 149, PAHC.

47. J.W.P to Eugene Stead, August 26, 1970, 1, item 153, PAHC.

48. Eugene Stead, transcript from a panel discussion, cover letter from Harry Becker, July 26, 1967, 4, item 159, PAHC.

49. Eugene E. Stead to Evelyn Malkin, June 15, 1967, 1, item 149, PAHC. Malkin was chair, Department of Nursing, California State College, Los Angeles.

50. See Patricia D'Antonio, "Women, Nursing and Baccalaureate Education in the Twentieth Century," *Journal of Nursing Scholarship* 36 (4) (2004): 379–384.

51. Dorothy Novello, "Workshop Report," *Pennsylvania Medicine* 71 (7) (July 1968): 51–55, quote on 55.

52. Stead to Malkin, June 15, 1967, PAHC. Other physician assistant programs accepted nurse applicants from the beginning, and the Duke program began to admit women by the late 1960s.

53. Berg, "More than a Nurse," 59–61.

54. Ruth B. Freeman to Eugene E. Stead, October 13, 1964, 2, item 144, PAHC.

55. Ibid., 2.

56. Eugene E. Stead to Ruth B. Freeman, October 20, 1964, 1, item 144, PAHC.

57. AAMC, "Women Applicants, Enrollees and Graduates," http://www.aamc.org/members/wim/statistics/stats99/99table1.pdf (accessed July 4, 2007).

58. William McClure, "A 'Medic' in General Practice," *Medical Economics*, May 15, 1967, 72–78.
59. Evelyn Malkin to Eugene E. Stead, June 8, 1967, 1–2, item 149, PAHC.
60. American Medical Association, 1969–1978, *Digest of Official Actions of the American Medical Association* (Chicago: AMA, 1980), 282. See also AMA, Committee on Nursing, "Medicine and Nursing in the 1970s: A Position Statement," *Journal of the American Medical Association* 213 (11) (1970): 1881–1883.
61. Walter C. Bornemeier, "Rx for the Family Doctor Shortage," *Reader's Digest*, July 1970, 104.
62. Staff, "AMA Unveils Surprise Plan to Convert R.N. into Medic," *American Journal of Nursing* 70 (1970): 724–727. See also Staff, Western Council on Higher Education for Nursing, "AMA Urges Major New Role for Nurses," *News* 1 (3) (Spring 1970): 1.
63. "AMA Unveils," 725.
64. "Nursing Acceptance of Physician Assistants," 1971, 1, item 198, PAHC. Original materials from the Allied Health Records. This is a compilation of the raw data from a survey conducted in 1971.
65. "Nursing Acceptance of Physician Assistants," 2, PAHC.
66. Ibid.
67. Dorothy Mereness, "Recent Trends in Expanding Roles of the Nurse," *Nursing Outlook* 18 (May 1970): 30–33, quote on 31.
68. ANA Board of Directors, minutes, January 19–23, 1970, 11, 15, box 75, folder 13. From the ANA Collection in the Howard Gotlieb Archival Research Center at Boston University, Boston (ANA Collection).
69. John Harley Warner, "Grand Narrative and Its Discontents: Medical History and the Social Transformation of American Medicine," in special issue: "Transforming American Medicine: A Twenty-Year Retrospective on the Social Transformation of American Medicine," *Journal of Health Politics, Policy and the Law* 29 (4–5) (August–October 2004): 756–780.
70. ANA, "Nurses, in the Extended Role, Are Not Physician Assistants," July 9, 1973, 3, National Joint Commission Papers, Shirley Smoyak Collection, Barbara Bates Center for the Study of the History of Nursing, School of Nursing, University of Pennsylvania, Philadelphia, (Smoyak Collection).
71. C. H. William Ruhe to William Stead, December 21, 1970, 1, item 153, PAHC.
72. The informal moratorium was supported by the DHEW, the American Hospital Association, the ANA, and the AMA. Board of Directors, minutes, May 26–28, 1971, 6, box 488, ANA Collection.
73. PAHC, Eugene A. Stead to Henry T. Ricketts, August 27, 1970, 1, item 153. Stead was complaining about the report by Joseph Kadish and James W. Long, "The Training of Physician Assistants: Status and Issues," *Journal of the American Medical Association* 212 (6) (May 11, 1970): 1047–1051. Kadish was from the AMA's Division of Allied Health Manpower, and Long from the Bureau of Health Professions Education and Manpower, NIH. Programs were starting, but not as fast as Stead wanted.
74. Stead to Ricketts, August 27, 1970, 1, PAHC. The North Carolina State Medical Society officials agreed to allow supervision via telephone.
75. No educational standards existed until January 1, 1972, when the AMA published those for assistants in orthopedic and primary care. The states were also moving rapidly to enact exceptions to their medical practice acts to permit physicians to delegate traditional functions to nonphysicians. See U.S. Bureau of Health Manpower

Education, *Selected Training Programs for Physician Support Personnel* (Washington, DC: DHEW, PHS, revised May 1972); Kadish and Long, "The Training of Physician Assistants," 1047–1051; "Progress and Problems in Training and Use," iv, viii–x.

76. Richard A. Smith, MD, MPH, Biographies, 1, PAHC. http://www.pahx.org/smithBio.html (accessed September 28, 2004).

77. Richard A. Smith, MD, MPH, Biographies, 1, PAHC. See also Fitzhugh Mullan, "Carl Toney, PA, Building a New Profession in Portland, Maine," *Medscape General Medicine* (March 2, 2001): 3. http://www.medscope.com/viewarticle/408105 (originally accessed March 3, 2001). Toney graduated from Duke University in 1979.

78. The program was funded via the National Center for Health Services Research and Development (NCHSRD). See Robert G. Harmon, Steven Turnipseed, Sharon Schlittenhard, and Andrew Penman, "Training Physician Assistants for the Pacific Northwest: The MEDEX Northwest Ten-Year Experience," *Western Journal of Medicine* 138 (2) (February 1983): 280–284.

79. DHEW, NCHSRD, *Report on Licensure and Related Health Personnel Credentialing, the Physician's Assistant,* Appendix B (Washington, DC: Government Printing Office, June 1971), 198.

80. These programs included Charles R. Drew Postgraduate Medical School, Los Angeles; Howard University College of Medicine; Dartmouth Medical School; University of North Dakota School of Medicine; University of Washington School of Medicine; University of Hawaii School of Medicine; Penn State University College of Medicine; Medical University of South Carolina; and University of Utah College of Medicine. Almost all of the programs trained general practice or family practice MEDEXs except for the Howard University program, which placed trainees with emergency room physicians and focused on inner-city placements in urban Washington, DC. See David Lawrence, William Wilson, and C. Hilmon, "Employment of MEDEX Graduates and Trainees: Five-Year Progress Report for the United States," *Journal of the American Medical Association* 234 (2) (1975): 174–177.

81. Although this represented only forty-one women, their proportion gave credence to the fears of nursing leaders that the programs could potentially co-opt their constituency. H. B. Perry, "An Analysis of the Specialty and Geographic Location of Physician Assistants in the United States," *American Journal of Public Health* 68 (October 1978): 1019–1021.

82. For examples, see Jones and Cawley, "Physician Assistants," 1266–1272; Harmon, "Training Physician Assistants," 280–284; Office of Statewide Health Planning and Development and the Center for California Health Workforce Studies at the University of California, San Francisco, *Nurse Practitioners, Physician Assistants and Certified Nurse Midwives in California* (San Francisco: office of Statewide planning, Spring 2000), 1–3, Smoyak Collection.

83. Harmon, "Training Physician Assistants," 280–284, stats on 283.

84. Perry, "An Analysis of the Specialty," 1019–1021; Congressional Budget Office, *Physician Extenders: Their Current and Future Role in Medical Care Delivery* (Washington, DC: Government Printing Office, April 1979).

85. The AMA and Malcolm C. Todd, "The Physicians' Assistant—A Progress Report," 1971, 1, item 184, Miscellaneous Correspondence, 1970–1974 Collection and Subject Files, PAHC. Todd was the chairman of the Council on Health Manpower. For the guidelines, see T. C. Points, "Guidelines for Development of New Health Occupations," *Journal of the American Medical Association* 213 (7)

(August 17, 1970): 1169–1171. The guidelines included sixteen categories such as career mobility, salary, and need.

86. Eugene Stead, transcript from a panel discussion, cover letter from Harry Becker, July 26, 1967, 3, item 159, PAHC..

87. Ibid.

88. R. A. Smith et al., "A Strategy for Health Manpower: Reflections on an Experience Called MEDEX," *Journal of the American Medical Association* 217 (10) (September 6, 1971): 1362–1367.

89. D. Robert Howard to Ira L. Myers, November 13, 1971, 2–3, item 63, D. Robert Howard—Miscellaneous Correspondence and Subject Files, 1968–1972, PAHC. In the letter, Howard outlines the various options and changes in the name. Howard was the director of the Duke University physician assistant program, and Myers was the secretary of the Alabama Board of Medical Examiners.

90. Ibid. The first volume was published in April 1971. The registry chose "associate" as its terminology because the term PA [initials] had become "totally generic and could not be protected by a patent," quote on 2.

91. Ibid.

92. "Walter Bornemeier to Eugene Stead," November 17, 1970, 1, item 155, PAHC.

93. C. H. William Ruhe to Eugene A. Stead, December 21, 1970, 1, item 155, PAHC. Ruhe's letter is two pages long, single spaced, laying out the logistics of the council structure, implying that Stead simply did not understand the intricacies of the AMA.

94. Ibid., 2; Todd, "The Physicians' Assistant—A Progress Report", 2. The AAMC was also working on the physician assistant issue through its Liaison Committee on Medical Education.

95. See Malcolm C. Todd and Donald F. Foy, "Current Status of the Physician's Assistant and Related Issues," *Journal of the American Medical Association* 220 (13) (1972): 1714–1720.

96. Stead uses the phrase "analysis paralysis" in Stead to Ricketts, August 27, 1970, 1, item 153, PAHC.

97. The Veterans Administration, Department of Medicine and Surgery, "Status Report on Physician Assistant Programs for Physicians Associates and MEDEX: Developing a New Health Profession of Physician Manpower," February 3, 1971, item 75, D. Robert Howard—Miscellaneous Correspondence and Subject Files, 1968–1972, PAHC.

98. Eugene Stead to C. H. William Ruhe, January 7, 1971, 1, item 155, PAHC.

99. Stead to Bornemeier, January 7, 1971, 1, PAHC.

100. Ruhe to Stead, December 21, 1970, 2, PAHC.

101. Ibid.

102. Targeted federal funding for physician assistant education began in 1971 through the 1971 Comprehensive Manpower Training Act. The AMA was not entirely enthusiastic about the funding but did not campaign against inclusion of money for physician assistant programs. See Gary L. Appel and Aaron Loivin, *Physician Extenders: An Evaluation of Policy-Related Research* (Washington, DC: National Science Foundation, 1975), 28.

103. AMA, Committee on Allied Health Education and Accreditation, *Essentials and Guidelines for an Accredited Educational Program for the Physician Assistant* (Chicago: American Medical Association, 1971). The guidelines were revised in 1978, 1985, 1990, and cyclically since then. See also P. Eugene Jones and James F. Cawley,

"Physician Assistants and Health System Reform," *Journal of the American Medical Association* 271 (16) (April 27, 1994): 1266–1272.

104. The first programs included Aldesson-Broaddus College in Phillipi, WV; Bowman-Grey School of Medicine, Wake Forest University, Winston-Salem, NC; Brooklyn Hospital, New York City; and the Duke University School of Medicine, Durham, NC. See First Training Programs for PAs Approved, AMA, news release, September 12, 1972, item 121, Subject file (RDC), PAHC.

105. Comptroller General of the United States, *Report to the Congress: Progress and Problems in Training and Use of Assistants to Physicians*, GAO Pub. # MWD-75–35 (Washington, DC: Government Printing Office, 1975), 27.

106. American Academy of Physician Assistants, "How the PA Sees His Place in Medicine," *Patient Care* 1 (August 1973): 131–132; *Nurse Practitioners, Physician Assistants and Certified Nurse Midwives in California*, 1–3. California reported a greater proportion of physician assistants and nurse practitioners working in primary care/family practice than the national data show.

107. Jones and Cawley, "Physician Assistants and Health System Reform," 1266–1272, statistics on 1268.

108. John Harley Warner discusses the need to think about the relationship between practice and identity in "Grand Narrative and its Discontents," 756–780.

109. For examples, see US DHEW, *Progress and Problems in Training*, 11; Gary L. Appel and Aaron Loivin, *Physician Extenders: An Evaluation of Policy-Related Research* (Washington, DC: National Science Foundation, 1975,) 28; Harold C. Sox, "Quality of Patient Care by Nurse Practitioners and Physician's Assistants: A Ten-Year Perspective," *Annals of Internal Medicine* 91 (3) (1979): 459–468; T. Elaine Adamson, "Critical Issues in the Use of Physician Associates and Assistants," *American Journal of Public Health* (September 1971): 1776 (this is a DHEW-funded study done at Duke and at the Kaiser Foundation clinics in San Francisco and Oakland, CA, to see delegation patterns as recorded by independent observers); Harold M. Goldstein and Morris A. Horowitz, *Restructuring Paramedical Occupations: A Case Study I*, U.S. Department of Labor, Contract #41–9-004–23 (Boston: Northeastern University Press, 1971); Uwe Reinhardt, "A Production Function for Physician Services," *Review of Economics and Statistics* 54 (1) (February 1972): 54–58. Lists of studies found in National Academy of Sciences, IOM, "Study Proposal: An Analysis of the Functions and Roles of Primary Health Care Manpower," final draft with cover letter to A. Alan Fisher from Karen Grimm (staff officer), February 4, 1974, 1, Smoyak Collection.

110. Pennsylvania State Board of Medical Examiners and Licensure, minutes, January 8, 1977, 16, Office of the Commissioner of Professional and Occupational Affairs, Harrisburg, PA.

111. Jones and Cawley, "Physician Assistants and Health System Reform," 1266–1272. In 2007 physician assistants could prescribe in all fifty states, the District of Columbia, and Guam, and 139 programs were accredited by the accreditation review committee. Most programs are twenty-six months in length. See American Association of Physician Associates Web site, http://www.aapa.org/glance.html (accessed September 17, 2007).

112. This quote was part of the discussion at an invitational institute on primary care sponsored by the AAMC in 1974. See Staff, "FP Leaders, Academicians at Odds over Primary Care," *Hospital Practice* 9 (12) (December 1974): 97, 101–102, 106–108, quote 106.

113. Ibid. This article describes the battle between family practice physicians, pediatricians, and internal medicine physicians over who should control primary care provision.

Chapter 5   The AMA and ANA under Siege

1. Grant McConnell, *Private Power and American Democracy* (New York: Knopf, 1966), 5. In this regard, they were very similar to other professional groups in health care and beyond.
2. Ibid.
3. Oliver Garceau, *The Political Life of the American Medical Association* (Hamden, CT: Archon Books, 1961), 4.
4. See also chapter 7. For an example of the ANA's work to present nurse practitioners as a viable solution to health system demand, see Constance Holleran to Rep. Paul Rogers, May 6, 1971, AAP Miscellaneous, 1969–1985, American Nurses' Association (ANA) Archives, Silver Springs, MD (ANA Archives). Holleran was the director of government relations of the ANA, and Rogers was the 6th Congressional District representative from the state of Florida.
5. See Shirley Smoyak, "Specialization in Nursing: From Then to Now," *Nursing Outlook* 24 (11) (November 1976): 676–681.
6. Ibid, quote 681.
7. Julie Fairman and Joan Lynaugh, *Critical Care Nursing: A History* (Philadelphia: University of Pennsylvania Press, 1998). See also Barbara Callaway, *Hildegard Peplau: Psychiatric Nurse of the Century* (New York: Springer, 2002).
8. In 1944, the ANA, the National League for Nursing Education (NLNE), and the National Organization for Public Health Nursing (NOPHN), later joined by the Association of Collegiate Schools of Nursing (ACSN), the American Association of Industrial Nurses (AAIN), and the National Association of Colored Graduate Nurses (NACGN), undertook a joint survey of their organizational structures, functions, and resources to determine if there was a better way to more strongly promote professional nursing. The structure study, as it was called, resulted in a two-organization structure for professional nursing—an already existing organization, the ANA, and a new organization, the National League for Nursing (NLN), in 1952. The NLN was a conglomeration of the NLNE, NOPHN, and the ACSN. The NACGN voluntarily disbanded in 1951, and the AAIN remained independent. See Edith Lewis, "How It All Came About," *Nursing Outlook* 25 (2) (February 1977): 96–97.
9. Issues of *Trained Nurse* were devoted to the interests of its over 200,000 readers and focused primarily on workplace conditions such as wages and hours, and ways to increase efficiency. See Susan Reverby, *Ordered to Care: The Dilemma of American Nursing 1850–1945* (New York: Cambridge University Press, 1987), 137–142.
10. The ANA house of delegates did not approve a resolution on the nurse practitioner until 1970, although they discussed the issue from 1965 on. See ANA Board of Directors, minutes, January 19–23, 1970, 15, box 75, file 13, from the ANA Collection in the Howard Gotlieb Archival Research Center at Boston University (ANA Collection).
11. Board of Directors, minutes, January 23–27, 1968, 37, box 75, file 9, ANA Collection. At this meeting a motion carried that "the first priority of the Association be given to nursing practice," (37). The next priorities were assigned to economics and general welfare, nursing education, and nursing service, in that order.

12. The committee consolidated education and practice even more in 1960 by adding a third goal that promoted the baccalaureate degree as the basic educational foundation for nursing education. By tying practice to basic education level, the committee inserted the ANA into the entry-into-practice debate. See Helen C. Hanson, "Supplemental Report," *Proceedings of the 42nd Convention of the American Nurses' Association*, May 2–6, 1960 (New York: ANA, 1960), 54–55.

13. Ibid., 54.

14. ANA, "Historical and Philosophical Development of Sections, Branches and Conference Groups within the ANA," September 29, 1958, file 1 box 127, ANA Collection. See also Directors of Conference Groups, minutes, October 24, 1962, file 4, box 127, ANA Collection.

15. Kimi Taguchi Hara to maternal and child nurse practitioners, memo #1, August 1963, 1, box 128, file 1, ANA Collection. Five different conferences took place by 1960: community health, geriatric, maternal and child health, medical-surgical (which may have incorporated operating-room nursing), and psychiatric and mental health nursing.

16. The Congress for Nursing Practice replaced the Council of Division Chairmen in 1968. Five councils on nursing practice were established starting in 1972: councils of advanced practitioners in medical-surgical nursing, psychiatric and mental health nursing, family nurse practitioners, and advanced practitioners in nursing of children. See Board of Directors, minutes, September 19–21, 1973; January 30–February 1–2, 1973; and April 22–26, 1972. All from box 488, no file number, ANA Collection. See also Lyndia Flanagan, compiler, *One Strong Voice: The Story of the American Nurses' Association* (Kansas City, MO: American Nurses Association, 1976).

17. U.S. Department of Health, Education and Welfare, Surgeon General's Consultant Group on Nursing, *Toward Quality in Nursing: Needs and Goals*, PHS Pub. #992 (Washington, DC: Government Printing Office, 1963).

18. ANA, *Educational Preparation for Nurse Practitioners and Assistants of Nurses: A Position Paper* (New York: ANA, 1965), 4. The word "practitioners" in the report title referred to nurses who practiced, not nurse practitioners.

19. Flanagan, *One Strong Voice*, 244.

20. In order to prevent a severe backlash by the American Hospital Association and the AMA, which were worried about hospital staffing during a time of severe nursing shortages, the ANA continued to try to recruit students into the diploma programs despite its stand on baccalaureate education. But they planned to follow this strategy only until there were sufficient numbers of university/college programs. See ANA Board of Directors, minutes, September 12, 1967, 12, box 75, file 8, ANA Collection.

21. Mathilda Scheuer, "Supplemental Report," *Proceedings of the 41st Convention of the ANA* (June 9–13, 1958) (New York: ANA, 1958), 74.

22. "ANA Board Approves a Definition of Nursing Practice," *American Journal of Nursing* 55 (1955): 1474.

23. Flanagan, *One Strong Voice*, 218; Dorothy V. Moses, "Report of the Committee on Standards of Geriatric Nursing Practice," *Proceedings of the 46th Convention of the ANA*, (May 13–17, 1968) (New York: ANA, 1968), 72.

24. "ANA Board Approves a Definition of Nursing Practice," 1474.

25. This requirement for academy fellowship did not endure. The academy was founded in 1973 under the auspices of the ANA.

26. Mary E. Beam, "Report of the Intersection Committee on Recognition of Superior Performance," *Proceedings of the 42nd Convention of the ANA*, May 2–6, 1960 NY: ANA, 1960), 87–88.

27. Ibid., 25–26.

28. Hazel Gill to officers of the conference groups, memo, July 15, 1960, 1, box 128, file 1, ANA Collection. The 1960s were a very important time for the reorganization of the ANA as well as the state nurses' associations (SNA). They tried to mirror the national effort, but they were still primarily concerned with workplace issues, such as work conditions, and providing representation to the House of Delegates. But by the end of the 1960s, there were twenty-four state councils on practice, twenty-six standing committees, and one commission. See ANA Committee on Interrelationships, report, April 1972, 6, series 3, box 6, file 70–72, Jessie Scott Collection, Barbara Bates Center for the Study of the History of Nursing, Philadelphia, (Scott Collection).

29. Mathilde Scheuer, address to the 43rd convention, ANA, Detroit, May 14–18, 1962. Reprinted in Flanagan, *One Strong Voice*, 548–555. In 1962 at the ANA Biennial Convention twenty-one clinical sessions extended over two and a half days. Each session was published as a monograph in 1962 by the ANA and sold for one dollar. See Dorothy Smith, "Education and Nursing," memo to the faculty, December 17, 1962, 1–12, box 6, file 19, Smith Collection.

30. Frances Reiter, "The Improvement of Nursing Practice," in *Improvement in Nursing Practice: Speeches Presented at the American Nurses' Association Section, Regional Conferences for Professional Nurses* (New York: ANA, 1961), 11. Reiter gave the speech in 1961 but was commenting on the program for the upcoming 1962 ANA Biennial Convention in Detroit.

31. Taguchi Hara, to maternal and child nurse practitioners, memo #2, June 1964, 1, box 128, file 2, ANA Collection.

32. The letters and postcards are found in boxes 127 and 128, various files, ANA Collection.

33. Scheuer, as reproduced by Flanagan, *One Strong Voice*, 553.

34. Board of Directors, minutes, January 26–29, 1971, 26, box 75, file 15, ANA Collection.

35. For Peplau's personal account, see Callaway, *Hildegard Peplau*, 348. See also Peplau's Executive Director's Report to the Board of Directors, January 19–23, 1970, file 13, box 75, ANA Collection. This report documents the severe financial straits of the organization. She noted she was forced to decrease program staff from sixty-nine to forty-seven people, and support staff from eight-six to sixty-seven people. Financial problems also noted in minutes of the special meeting of the ANA board of directors, February 12, 1970, 1, box 75, file 13, ANA Collection. Part of the ANA's debt encompassed a $300,000 loan from the membership account. The executive board also considered but did not seek a loan from the American Journal of Nursing Corporation, in which it had a financial stake.

36. Directors of Conference Groups, minutes, October 24, 1962, 3, box 127, file 4, ANA Collection.

37. Board Meeting of the Officers, MCHN, minutes, November 15–16, 1962, 2, 1964–66 History Book, box 128, ANA Collection.

38. Board Meeting of the Officers, MCHN, minutes, April 10–12, 1965, History Book. Pitocin is a powerful drug used to stimulate uterine contractions during obstetrical deliveries.

39. Joan Lynaugh, "400 Postcards," *Nursing Research* 39 (1990): 252–253.

40. Margaret Dolan, president, to the ANA Board of Directors, memo, February 24, 1964, box 128, file 1; also Judith Whitaker to the MCHN division, March 25, 1965, History Book.

41. Henry K. Silver and James A. Hecker, "The Pediatric Nurse Practitioner and the Child Health Associate: New Types of Health Professional," *Journal of Medical Education* 45 (1970): 171–176.

42. The original names were the American Association of Coronary-Care Nurses (AACN) and American Association of Nephrology Nurses and Technicians (AANT).

43. This terminology is used at various times by the ANA to describe emerging independent groups. See, for example, Board Meeting of the Officers, MCHN, minutes, October 27–29, 1965, box 128, History Book.

44. Board Meeting of the Officers, MCHN, minutes, October 15–16, 1964, 2; February 10–13, 1965, 3, History Book.

45. ANA committee on interrelationships, April 1972, 7, Scott Collection.

46. Ibid.

47. The committee went as far as to suggest additional fees for specialized services pertaining to newsletters and educational conferences. This type of fee structure eventually happened, but not in the 1970s.

48. Board of Directors, minutes, September 12, 1967, 13, box 75, file 8, ANA Collection.

49. Judith Whitaker and Jo Eleanor Elliott to Frank Lock and Robert Kimbrough, February 16, 1965, attached to memo 4, June 1965, ANA Conference on MCH Nursing, 2, box 128, file 2, ANA Collection.

50. Officers of ANA Conference on MCH Nursing to Maternal and Child Nurse Practitioners, attached to memo 4, 3.

51. Ibid.

52. Kimbrough to Elliott, March 18, 1965, attached to memo 4, June 1965, 3.

53. Lock to Elliott, March 18, 1965, attached to memo 4, June 1965, 3.

54. Willis E. Brown, "Postgraduate Education for Nurses in Obstetric, Gynecological and Neonatal Nursing Care," *Hospital Topics*, December 1964, 81–85.

55. Questionnaire dated March 1, 1965, Board Meeting of the Officers, MCHN, minutes, October 27–29, 1965, History Book.

56. Judith Whitaker to the MCHN Conference Group, memo, March 25, 1965, box 128, ANA Collection.

57. Board Meeting of the Officers, MCHN, minutes, April 10–12, 1965, 2, History Book.

58. Margaret McDermott, "Report of Visit to ACOG," April 7, 1965, History Book.

59. The Nurses' Association of the American College of Obstetricians and Gynecologists (NAACOG) issued its first statement on the role of the obstetric and gynecological nurse practitioner in 1972. See Joellen W. Hawkins and Linda L. Bellig, "Evolution of Advanced Practice Nursing in the United States: Caring for Women and Newborns," *Journal of Obstetric, Gynecologic, and Neonatal Nursing* 29 (1) (January/February 2000): 83–89.

60. ANA, Committee on Interrelationships, April 1972, 9, Scott Collection. The ANA attempted to work with these groups but never achieved the desired integration they wanted.

61. In 1966 the ANA and the NLN approved a joint statement describing their working relationship. This document is reprinted in Flanagan, *One Strong Voice*, 651–652. A similar statement was adopted in 1970 and affirmed in 1973, also reprinted in ibid., 652–653.

62. Rosemary Stevens uses these words to describe the dilemma of the AMA during this time. See *American Medicine and the Public Interest*, Updated Edition with a New Introduction (Berkeley: University of California Press, 1998), 530–534, quote on 533.

63. Sydney A. Halpern, "Dynamics of Professional Control: Internal Coalitions and Crossprofessional Boundaries," *American Journal of Sociology* 97 (4) (January 1992): 994–1021. Halpern discusses the influence of interdependencies between groups within one profession on the boundaries of neighboring professions.

64. Charles L. Leedham, "The AMA Position," *Pennsylvania Medicine* 71 (7) (1968): 55–56.

65. These conferences continued for at least three more years and eventually adopted a regional format.

66. ANA and the AMA, "Introduction," Proceedings of First National Conference for Professional Nurses and Physicians Sponsored by the American Nurses' Association and the American Medical Association, Williamsburg, Virginia, February 13–15, 1964, v.

67. Leedham, "The AMA Position," quote on 55.

68. Board of Directors, minutes, January 27, 1964, 3, box 75, file 5, ANA Collection.

69. See Callaway, *Hildegard Peplau*, 328. The language of "docs" and "girls" is not found in the published conference proceedings. Callaway is drawing her data from the unedited transcripts of the conference. See ANA and the AMA, "Medical and Nursing Practice in a Changing World."

70. For a discussion of the insufficiency of language and the lack of fit between language and women's experiences, see Marjorie L. DeVault, *Feeding the Family: The Social Organization of Caring as Gendered Work* (Chicago: University of Chicago Press, 1991), 5.

71. Although these conferences preceded the formal nurse practitioner role, the discussion touched on the expanding work boundaries of nurses, primarily in hospitals, and occasionally in clinics and private practices that were not yet labeled nor legally sanctioned. The discussions ranged from cultural behaviors (e.g., standing for physicians) to clinical behaviors (e.g., should nurses be legally responsible for giving immunizations?).

72. See ANA and the AMA, "Medical and Nursing Practice in a Changing World."

73. Board of Directors, minutes, January 23–28, 1967, 33, box 75, file 7, ANA Collection.

74. Throckmorton also served on the AMA Department of Investigation and the Department of Ethics, known as the "quack-busting" department. See Howard Wolinsky and Tom Bruce, *The Serpent on the Staff: The Unhealthy Politics of the American Medical Association* (New York: G. P. Putnam's Sons, 1994), 126.

75. This program consisted of large grants to health care institutions and independent community corporations to develop comprehensive health centers in low-income communities. By 1970 there were over seventy such centers. See US DHEW, Public Health Service, *A Conceptual Model of Organized Primary Care and Comprehensive Community Health Services*, PHS Pub. #2014 (Rockville, MD: US DHEW, US PHS, 1970).

76. Matthew Marshall, "OEO Neighborhood Health Centers, The Poor and You," *Pennsylvania Medicine* 71(12) (1968): 44–45, quote 45.

77. Staff, "AMA News," *Pennsylvania Medicine* 72 (9) (1972): 55.

78. House of Delegates, Pennsylvania Medical Society, Proceedings of the House of Delegates, 119th Annual Session, Pittsburgh, PA, September 26–28, 1968, Resolution 68–31, "Unscientific Practices and Practitioners in Pennsycare," published in *Pennsylvania Medicine* 72 (1) (1969): 78. The AMA formed the committee on quackery in 1963, under its Division of Investigation, and its prime mission was to eliminate chiropractics. The committee operated throughout the 1970s and was

disbanded in 1984; http://www.chirobase.org/08Legal/AT/at02.html (accessed October 13, 2006).

79. In 1987 the AMA was enjoined in the case of *Wilk et al. v. AMA et al.* from restricting AMA members, institutions, or hospitals from associating with chiropractors; http://www.chirobase.org/08Legal/AT/at02.html (accessed October 13, 2006). The American College of Surgeons and the American College of Radiology were initially defendants in the case but settled shortly before Justice Susan Gezendanner issued her ruling. Both organizations made payments of $200,000 to a particular chiropractic institution and to defray the court costs of the plaintiffs.

80. For example, see John Bird, "Your Doctor and the AMA," *The Saturday Evening Post* 239 (1) (January 1, 1966): 13–17, 37–38. This was one of many pieces written with assistance from the AMA to improve its image.

81. Stevens, *American Medicine and the Public Interest*, 530–534.

82. Wolinsky Bruce, *The Serpent on the Staff.*

83. See Proceedings of the AMA House of Delegates, June 21–25, 1970, 49.

84. Esselstyn was a surgeon and executive director of the Community Health Association in Detroit, a large and early prepaid group practice. Standard was a professor at New York University. See Bird, "Your Doctor," 13–17, 37–38.

85. Wolinsky and Bruce, *The Serpent on the Staff*, 126.

Chapter 6   Coming Together, Breaking Apart

1. James A. Morone, "Morality, Politics, and Health Policy," in *Policy Challenges in Modern Health Care*, ed. David Mechanic, Lynn B. Rogut, David C. Colby, and James R. Knickman (New Brunswick, NJ: Rutgers University Press, 2005), 13–25.

2. National Commission for the Study of Nursing and Nursing Education (NCSNNE), *Abstract for Action* (New York: McGraw-Hill, 1970).

3. Ibid., 289.

4. DHEW, *Extending the Scope of Nursing Practice: A Report of the Secretary's Committee to Study Extended Roles for Nurses* (Washington, DC: Government Printing Office, 1971).

5. Jerome Lysaught, telephone interview by Julie Fairman, October 29, 1999, lines 230–234.

6. The idea of a joint practice commission was part of the AMA Committee on Nursing, position statement, "Medicine and Nursing in the 1970s: A Position Statement," *Journal of the American Medical Association* 213 (11) (1970): 1881–1883. The ANA also incorporated the idea of joint practice into a position statement, "Regarding the Changing Role of the Nurse in Ambulatory Child Care," meeting of the American Academy of Pediatrics and the MCHN division of the ANA, July 31, 1970, attachment 3, 2, Liaison Committee Collection, ANA Archives, Silver Springs, Maryland (ANA Archives). The ANA published a summary report of the NCSNNE in the *American Journal of Nursing* 70 (2) (February 1970): 279–294.

7. See attachment 1, "Memorandum of Agreement of AMA and ANA Boards on Establishing the NJCP in 1971," NJPC Papers, Shirley Smoyak Collection, Barbara Bates Center for the Study of the History of Nursing, Philadelphia, (Smoyak Collection). Smoyak, an advanced practice psychiatric mental health nurse and nurse educator, was a member of the commission over its entire life.

8. "Memorandum of Agreement of AMA and ANA Boards," Smoyak Collection.

9. The eight physicians were to include one or two practitioners who were members of the AMA Committee on Nursing and the remainder to be practitioners designated

by the AMA from their broad-based sections on practice. The nursing appointees were originally intended to come from within the ANA—three members from the Congress on Nursing and one representative from each ANA Division on Practice. Elizabeth Carter to Shirley Smoyak, November 10, 1971, 2, Smoyak Collection. Carter was the program coordinator, Division on Psychiatric and Mental Health Nursing, of the ANA. The 1973 bylaws indicated that each commissioner had to be a member of the AMA or the ANA and that at least five had to be active practitioners (50 percent or more of "his" time in direct patient care). NJPC, bylaws, approved July 27, 1973, 3, Smoyak Collection. Male pronouns are used consistently in the documents to refer to physicians, and female pronouns to nurses.

10. Sidney H. Willig, J.D., "Legal Aspects of Medical and Nursing Practice," a presentation to the National Joint Practice Commission, September 15, 1978, 44, Smoyak Collection. Willig was a law professor at Temple University, Philadelphia, and a nationally known expert on practice act legislation.

11. The original nurse practitioner members of the NJPC were Genrose J. Alfano (New York), Patricia Devine (Kansas), Marilyn J. Howe (Ohio), Nancy Melvin (Arizona), Anna Sherlock (Arizona), Shirley Smoyak (New Jersey), Virginia Stone (North Carolina), and Barbara Taylor (Massachusetts). The physician members were Thomas Dillon (New York) (replaced by Daniel Beacham from Louisiana), A. Alan Fischer (Indiana), Robert Hoekelman (New York), Joseph Marshall (Idaho), William Muller Jr. (Virginia), Robert Murray (Texas), Otto Page (Oregon), and James Walker (Florida).

12. Shirley Smoyak, interview with Julie Fairman New brunswick, NJ, October 21, 1999, lines 205–208.

13. NJPC, minutes, April 6–7, 1972, Chicago, 2, Smoyak Collection. The ANA/AMA contribution eventually reached $25,000 each before the commission disbanded.

14. NJPC, minutes, January 21, 1972, St. Louis, MO, 3, Smoyak Collection.

15. Smoyak interview, October 21, 1999, lines 233–243.

16. Ibid., lines 249–255, 268–271; NJPC, minutes, January 21, 1972, 4, Smoyak Collection. They used the nominal group process. See Andre L. Delbecq and A. H. Van deVen, "A Group Process Model for Problem Identification and Program Planning," *Journal of Applied Behavioral Science* 7 (July/August 1971): 466–491.

17. NJPC, January 21, 1972, 3, Smoyak Collection. This was the only meeting at which names were used in the narrative. A reporter from the *American Journal of Nursing* published quotes from the first meeting without authorization, and the commission halted the practice. See Smoyak interview, October 21, 1999, lines 904–905.

18. NJPC, January 21, 1972, 4, Smoyak Collection.

19. NCSNNE, "The National Joint Practice Commission: New Bottles, New Wine," self-published pamphlet, circa 1972.

20. NJPC, minutes, November 10–11, 1972, 5–6, Smoyak Collection.

21. Ibid., 6.

22. Robert Hoekelman to Hugh H. Hussey, "The National Joint Practice Commission," August 6, 1973, 11, Smoyak Collection. William Schaffrath, PhD, was the first and only director. He had experience in health care management and at one time served as the executive director of the District of Columbia Nurses' Association.

23. For example, see the Tennessee Hospital Association, the Tennessee Medical Society, and the Tennessee Nurses' Association, "Joint Statements on Patient Care," approved 1968, Smoyak Collection.

24. Jerome Lysaught, "Putting the *Abstract* into Action: Implementation Activities at the State Level," manuscript, 1974, 1–26, Smoyak Collection, quote on 25.

25. Richard E. Flood, "Background and Present Interests of the NPC and the West Virginia Liaison Committee," *NJPC Bulletin* 3 (1) (November 1975): 3–4, Smoyak Collection.
26. Lysaught, "Putting the *Abstract* into Action," 11.
27. Mary McCann Spicer to Genrose Alfano, February 28, 1978, Smoyak Collection. Spicer was the executive director of the Maryland Nurses' Association. Alfano was the chairperson of the NJPC. The medical society directly appointed its members to the State Board of Medical Examiners, thus they were able to shape the practice act debates. The Pennsylvania Medical Society was also able to influence legislation in this way. On the other hand, the Maryland Nurses' Association gave the governor a list of potential appointees from which the governor chose the State Board of Nursing Examiner membership. All on the list could have been association members.
28. The AMA-ANA sponsored the first national conference for professional nurses and physicians in Williamsburg, Virginia, in 1964. See James W. Walker, "NJPC Involvement with the State JPC's," manuscript dated 1972, 1, Smoyak Collection.
29. Ibid.
30. Ibid.
31. Ibid.
32. Data available only for the first year and a half of monthly meetings. See NJPC, "Commissioners' Record of Attendance," April 10, 1972, to December 1974, Smoyak Collection.
33. Smoyak interview, October 21, 1999, lines 831–836.
34. Ibid., lines 922–923.
35. Ibid., lines 418–431.
36. Ibid., lines 366–389.
37. Robert Hoekelman, "Nurse Physician Relationships: Problems and Solutions," commencement address given to graduates of the pediatric and medical nurse associate training programs, Rush Presbyterian–St. Luke's Medical Center, Chicago, June 16, 1974, 8, Smoyak Collection.
38. Virginia C. Hall, *Statutory Regulation of the Scope of Nursing Practice—A Critical Survey* (Washington, DC: National Joint Practice Commission, 1975).
39. For listings of court cases, see the National Academy of Sciences, Institute of Medicine (IOM), staff paper prepared by Neil Weisfeld and M. S. Hyg, "Legal Liability of Primary Care Manpower," January 11, 1977, Smoyak Collection. For exemplars of research on the subject see Eli P. Bernzweig, "The Malpractice Problem and the Use of Physician Assistants," US DHEW, Secretary's Commission on Medical Malpractice, *Report to the Secretary*, vol. 2, DHEW Pub. #OS 73–89 (Washington, DC: Government Printing office, 1973); Sidney H . Willig, "The Medical Board's Role in Physician Assistancy," *Bulletin of the Federation of State Medical Boards* 58 (1971): 171; Edward H. Forgotson and Ruth Roemer, "Government Licensure and Voluntary Standards for Health Personnel and Facilities: Their Power and Limitation in Assuring High-Quality Health Care," *Medical Care* 6 (1968): 350–354.
40. Arlene Keeling, *Nursing and the Privilege of Prescription, 1893–2000* (Columbus: Ohio State University Press, 2007).
41. Barbara Safriet makes this argument in the classic paper, "Health Care Dollars and Regulatory Sense: The Role of Advanced Practice Nursing," *Yale Journal on Regulation* 9 (417) (1992): 417–488.
42. ANA, Nursing Practice Department, "1973 Legislation Survey," August 13, 1973, 14, Smoyak Collection.

43. "ANA Board Approves a Definition of Nursing Practice," *American Journal of Nursing* 55 (1955): 1474.

44. ANA, "1973 Legislation Survey," Smoyak Collection.

45. Disciplines outside of health care, particularly in the law profession, were also interested in the changing roles of various health professions before the commission formed. See Rick J. Carlson, "Health Manpower Licensing and Emerging Institutional Responsibility for Quality of Care," *Law and Contemporary Problems* 35 (1970): 849, 876–878; Edward H. Forgotson and John L. Cook, "Innovations and Experiments in Uses of Health Manpower—The Effects of Licensure Laws," *Law and Contemporary Problems* 32 (1967): 731, 744–748.

46. For cases and statutes, see Virginia Hall to Howard Jacobson, memo, May 11, 1972, 14–15, Smoyak Collection. Hall was an attorney consulted by Jacobson, the medical director of the Macy program, for clarification of the position under Massachusetts law of its graduates to practice with other health personnel and in institutions that hired them. The Macy program was a joint Harvard Medical School and Boston College School of Nursing effort funded by the foundation to prepare clinical nurse specialists in maternity and pediatric ambulatory services. The program began in 1970, and the first class graduated in June 1973. See T. Chopoorian and Howard N. Jacobson, "Joint Boston College School of Nursing–Harvard Medical School Program (the Macy Program), Progress Report 1973–1974," April 9, 1974, Boston, Smoyak Collection.

47. Pennsylvania State Board of Medical Examiners and Licensure, minutes, January 8, 1977, 16, Office of the Commissioner of Professional and Occupational Affairs, Harrisburg, PA.

48. NJPC, "Statement on Medical and Nurse Practice Acts," Smoyak Collection.

49. Hal Higdon, Ron Offen, and Jack Starr, *Together: A Casebook of Joint Practices in Primary Care*, ed. Berton Roueché (Chicago: Educational Publications and Innovative Communications for the NJPC, 1977).

50. See "Suite 511" and "Standing Orders in the Mountains" in Higdon, Offen, Starr, *Together*, 1–11, 123–132.

51. Ibid.

52. The R. W. Johnson Foundation funded the casebook in 1975 by granting $79,475. *NJPC Bulletin* 1 (1) (May 1975): 10.

53. NJPC, minutes, "Comments on the ANA Liaison Report," December 15, 1974, 6, Smoyak Collection.

54. NJPC executive committee, minutes, September 9, 1978, Smoyak Collection. William Schaffrath offered this information.

55. Max H. Parrott, "Introduction," in Higdon, Offen, and Starr, *Together*, ix.

56. Ibid.

57. Ibid.

58. For an example, see review of *Together* by Barbara Resnick, *Nursing Outlook*, September 1977, 595. *Outlook* is the official journal of the American Academy of Nursing. A search of the nursing and medical databases by University of Pennsylvania librarian Sherry Morgan did not produce any additional reviews of *Together*. There is no mention of the casebook in the ANA executive board minutes nor the practice division minutes, 1973–1975, in the ANA Collection in the Howard Gotlieb Archival Research Center at Boston University (ANA Collection).

59. Smoyak interview, October 21, 1999, lines 665–669. The importance of the unused material is also noted in the NJPC, minutes, December 5, 1974, 14, Smoyak Collection.

60. The AMA trustees also proposed a reduction of forty-seven staff, requested the House of Delegates to increase dues from $110 to $200, and wanted a cutback the number of issues of some of its journals. The dues increase was eventually put on hold, but members were charged a $60 assessment. While the AMA was cutting its administrative costs, it was also planning to build an association campus adjacent to its headquarters in Chicago. This campus would house other specialty associations and the AMA's current committees and staff. See AMA, report by the AMA liaison, minutes, NJPC, December 5, 1974, 2-3, Smoyak Collection.

61. Robert Hoekelman to James H. Sammons, December 16, 1974, Smoyak Collection. This letter acknowledges the importance of the NJPC in light of the AMA's action to dissolve its Committee on Nursing and the ANA Liaison Committee. Sammons was the executive director of the AMA.

62. Nicholas Griffin to James Sammons, "Memo on New Health Practitioners," December 2, 1977, Smoyak Collection. Griffin was secretary of the AMA Council on Medical Services.

63. NJPC, "Statement on Nursing Staffs in Hospitals," September 1977, Smoyak Collection.

64. NJPC, "Discussion of the Working Paper," attachment 3B to minutes, March 7-8, 1975, Smoyak Collection.

65. See NJPC, "Draft Statement on "Nurse/Physician Relationships in Hospitals," attachment 3A to minutes, March 7-8, 1975, Smoyak Collection. This initial draft statement was separated into two individual statements, 3 and 4, by June 1977.

66. JCAH, "Nursing Service Principles from the Accreditation Manual for Hospitals," updated version, 1973, 51; JCAH, "Medical Service Principles from the Accreditation Manual for Hospitals," updated version, 1973, 35. See also "Discussion of Working Paper," March 7-8, 1975, 13. All from Smoyak Collection. It is unclear who drafted the original NJPC statement. The transcribed discussion only lists the writer as "N" for nurse, but William Schaffrath probably drafted part of the document.

67. NJPC, "Draft Statement on "Nurse/Physician Relationships," 1, Smoyak Collection.

68. Ibid. This language is absent from the final version—nursing is still responsible, but the nursing staffs "exercise the responsibility for the quality of nursing care."

69. James Sammons to William Schaffrath, October 20, 1975, Smoyak Collection.

70. Sammons to Schaffrath, October 20, 1975, Smoyak Collection.

71. Betty Erlandson to Shirley Smoyak, December 30, 1975, Smoyak Collection. Erlandson was the program coordinator for the ANA Congress on Nursing Practice. The AMA response came from the board of trustees through the executive director, indicating the higher level of attention given by the AMA. The ANA response came through the Congress on Nursing Practice rather than the Board of Directors, although probably with the board's consent.

72. A. Alan Fischer to William Schaffrath, August 5, 1977, attached to William Schaffrath memorandum of June 12, 1979, Smoyak Collection.

73. NJPC, minutes, June 17, 1977, 3, Smoyak Collection.

74. American Hospital Association, "A Patient's Bill of Rights" (Chicago: American Hospital Association, 1972). Smoyak Collection.

75. The NJPC, "Statement on Joint Practice in Primary Care: Definition and Guidelines," September 1977, Smoyak Collection.

76. The NJPC, "Statement on the Definition of Joint or Collaborative Practice in Hospitals," September 1977, Smoyak Collection. Italics in pamphlet.

77. American Academy of Family Physicians, "Position Statement on Family Nurse Practitioners," adopted by the board of directors, July 20, 1974, 1–2, Smoyak Collection.

78. George T. Wolff to A. Alan Fischer, July 27, 1977, 1, Smoyak Collection. Fischer was the American Academy of Family Physicians Liaison to the NJPC. The concerns are spelled out in this letter and in the minutes of the academy board, July 16–17, 1977, 55–56, Smoyak Collection.

79. See NJPC, minutes, June 17–18, 1977, 3–5, Smoyak Collection.

80. Nicholas Griffin to James Sammons (for the AMA Board of Trustees), memo, "New Health Practitioners," December 2, 1977, 2, Smoyak Collection. For examples, see AMA, "Guidelines to Assist in Development of New Health Occupations," Proceedings, House of Delegates, AMA, 120th Annual Convention, Atlantic City, NJ, June 20–14, 1971, 84. Griffon was the secretary of the Council on Medical Service. The guidelines were written in 1969. The Council on Manpower was also working with individual medical specialties to develop functional models and the appropriate role of physician support personnel in that specialty (85). For the specialty medical organization guidelines on nurse practitioners, see, for example, the AAFP's "Position Statement on Family Nurse Practitioners," Smoyak Collection.

81. Bernadine Z. Paulshock, "I Don't Want to be 'Role-realigned'," *Medical Economics,* April 18, 1977, 114–123, quote on 123. Paulshock was an internist in Delaware and sent this article to Shirley Smoyak in November 1977. In her letter to Smoyak she thanks her for coming to Delaware to talk about the NJPC and notes "[I] do not expect you to care for it [the paper]." Bernadine Z. Paulshock to Shirley Smoyak, November 29, 1977, Smoyak Collection.

82. Griffin to Sammons, December 2, 1977, 2.

83. NJPC, Long Range Goals Committee, minutes, September 14, 1978, 1, Smoyak Collection.

84. NJPC, Director's Annual Report, August 1, 1977, to July 31, 1978, 2, Smoyak Collection.

85. Handwritten notes taken by commissioner Shirley Smoyak during NJPC meeting, September 14, 1978, 2, Smoyak Collection. There is also a note re discussion by Jackson Riddle, the AMA staff liaison person, that the AMA board was concerned with the compatibility of the NJPC statements with the AMA. "Sammons doesn't want NJPC to follow in JCAH's foot steps. NJPC should respond to parent organizations." He is referring to the proposed JCAH's bylaw changes in the mid-1970s that would have made it independent of the AMA. Ritter added, "Well, JCAH didn't change its by-laws—but we changed our 6 commissioners and we accomplished what we wanted." (Quotes used by Smoyak.)

86. NJPC, Director's Annual Report, August 1, 1977, to July 31, 1978, 3, Smoyak Collection.

87. "Comment from Commissioners," attached to Willig, "Legal Aspects of Medical and Nursing Practice," ii.

88. "Comment from Commissioners," iii.

89. AAP, "Summary of Responses and Proposed AAP Position to Three Statements on Nurse-Physician Collaboration by the National Joint Practice Commission on Medicine and Nursing," January 1978, 1, Smoyak Collection.

90. Ibid., 3.

91. Ibid.

92. NJPC, Executive Committee, minutes, December 6–7, 1979, attachment A, Smoyak Collection.

93. James Sammons, "Remarks to the NJPC," March 9, 1978, attachment to NJPC minutes, September 15–16, 1978, Smoyak Collection.

94. Sammons, "Remarks to the NJPC."

95. Ibid.

96. NJPC, minutes, February 9, 1979, 7, Smoyak Collection.

97. William B. Schaffrath to the NJPC and Liaison Staff, "Review of Published JPC Statements," June 12, 1979, 1, Smoyak Collection.

98. NJPC, minutes, May 18, 1979, 5, Smoyak Collection.

99. NJPC, Executive Committee, September 6, 1979, attachment A, Smoyak Collection. At this point the committee itself was calling the statements "inflammatory."

100. The commission had money for projects rather than operational expenses. For example, in 1977 during the height of the controversy over the statements, the commission received almost a million dollars from the W. K. Kellogg Foundation for a hospital demonstration project for joint practice, primary nursing, and patient-centered records. NJPC, minutes, July 15, 1977, 9, Smoyak Collection.

101. NJPC, minutes, June 5, 1980, 5, Smoyak Collection.

102. Ibid., May 7, 1980.

103. Prospective Payment is a system of Medicare reimbursement, part A, that bases payment on admission medical diagnosis. This was a shift in patients' charges from those traditionally based on reasonable and acceptable charges. See http://www.nber.org/data/pps.html (accessed October 10, 2006).

104. Richard Chamberlin, "Report of the Chairperson," May 9, 1980, Smoyak Collection.

Chapter 7   Triangulating Specialty Practice

1. Evelyn Barbee, "Racism in Nursing," *Medical Anthropology Quarterly* 7 (4) (December 1993): 346–362.

2. Joan Lynaugh, personal communication, January 2, 2003.

3. Frances Hughes et al., "Nurse Practitioner Research: An Historical Analysis," in *Nurses, Nurse Practitioners*, ed. Mathy D. Mezey and Diane O. McGivern (New York: Springer), 84–108.

4. John P. Connelly, "Nurses and Physicians Collaborate," *Pediatrics* 47 (6) (1971): 996–98.

5. Over six thousand pediatricians responded to the survey, which accounted for over 90 percent of the active, board-certified practicing pediatricians in the country. This was a remarkable return that indicated the high level of interest generated by the issues. See Alfred Yankauer, John P. Connelly, Pricilla Andrews, and Jacob J. Feldman, "The Practice of Nursing in Pediatric Offices—Challenge and Opportunity," *New England Journal of Medicine* 282 (15) (April 9, 1970): 843–847, statistics on 843.

6. Alfred Yankauer, John Connelly, and Jacob Feldman, "Pediatric Practice in the United States with Special Attention to Utilization of Allied Health Worker Services," *Pediatrics* 45 (3) (1970): 521–554.

7. The AAP also established an Office of Allied Health Manpower in 1969 and one of its first functions was to meet with the ANA in June 1969. See ANA, Board of Directors, minutes, April 29, 30; May 1, 1970, from the ANA Collection in the Howard Gotlieb Archival Research Center at Boston University (ANA Collection).

8. American Academy of Pediatrics, "News," *American Academy of Pediatrics Newsletter* 20 (1969). See also Dorothy G. Fiorino, "An Historical Study of the

National Association of Pediatric Nurse Associates/Practitioners (NAPNAP), 1973–1978," master's thesis, Wright State University, Dayton, Ohio, 1980.

9. ANA position paper prepared by Sonia Loir, "The Responsibility of the Nursing Profession for Preparing the Nurse of the Future for Pediatric Patient Care," April 10, 1970, AAP Misc., ANA Archives, Silver Springs, MD (ANA Archives). Loir also participated in an AAP-sponsored meeting two days later, where she presented her remarks. She noted in her records of the meeting that many of the nurses in the room criticized the ANA's position on the guidelines. She told the group the ANA first received copies of the guidelines on December 22, 1969; endorsement was requested immediately, and the ANA did not have time to survey its membership. See Sonia Loir, report, April 12, 1970, 2, ANA Representatives to AAP Meetings Collection (ANA Rep), ANA Archives.

10. AAP and the ANA, "Guidelines on Short-term Continuing Education Programs for Pediatric Nurse Associates," *Pediatrics* 47 (6) (1971): 1075–1079.

11. ANA, Board of Directors, report of the Division on MCHN, September 9, 12–14, 1997, 5–6, box 75, file 14, ANA Collection.

12. AAP and the ANA, "Guidelines," 1075–1079.

13. Data from table 4, viii, US DHEW, PHS, BHME, *Selected Training Programs for Physician Support Personnel*, DHEW Pub. #NIH 72–183 (Washington, DC: Government Printing Office, revised May 1972).

14. AAP and ANA, "Guidelines," 1075, 1076.

15. Ibid.

16. For the AMA standpoint, see AMA, Committee on Nursing, "Medicine and Nursing in the 1970s: A Position Statement," *Journal of the American Medical Association* 213 (11) (1970): 1881–1883.

17. The physicians included Bruce Graham, chairman, District 5, AAP; Bruce Mayer, private pediatrician, Columbus, OH; Donald Frank, AAP Manpower Committee member and director of the University of Cincinnati pediatric nurse associate program; Robert Heavenrich, president of the AAP. The nurses included Gloria Rookard and Sue Hooverman, president and vice president, respectively, of the Ohio Pediatric Nurse Associates; Marianne Kainz, chair, California Pediatric Nurse Practitioners; Sally Walsh, president of the Pediatric Nurse Associates of Greater New England; Carole Passarelli, president of the Connecticut Pediatric Nurse Associates; Sharon Elsass, Suzanne Brunner, and Janet McCleery, pediatric nurse associates from Ohio; Irashel Fitzgerald from California; Marie Brown from Colorado; Rita Lewis, U.S. Air Force (Texas); and Judy Birchenough from Massachusetts. NAPNAP, Planning Committee, minutes, May 2 1973, from the personal collection of Barbra Dunn, Richmond, VA (Dunn Collection). Dunn is a pediatric nurse practitioner who held many leadership positions within NAPNAP, including the presidency from 1975 to 1977.

The terms "pediatric nurse practitioner" and "pediatric nurse associate" will be used interchangeably according to their use in the documents. Pediatric nurse associate was the preferred term of the American Academy of Pediatrics.

18. Robert Heavenrich to Janet McCleery, May 30, 1973, NAPNAP Collection, Center for Nursing Historical Inquiry (CNHI), School of Nursing, University of Virginia (NAPNAP Collection). His claim was supported by Robert Frazier, executive director of the AAP. See Robert G. Frazier to Eileen Jacobi, June 14, 1973, AAP miscellaneous collection, 1969–1985, ANA Archives.

19. Frazier to Jacobi, June 14, 1973.

20. The preorganization meeting was supported and organized through the efforts of Ann McRedmond, the nursing consultant from Ross Laboratories, who reached interested nurses via the company newsletter, "Pediatric Nursing Current," and the AAP, which also made their mailing lists available to the organizers. Other industry support came from Carl Spaulding of Johnson and Johnson. The Schering Corporation supplied $1,500 to defray initial travel expenses of the participants. NAPNAP, Planning Committee, May 2, 1973.

21. This was not a formal affiliation until later—NAPNAP was an independent organization but chose to align itself politically and ideologically with AAP rather than the ANA.

22. See Julie Fairman and Joan Lynaugh, *Critical Care Nursing: A History* (Philadelphia: University of Pennsylvania Press, 1998), and Nancy Hoffart, "A Professional Organization for Nephrology Nurses," *ANNA Journal* 16 (3) (1989): 197–199.

23. Heavenrich to McCleery, May 30, 1973, NAPNAP Collection.

24. Sonia Loir noted in her report of her participation on the April, 1970, AAP panel that she was verbally attacked by many of the nurses in the crowd who accused the ANA of being against both nurse practitioners and diploma nurses. See Loir, "Report," April 12, 1970, 1–2.

25. Sally Walsh, NAPNAP Archive interviews, March 17, 1995, videotape 1, CNHI. Barbara Dunn conducted the interviews in 1995.

26. ANA, Board of Directors, President's Report, minutes, January 25–28, 1972, 3, box 488, ANA Collection.

27. ANA, Board of Directors, report of Nursing Practice Department, minutes, January 26–29, 1971, box 75, file 15, 10, ANA Collection. Pearl Dunkley was acting director of the department.

28. Dorothy M. Saller and Dorothy Talbot, "Federation of Nursing Specialty Organizations and ANA; A History," manuscript, series 1: administrative subseries, AAP/ANA/NAPNAP correspondence, NAPNAP Collection.

29. Rap sessions documented in "Notes on PNP Rap Session, ANA Meeting," May 2, 1972, series 1, NAPNAP Collection. The presence of this note in the NAPNAP files indicates someone from the organization was at the session and recorded the discussion. For quote, see Hildegard Peplau, "A Time to Stand Up and Be Counted," speech to the house of delegates, 48th convention, Detroit, April 30 to May 5, 1972, 584–592, in Lyndia Flanagan, compiler, *One Strong Voice: The Story of the American Nurses' Association* (Kansas City, MO: ANA, 1976), quote on 589.

30. ANA, Board of Directors, report of independent practitioners, September 19–21, 1973, box 488, 19, ANA Collection.

31. Meeting of presidents and executive directors of organizations of registered nurse practitioners with the president and executive director of ANA, November 17, 1972, minutes, as noted by Saller and Talbot, "Federation of Nursing Specialty Organizations and ANA." It should be noted that Saller and Talbot use the language of nurse practitioner organizations, but they were probably all some sort of specialty organizations that included both nurse practitioners and non-nurse practitioners. Nurse practitioners tended to find organizational homes in the specialty organizations.

32. Saller and Talbot, "Federation of Nursing Specialty Organizations" See also Fairman and Lynaugh, *Critical Care Nursing*, 102–105.

33. The group of nurse practitioner organizations that met in November with the ANA agreed to merge into one group. This joint group eventually became the contemporary

National Federation of Specialty Nursing Organizations in June 1973. NAPNAP became a member in 1974. The original founding members included: American Association of Critical-Care Nurses, American Association of Industrial Nurses, American Association of Nephrology Nurses and Technicians, American Association of Nurse Anesthetists, American Association of Neurosurgical Nurses, American College of Nurse-Midwives, American Nurses' Association, American Urological Association Allied, Association of Operating Room Nurses, department of school nurses of the National Education Association, National Emergency Department Nurses Association, Nurses Association of the American College of Obstetricians and Gynecologists, and public health nursing section of the American Public Health Association.

34. NAPNAP, minutes, August 15, 1973, Dunn Collection. Actually, the ANA Board of Directors approved the Pediatric Nurse Practitioner Council earlier in October 1972 (ANA, Board of Directors, minutes, October 5, 6, 1972, box 488, ANA Collection). Essentially, the ANA approved the council before they told the ANA-AAP liaison committee about it in November 1972. The ANA also created the Council of Advanced Practitioners in psychiatric mental health nursing in 1972 (ANA, Board of Directors, report of the Division on Psychiatric and Mental Health Nursing, minutes, April 22–26, 1972, box 488, 18). Five nurse practitioner councils were created between 1972 and 1974: advanced practitioners in medical-surgical nursing, advanced practitioners in psychiatric and mental health nursing, family nurse practitioners, and advanced practitioners in nursing of children (also called the council of pediatric nurse practitioners). See Flanagan, *One Strong Voice*, 211.

35 "Message from the Chairman," *Pediatric Nurse Practitioner* 1 (1) (1973): not paginated, box 6, NAPNAP Collection. By this time there was also a Family Nurse Practitioner (FNP) Council, and in 1974, much debate about adult nurse practitioners joining the FNP Council. The council voted to change the name to Primary Care Nursing Practice Council. The name change later created problems with the Pediatric Nurse Practitioner Council, which also believed primary care to be its realm. "Family Nurses Meet to Organize," *ANA Convention Journal*, June 12, 1974, Kathryn Jacquette Collection, University of Virginia, School of Nursing, Center for Nursing Historical Inquiry (Jacquette Collection).

36. Patricia Stewart to Janet McCleery, March 30, 1973, series 1, NAPNAP Collection. Stewart was also the first chair of the Pediatric Nurse Practitioner Council. See also NAPNAP, minutes, affiliation meeting, August 15, 1973, series 1, NAPNAP Collection. Anne McRedmond also knew about the council in June 1973. See Barbara E. Bishop to Anne McRedmond, June 21, 1973, AAP Misc., ANA Archives. For Redmond's involvement in the first NAPNAP meeting, see note 20.

37. Although the ANA did not guarantee pediatric nurse practitioner representation on the executive committee, Patricia Stewart, a pediatric nurse practitioner from Fresno, California, was chairman of the interim executive committee of the ANA Council on Pediatric Nurse Practitioners. See NAPNAP, minutes, August 15, 1973, Dunn Collection. See also ANA, Board of Directors, "Exhibit III," May 1–3, 1973, box 488, ANA Collection. According to this document, the councils reported to the divisions and were, by nature of their definition, temporary, according to the particular interest of a particular group, and they had an ad hoc character. The councils, as NAPNAP realized, were not guaranteed representation on the division executive committee. To NAPNAP, the councils seemed more like special interest groups than policy-making groups.

38. ANA-NAPNAP-AAP Task Force, "Message from the Chairman," *Pediatric Nurse Practitioner* 1 (1) (1973). In contrast, as an independent organization NAPNAP could publish its own newsletter and did so before the first official meeting of the organization. Johnson and Johnson Baby Products agreed to fund a newsletter for 1974. Rita Lewis was the first editor and Jean Splann was the managing editor of *Pediatric Nurse Practitioner.*

39. NAPNAP, minutes, August 15, 1973, Dunn Collection. Also see Barbara Dunn, telephone interview by Julie Fairman, May 31, 2003, lines 476–481. Once NAPNAP was organized and affiliation determined, the president of NAPNAP became a member of the AAP Pediatric Manpower Committee.

40. For the vote, see First National Meeting of NAPNAP, minutes, October 23, 1973, Dunn Collection. See also letter requesting space from the AAP for the first meeting, Janet McCleery to Robert Frazier, April 20, 1973, NAPNAP Collection. It is unclear how many pediatric nurse practitioner/assistants were at the meeting, but within the year membership climbed to 496, or about 30 percent of all eligible pediatric nurse practitioners. Statistics are found in a 1983 document, "NAPNAP: The First Decade," manuscript, series 1, NAPNAP Collection.

41. First National Meeting of NAPNAP, minutes.

42. Walsh, March 17, 1995, tape #1, CNHI.

43. Margaret Hicks, NAPNAP Archive interviews, March 17, 1995, tape #1, CNHI. Hicks held multiple leadership posts in NAPNAP and was president 1978 to 1979.

44. Patricia McAtee to Janet McCleery, June 1974, series 1, NAPNAP Collection.

45. The state organizations served as the collective bargaining units of the organization, and economic welfare, at least for the generalists, at times trumped clinic practice issues as their priority. See ANA, Board of Directors, minutes, January 30, February 1–2, 1973, box 488, 18–19, ANA Collection. See also the press release, ANA, Board of Directors, "ANA Launches Massive Organization Campaign, Organizing 800,000 Nurses for the Purposes of Collective Bargaining," minutes, January 29, February 2, 1974, box 488, ANA Collection.

46. McAtee to McCleery, June 1974, NAPNAP Collection.

47. See ANA Report, "Continuing Education," September 1971, box 6, series 3, file "ANA Study to Evaluate Effectiveness of Types of Nursing Programs," 1, Jessie Scott Collection, Barbara Bates Center for the Study of the History of Nursing, School of Nursing, University of Pennsylvania, Philadelphia (Scott Collection). The programs, to be three in number, were jointly planned by the ANA-AAP liaison committee.

48. ANA, "Nurses, in the Extended Role, Are Not Physician Assistants," July 9, 1973, 3, National Joint Commission Papers, Shirley Smoyak Collection, Barbara Bates Center for the Study of the History of Nursing, School of Nursing, University of Pennsylvania, Philadelphia (Smoyak Collection). Emphasis in original.

49. ANA, "Scope of Practice for Pediatric Nurse Practitioners," NAPNAP Collection.

50. ANA, "Certification Program for the Pediatric Nurse Practitioner in Ambulatory Health Care"; "Accreditation of Continuing Education Programs Preparing Nurses for Expanded Roles"; and "Scope of Practice for Pediatric Nurse Practitioners." All three statements found in the NAPNAP Collection.

51. Flanagan, *One Strong Voice*, 232–233. Flanagan notes that the interim boards were to exist only through the initial work of developing standards and criteria. Eventually, they would be composed of certified nurse practitioners appointed by the board. It is difficult to understand exactly who was the focus of certification, as the term "nurse practitioner" had been used for decades to indicate the practicing generalist nurse.

52. There are references to an explicit ANA certification program in the board of directors' minutes as early as January 1972, when Peplau cites the emergence of "splinter groups" as one reason to move "expeditiously with its certification program." See ANA, Board of Directors, minutes, January 25–28, 1972, box 488, 5, ANA Collection. The board was still referring to practicing nurses at any level as "nurse practitioners" and did not formally change their language until 1973. In May 1974 the ANA administered the first certification exam in both geriatric nursing and pediatric nursing in ambulatory care.

53. Eileen Jacobi, "Memo to PNP/A," 2–3, from the Luther Christman Collection in the Howard Gotlieb Archival Research Center at Boston University, Boston (Christman Collection). Jacobi quotes directly from the minutes of the ANA-AAP Liaison Committee minutes.

54. Ibid., 3–4, Christman Collection. Those present at the meeting included AAP representatives Robert Burnett, John Connelly, Donald Frank, Robert Hoekelman, and ANA representatives Pearl Dunkley, Jeannette Sasmor, Iris Shannon, Arlene Burrough, and M. Elaine Whitman. See also similar statements in "ANA and Pediatricians Resume Dialogue," *American Journal of Nursing* 75 (1) (1975): 7–9.

55. See Jacobi, "Memo to PNP/A," 5, Christman Collection. The same data are presented in "ANA and Pediatricians," 7–9. See also Barbara Bishop to Robert Frazier, January 3, 1974, AAP Misc., ANA Archives.

56. See Jacobi, "Memo to PNP/A," 4, Christman Collection.

57. Ibid., 5.

58. This notification came in the AAP *Newsletter*, June 15, 1972. See Eileen Jacobi to J. M. Arena, AAP Misc., ANA Archives. In this letter, Jacobi notes the ANA concern over the AAP certification exam notification, which was "contrary in principle and intent" to the agreements worked out in the last liaison meeting, April 15, 1972. Arena was president of the AAP.

59. Robert Frazier to Eileen Jacobi, August 24, 1972, AAP Misc., ANA Archives. This is also noted in a memo from Robert Frazier to Wesley Duiker, August 23, 1972, AAP Misc., ANA Archives. Duiker was the AAP staff person.

60. This announcement by Hoekelman is noted by Fiorino, "An Historical Study of the National Association" 145–146. See also NAPNAP, first national meeting, minutes, October 23, 1973, 4, Dunn Collection. Henry Silver also tangentially refers to the AAP ad hoc committee recommendations in a memo to graduates of the University of Colorado NP program on September 6, 1973, The Loretta Ford Personal Collection, Wildwood, FL (Ford Collection).

61. NAPNAP, minutes, first national meeting, 4, Dunn Collection.

62. NJPC, "Statement on Certification of Nurses and Physicians," February 1974, Smoyak Collection. For the lack of NAPNAP response, see Fiorino, "An Historical Study of the National Association," 145–147.

63. Janet McCleery to WR, February 19, 1974, series 1: administrative, file 1/74–12/74, NAPNAP Collection.

64. AAP to Fellows, January 16, 1974, NAPNAP Collection; AAP to pediatric nurse associates, January 16, 1974, NAPNAP Collection.

65. This version of the scope was originally entitled "AAP Scope of Practice." See AAP (cc to Janet McCleery), draft of AAP scope of practice, January 4, 1974, NAPNAP Collection. It became a joint statement by December 1974. See Scope of Practice statement for pediatric nurse associates/practitioners, December 12, 1974, NAPNAP Collection.

66. AAP, Scope of Practice, December 12, 1974, NAPNAP Collection.
67. ANA, "Scope of Practice for Pediatric Nurse Practitioners," Jacquette Collection.
68. SJ to Mary Kaye Willian, March 5, 1975, correspondence, NAPNAP Collection.
69. LP to Mary Kaye Willian, April 9, 1975, correspondence, NAPNAP Collection.
70. JJ to Mary Kaye Willian, May 5, 1975, correspondence, NAPNAP Collection.
71. Avrum L. Katcher to Robert Frazier, April 24, 1975, correspondence, NAPNAP Collection.
72. AAP, Committee on Pediatric Manpower, minutes, November 3–4, 1974, correspondence, NAPNAP Collection.
73. An original draft of the letter, January 4, 1974, is entitled "Draft of AAP Scope of Practice Statement." The January 16 letter has no such title. The original letter is much more aggressive in tone (AAP, "Draft," NAPNAP Collection).
74. AAP to Fellows, January 16, 1974, NAPNAP Collection. The AAP did not address the scope issues as aggressively in the letter to pediatric nurse practitioners (AAP to pediatric nurse associates, January 16, 1974, NAPNAP Collection). In the letter the rhetoric on physician supervision of nursing practice is missing. In an original draft of the letter ("AAP, Draft," NAPNAP), the AAP also issued an indirect threat to nurses and ordered their members to "withdraw support from the graduate who is unilaterally certified [e.g., only ANA certified]." This is missing from the final versions of the letters. The original draft was written by AAP vice president John C. MacQueen from the Department of Pediatrics, University of Iowa, but the final letter was signed and initialed by Robert Frazier.
75. AAFP, "Position Statement on Family Nurse Practitioners," adopted by the AAFP board of directors, July 20, 1974, Smoyak Collection. In a later discussion of the position paper by the NJPC in March 1975 the transcripts indicate the AAFP developed the statement in a joint study group sponsored by the AMA and advised by "pediatricians." See NJPC, "Discussion of the Statement on the FNP," edited transcript, March 8, 1975, 1, Smoyak Collection.
76. AAP to Fellows, January 16, 1974, NAPNAP Collection.
77. NAPNAP, Executive Council, minutes, January 16, 1974, 5, Dunn Collection. The minutes note NAPNAP's lack of advance knowledge of the AAP letter.
78. AAP staff and NAPNAP, executive session, January 31, 1974, series 1, NAPNAP Collection. The minutes of the April 22, 1974, meeting of the NAPNAP executive council note that three levels of certification were discussed at the January 31 meeting, including level 3, designated ANA certification. Although it is unclear why the ANA certification was included in the leveling (1–3), it may indicate a less than unanimous stance by NAPNAP on who should certify the pediatric nurse practitioner.
79. WR to Janet McCleery, February 2, 1974, NAPNAP Collection.
80. DHEW, Comptroller General of the U.S., Report to Congress, *Progress and Problems in Training and Use of Assistants to Primary Care Physicians* (Washington, DC: Government Printing Office, 1976), B-164031(5). See also "ANA and Pediatricians Resume Dialogue," 7–9.
81. Jacobi, "Memo to PNP/A," 4, Christman Collection.
82. Nine nurse practitioners from Jacobi Hospital, Bronx, NY, to Janet McCleery, January 14, 1974, series 1, NAPNAP Collection.
83. DN to Robert Frazier, January 23, 1974, series 1, NAPNAP Collection.
84. JF to Robert Frazier, January 21, 1974, series 1, NAPNAP Collection.
85. WR to Janet McCleery, February 2, 1974, series 1, NAPNAP Collection.

86. EL to Janet McCleery, February 1, 1974, series 1, NAPNAP Collection.
87. Janet McCleery to Ellen Laase, February 19, 1974, series 1, NAPNAP Collection.
88. Barbara Dunn to Janet McCleery, February 2, 1974, series 1, NAPNAP Collection.
89. Janet McCleery to Barbara Dunn, February 12, 1974, series 1, NAPNAP Collection.
90. Dunn to Janet McCleery, February 19, 1974, NAPNAP Collection.
91. McCleery to Dunn, February 12, 1974, series 1, NAPNAP Collection.
92. WR to McCleery, February 2, 1974, NAPNAP Collection.
93. PS to Janet McCleery, February 3, 1974, series 1, NAPNAP Collection.
94. Patricia Stewart attended as a pediatric nurse practitioner consultant, but she also happened to be chair of the ANA Council of Pediatric Nurse Practitioners. She was asked by the group to take the concerns identified in the discussions back to the ANA. See report of the liaison committees of NAPNAP and AAP, March 1–2, 1974, NAPNAP Collection.
95. During its November 2–4, 1974, meeting, an ad hoc committee, consisting of two members from both the AAP and NAPNAP, Mary Kaye Willian, a pediatric nurse practitioner recently appointed to the liaison staff of AAP, and Lee Bennett from the USAF were appointed to draw up a format for an entry-level pediatric nurse practitioner certification exam. The ANA was invited to send two representatives to the ad hoc committee's next meeting in December 1974. AAP, Committee on Pediatric Manpower, minutes, November 3–4, 1974, 2, correspondence, NAPNAP Collection. The ANA did not participate.
96. ANA and AAP, "The Relationship between the PNP and the Pediatrician," NAPNAP Collection.
97. Her views are laid out in a handwritten letter to Janet McCleery, May 1974, correspondence, NAPNAP Collection.
98. Karen Fond to Mary Kaye Willian, November 1975, correspondence, NAPNAP Collection.
99. "News from NAPNAP," *Pediatric Nursing* 1 (1975): 20.
100. Walsh, NAPNAP Archives interviews, NAPNAP Collection. NAPNAP held its first independent meeting in 1980.
101. NAPNAP, Executive Board, minutes, October 31, 1981, box 2, file 15, NAPNAP Collection. The CHAMPUS demonstration project was a federally funded health care initiative to improve services for government employees and military personnel. Only ten claims for services by nurse practitioners were submitted in the first few months of the project in May 1981, and forty-four were submitted by September 30, 1981. The problems included lack of state practice acts that allowed independent practice as defined by CHAMPUS. See Karen Fond to Col. Kenneth Herman, July 27, 1981, box 2, file 15, executive board minutes, NAPNAP Collection.
102. NAPNAP, emergency session of the Executive Board, minutes, November 1, 1981, box 2, file 16, 1, NAPNAP Collection.
103. Ibid. The Association of Faculties of Pediatric Nurse Practitioner/assistant programs (AFPNP) began to loosely organize in March 1972 in Connecticut, and was an original member of the consortium in 1974 and later the national board.
104. NAPNAP, emergency session, November 1, 1981, NAPNAP Collection. See also NAPNAP, closed executive session, minutes, February 19, 1982, box 2, file 19, NAPNAP Collection.
105. NAPNAP, survey results attached to executive board minutes, March 24, 1983, 2, box 2, file 25, NAPNAP Collection.
106. NAPNAP, Executive Board, March 24, 1983, 2, NAPNAP Collection.

107. NAPNAP had more success than other nursing organizations in obtaining industry support. The NAPNAP seal was on each box of Pampers diapers, and the organization was instrumental in several federal child safety initiatives. Their public recognition factor was and remains high.

108. NAPNAP, Executive Board, minutes, June 27, 1983, box 2, file 27, 2, NAPNAP Collection.

109. Ibid. The AAP board voted down the resolution to withdraw support from NAPNAP in October 1983. See AAP, fall general meeting, president's report, October 23, 1983, 1, box 2, file 29, NAPNAP Collection.

110. NAPNAP, Executive Board, minutes, June 27, 1983, NAPNAP Collection.

111. NAPNAP, Executive Board, minutes, October 21, 1983, 3, box 2, file 28, NAPNAP Collection.

112. The board is now named the National Certification Board of Pediatric Nurse Practitioners and Nurses and is independent of NAPNAP.

113. AAP, Committee on Pediatric Workforce, policy statement. "Scope of Practice Issues in the Delivery of Pediatric Health Care," *Pediatrics* 111 (2) (February 2003): 426–435. Although the committee roster includes only physicians, a list of speaking points from the AAP Web site http://www.aap.org/workforce/spkgpts2%2D03.doc (accessed February 28, 2003) on the scope noted that both NAPNAP and the American Academy of Physician Assistants provided "thoughtful and constructive comments." NAPNAP requested withdrawal of its name from the portion of the statement noting participation. See Ruth M. Kleinpell, "Pediatric NPs Up in Arms over AAP Policy Statement," *Nursing Spectrum* 12 (7PA) (April 7, 2003): 6.

Chapter 8   Making Room in the Clinic

1. Drew E. Altman and Larry Levitt, "The Sad History of Health Care Cost Containment as Told in One Chart," commentary, Web exclusive, *Health Affairs* January 23, 2002, http://content.healthaffairs.org/cgi/content/full/hlthaff.w2.83v1/DC1 (accessed July 3, 2007).

2. Robert Aronowitz presents the idea of idiosyncrasy in his book, *Making Sense of Illness: Science, Society and Disease* (New York: Cambridge University Press, 1998).

3. Richard A. Cooper, Prakash Laud, and Craig L. Dietrich, "Current and Projected Workforce of Non-Physician Clinicians," *Journal of the American Medical Association* 280 (1998): 788–794; American Academy of Nurse Practitioners (AANP), *Scope of Practice* (Austin, TX: AANP, 1995); Richard A. Cooper, "Perspectives on the Physician Work-force to the Year 2020," *Journal of the American Medical Association* 274 (1995): 1534–1543. Recent scholars, including Richard Cooper, now project a shortage of physicians. See Richard A. Cooper, "Weighing the Evidence for Expanding Physician Supply," *Annals of Internal Medicine* 141 (2004): 705–714. In this analysis Cooper now calls for the expansion of allopathic medical schools. His perspective is still overgeneralized. The practice area of primary care, and specialties such as critical care medicine, cardiology, pulmonary medicine, and anesthesia are already experiencing shortages, as an oversupply of other specialists such as surgical subspecialists persist. See Gordon Morre and Jonathan Showstack, "Primary Care Medicine in Crisis: Towards Reconstruction and Renewal," *Annals of Internal Medicine* 138 (3) (2003): 244–247; Derek C. Angus, Mark A. Kelley, Robert J. Schmitz, Alan White, and John Poporich Jr., "Current and Projected Workforce Requirements for Care of the Critically Ill and Patients with Pulmonary

Disease," *Journal of the American Medical Association* 284 (21) (2000): 2762–2770. Alan Garber and Harold Sox reason that the supply of physicians in general is misunderstood and that "non-physician providers" such as nurse practitioners could be better utilized. See "Editorial: The U.S. Physician Workforce: Serious Questions Raised, Answers Needed," *Annals of Internal Medicine* 141 (9) (2004): 732–734.

4. GMENAC, Report of the Graduate Medical Education National Advisory Committee to the Secretary, Department of Health and Human Services, *Summary Report*, DHHS Pub. # (HRA) 81–651 (Washington, DC: GMENAC, 1981).

5. James Bryant, "Correspondence," *New England Journal of Medicine* 330 (21) (1994): 1535.

6. J. Greene, "Professional Issues: AMA Backs Limits on Scope of Non-Physician Practice," *American Medical News*, January 8, 2001 9–10.

7. The Quacktitioner also elicited over two thousand responses from nurses to an online advocacy site. See http://www.nursingadvocacy.org/news/2006/jan/11_mattel.html (accessed December 13, 2006) for discussion and responses.

8. Patricia D'Antonio and Julie A. Fairman, "Organizing Practice: Nursing, the Medical Model, and Two Case Studies in Historical Time," *Canadian Bulletin of the History of Medicine* 21 (2) (2004): 411–429.

9. Sandy Sherman and Sharon McRath to National Medical Specialties, Washington Representatives, "Endorsement of Citizens' Petition on Physician-Nurse Collaboration," June 5, 2000, http://www.nurse.org/acnp/news/ama.petition.pdf (accessed September 7, 2004).

10. AMA, "Citizens' Petition."

11. M. Coasdale, "Physician Task Force Confronts Scope of Practice Legislation," *American Medical News*, February 13, 2006, http://www.ama-assn.org/amednews/2006/02/13/pr10213.htm (accessed July 8, 2006).

12. American Academy of Nurse Anesthetists, "Coalition for Patients' Rights Calls on AMA to Cease Divisive Efforts to Limit Patients' Choice of Providers," http://www.aana.com/News.aspx?ucNavMenu_TSMenuTargetID=62&ucNavMenu_TSMenuTargetType=4&ucNavMenu_TSMenuID=6&id=3380 (accessed July 8, 2006).

13. James A. Morone, "Morality, Politics and Health Policy," in *Policy Challenges in Modern Health Care*, ed. David Mechanic et al. (New Brunswick, NJ: Rutgers University Press, 2005), 13–15.

14. See Accreditation Council for Graduate Medical Education (ACGME), "Statement of Justification," http://www.acgme.org/acWebsite/dutyHours/dh_impactStatement.pdf and "Frequently Asked Questions," http://www.acgme.org/acWebsite/dutyHours/dh_faqs.pdf (both accessed September 2, 2006).

15. Attending physician, personal communication, September 1, 2006.

16. Charles Rosenberg, "Banishing Risk: Or the More Things Change the More They Remain the Same," *Perspectives in Biology and Medicine* 39 (1) (Autumn 1995): 35.

17. Julie A. Fairman and Patricia D'Antonio, "Reimagining Nurses' Place in the History of Clinical Practice," paper presented at the Rosenberg Conference, Boston, June 10, 2004.

18. See the ANA, *The Scope of Practice of the Primary Health Care Nurse Practitioner* (Kansas City, MO: ANA, 1985), 6. Donna Diers, former dean of the Yale School of Nursing, used the term "half-fledged" in Donna Diers and S. Molde, "Nurses in Primary Care—The New Gatekeeper," *American Journal of Nursing* 83 (1983): 745.

19. See Cooper, "Weighing the Evidence," 705–714.

20. In 1998 the University of Pennsylvania, School of Nursing, developed LIFE (Living Independently for Elders). This program, based on earlier PACE models (Program of All Inclusive Care for Elders), provides health services in the community of West Philadelphia. Care is provided by a team of physicians, nurse practitioners, physical and occupational therapists, and many other providers. See http://www.lifeupenn.org/default.asp (accessed July 12, 2006).

21. Mary D. Naylor et al., "Comprehensive Discharge Planning and Home Follow-up of Hospitalized Elders: A Randomized Clinical Trial," *Journal of the American Medical Association* 281 (7) (February 17, 1999): 613–620.

22. American Nurses' Association, "The Nurse Practitioner Question," *American Journal of Nursing* 74 (12) (December 1974): 2188–2191, quote on 2191. This article reports on an interview with nursing leaders Loretta Ford, Mary Kohnke, Claire Fagin, Ellen Fahy, and Cathryne Welch.

23. Joan W. Scott makes this point about marginalization in "Feminism's History," *Journal of Women's History* 16 (2) (2004):10–29.

24. Ibid., quote on 13–14.

25. See American Association of Colleges of Nursing, "Percent Change in Enrollments in Baccalaureate Nursing Programs: 1994–2006," http://www.aacn.nche.edu/Media/ppt/94–06EnrChgs.ppt (accessed July 4, 2007). See also US DHHS, *The Registered Nurse Population: Preliminary Findings* (March 2004), http://bhpr.hrsa.gov/healthworkforce/reports/rnpopulation/preliminaryfindings.htm (accessed July 4, 2007), 3–4.

26. Between 1980 and 2004, nurses with master's degrees and doctorates grew 339 percent. The biggest proportion was those with master's degrees. See *The Registered Nurse Population*, 4.

27. Ibid. Also see Women Physicians' Congress, "Physicians by Gender," table 1, http://www.ama-assn.org/ama/pub/category/12912.html (accessed July 5, 2007).

28. American Association of Colleges of Nursing, "Position Statement on the Practice Doctorate in Nursing," October 2004. For programs, see http://www.aacn.nche.edu/DNP/DNPProgramList.htm (accessed July 3, 2007).

29. Afaf Meleis and Kathleen Dracup, "The Case against the DNP: History, Timing, Substance and Marginalization," *Online Journal of Issues in Nursing* 10 (3) (September 2005), www.nursingworld.org/okin/topic 28/tpc28_2.htm (accessed October 1, 2005).

30. Office of Technology Assessment, United States Congress, *NPs, Physician Assistants, and Certified Nurse-Midwives: A Policy Analysis*, HCS 37 (Washington, DC: Government Printing Office, 1986); Barbara Safriet, "Health Care Dollars and Regulatory Sense: The Role of Advanced Practice Nursing," *Yale Journal of Regulation* 9 (417) (1992): 417–488.

31. Institute of Medicine, *Health Professions Education: A Bridge to Quality* (Washington, DC: National Academies Press, 2003).

32. AMA House of Delegates, Resolution 211(A-06), "Need to Expose and Counter Nurse Doctoral Program Misrepresentation," accessed via http://www.ama-assn.org/ama1/pub/upload/mm/471/211a06.doc (accessed June 24, 2006).

33. Aronowitz, "Do Not Delay."

34. Milt Freudenheim, "Attention Shoppers: Low Prices on Shots in the Clinic off Aisle 7," *New York Times*, national edition, May 14, 2006, 1, 23. These clinics are usually run by clinic companies. The first in-store clinic opened in Minneapolis, Minnesota, in 2000. The industry leader, MinuteClinic, opened seventy-three retail

clinics in the United States by 2006 in Bartell Drugs, CVS pharmacies, Club Foods, and Target stores, and plans to have seven hundred operating by 2008. See Staff, "By the Numbers: Quick Fix," *Proto*, Summer 2007, 9.

35. The State of Pennsylvania, "Prescription for Pennsylvania," http://www.gohcr. state.pa.us/prescription-for-pennsylvania/Prescription-for-Pennsylvania.pdf (accessed July 7, 2007). Massachusetts and California are among the states generating independent health care reform proposals.

Index

Hudson, Charles, 95, 96, 101

Illinois, joint practice activities in, 141
Illinois, University of, Rockford School of
Medicine at, 38
Indiana State Nurses' Association, 124
information, demands for clinical, 121–122.
See also knowledge
Ingles, Thelma, 97, 99, 228n. 42
inner-city areas, physician shortage in, 35
Institute of Medicine (IOM), 92; on legal
liability of primary care, 145, 240n. 39;
2002 study of, 194
insurance, health care: for middle class, 33;
national, 114
intensive care, negotiation of practice
barriers in, 52
interim certification boards, 170–171,
248n. 51
internal medicine, and family practice, 95
Intersection Committee on Recognition of
Superior Performance, ANA, 120–121,
170
Iowa Medical Society, 130

Jacobi, Eileen, 176
job security, 115
Johnson, Amos, 101
Johnson, President Lyndon B., 36, 140,
213n. 65
Johnson administration, 51
Johnson, Robert Wood, Foundation. *See*
Robert Wood Johnson Foundation
Joint Commission of Associated Hospitals
(JCAH), on professional accountability,
150
joint practice: implementing, 136, 143–144;
issue of, 154; use of term, 155
joint practice commissions (JPCs), state,
141–142
joint practice conferences, regional, 154
Jourard, Sidney, 58
judgment, clinical, 205n. 45
jurisdictional dominance, concept of, 40,
211n. 36

Kaiser Permanante, 110
Kakosh, Marguerite E., 58

Kellogg Foundation. *See* W. K. Kellogg
Foundation
Kemp, C. Henry, 19
Kentucky, University of, 160; health centers
at, 37
Kimbrough, Robert, 125
Kinlein, M. Lucille, 41, 81
Kitzman, Harriet, 71, 72, 77
knowledge: and clinical practice, 117;
in clinical thinking, 21; nurses' vs.
physicians', 188; between nursing
and medicine, 15, 52
knowledge explosion, and health care
system, 7

Lambertson, Eleanor, 49
language: of accountability, 150–151; of
ANA, 118; of clinical thinking, 53; of joint
practice, 155; and Lysaught Commission,
48; for negotiating clinical practice, 48,
77, 90; of nursing, 73; patronizing, 129,
237n. 69
Lassman, Nate, 69, 70, 74
Leininger, Madeline, 52
Lewis, Edith, 50
licensure, 120; of new health personnel,
105; and physician assistants, 101
lifestyle, and chronic disease, 23
Lippincott Publishing Co., 77
Living Independently for Elders (LIFE)
program, 254n. 20
Lock, Frank, 125
Loir, Sonia, 245n. 9, 246n. 24
Lynaugh, Joan, 7, 15, 69, 77, 79, 81, 82, 83,
84; and collaborative practice, 70, 73, 74,
75–76
Lysaught, Jerome, 46, 47, 49, 136; and first
NJPC meeting, 139
Lysaught Commission, 47–49, 214n. 67,
214n. 72
Lysaught Report, 66, 136; reaction to, 49–50;
recommendations of, 50–51

Macy program, 241n. 46
managed care, impact of, 185
manpower funding initiatives, 134–135
Marcus Welby, M.D. (television series), 92,
226n. 23

professional organizations (*continued*)
practice, 188; conflict between medical
and nursing, 194; and expanded practice,
46; and local practice, 13; self-interests
of, 192
programs, clinically based, 46. *See also*
nurse practitioner programs
Programs of All Inclusive Care for Elders
(PACE), 254n. 20
prospective payment system (PPS), 4, 156,
184, 185
providers: changing environment for, 6;
collaborating, 8; control of, 188;
emergence of new, 87; in hierarchical
relationships, 14; teams of, 190
psychiatric clinical nurse specialists, 43,
212n. 47
psychiatry: collaborative practice in, 58;
nursing specialization in, 212n. 58
"psychology girls," 58, 217n. 20
public health nurses, 11; independence of,
18; negotiation of practice barriers by, 52
public health nursing, sharing of knowledge
in, 15
Public Health Service (PHS): graduate
study supported by, 51; nurse-run
practices supported by, 81
Public Health Service Act (1971), 51
public safety, rhetoric of, 183
Public Service Act (1956), Title VIII of,
213n. 66

quackery, AMA committee on, 132, 237n. 78
"Quacktitioner," 187
quality of care, and new practice models,
111–112

race: and NJPC, 140; and specialty nurse
practitioner organizations, 158
race, of nurse practitioners, 9
Rasmussen, Holier, 154
Reader, George, 71
reform, health care, and nurse practitioner
education, 193
reform programs, emergence of, 37–38
regional medical programs, creation of, 37,
210n. 27
reimbursement: control of, 188; for new
providers, 149

Reiter, Francis, 44, 58, 121
Reitz, J. Wayne, 57, 218n. 47
Rendell, Governor Edward, 195
responsibility: and clinical care, 1; for nurse
practitioners, 26–27
rhetorical force-multiplier, 14, 203n. 16
Ritter, Hubert A., 154
Robert Wood Johnson Foundation, 37, 146
Rochester, University of, 54, 160; health
centers at, 37, 68–84; nurse practitioner
program at, 83; shared governance at, 55
Rockefeller Foundation, 97
Rockford School of Medicine, of University
of Illinois, 38
Rogers, Martha, 46, 82
Ruhe, C. H. William, 108–109, 110
rural areas: delegation strategies in, 18;
during Depression, 22; federal funding of
nurses in, 51; nursing health conferences
in, 204n. 39; physician shortage in, 35;
public health in, 19
rural clinics, nurse practitioners in, 7
rural medical centers, clinical practice in,
33–34
Rush University Medical Center: health
centers at, 37; shared governance at, 55
Rutgers University: graduate nursing
programs at, 213n. 62; psychiatric
nursing at, 117
R. W. Johnson Foundation. *See* Robert Wood
Johnson Foundation

safety, patient, rhetoric of, 175, 188
salaries, as workplace issue, 115
sameness, idea of, 116
Sammons, James, 155, 156
Samuel Proctor Oral History Program
(SPOHP), 217n. 19
Schaffrath, William, 141, 156
Scheuer, Mildred, 121, 122
schools, nursing: hospital-based, 11; and
Lysaught Commission, 49–50. *See also*
education; medical schools
Schweer, Susan, 147
science, traditional focus on, 53. *See also*
education
screening centers, 23
Senate Subcommittee on Aging, 34

universities, nursing faculty at, 55–56. *See
also specific universities*
urban clinics, federal funding of nurses in,
51
urban medical centers, clinical practice in,
33–34

validation, sources of, 29–30
Veterans Administration, physician assistant
program of, 109–110
victimization, of nurses by physicians, 13
visiting nurses, 11

Walker, James, 139
Wallis, W. Allen, 214n. 67
Wallis, William A., 68
Wal-Mart, walk-in health clinics of,
194–195
Walsh, Sally, 165, 168
wars, sharing of knowledge in, 15
Washington, University of, MEDEX at,
106–107
Western Reserve University, health center
at, 66
West Virginia, joint practice activities in,
141

Whitaker, Judith, 125
Wilk et al v. AMA et al., 238n. 79
Williamsburg, VA, national conference for
nurses and physicians at, 129–130
Willian, Mary Kaye, 179
Willig, Sidney H., 137
W. K. Kellogg Foundation, 37, 47, 68, 156,
244n. 100; and NJPC funding, 140–141
Wolff, George T., 152
women: empowerment of, 12; in MEDEX
programs, 107, 230n. 80; and physician
assistant programs, 99, 100
women's movement, and nursing, 12
Wooden, Howard, 58
Woolf, Virginia, 200n. 9
workforce, nursing: cheap, 128; stratification
of, 43
workplace: duty-hours standards in, 189;
issues of, 115; for nurse practitioners, 191;
standards in, 115
Wyoming, joint practice activities in,
141–142

Yale University: graduate nursing programs
at, 213n. 62; health center at, 66
Young, Lawrence, 68

About the Author

Julie Fairman is the Class of 1940 Bicentennial Term Chair and an associate professor of nursing at the School of Nursing, University of Pennsylvania. She is also the director of the Barbara Bates Center for the Study of the History of Nursing and a Fellow of the American Academy of Nursing. She is the author of the book *Critical Care Nursing: A History* (1998).